Primary Care: The Art and Science of Advanced Nursing

Primary Care: The Art and Science of Advanced Nursing

Editor: Danna Carson

AMERICAN
MEDICAL PUBLISHERS
www.americanmedicalpublishers.com

AMERICAN
MEDICAL PUBLISHERS
www.americanmedicalpublishers.com

Cataloging-in-Publication Data

Primary care : the art and science of advanced nursing / edited by Danna Carson.
p. cm.
Includes bibliographical references and index.
ISBN 978-1-63927-452-9
1. Primary care (Medicine). 2. Primary health care. 3. Medical care. I. Carson, Danna.
RA427.9 .P75 2022
610--dc23

American Medical Publishers,
41 Flatbush Avenue,
1st Floor, New York,
NY 11217, USA

ISBN 978-1-63927-452-9 (Hardback)

Contents

Preface

This book was inspired by the evolution of our times; to answer the curiosity of inquisitive minds. Many developments have occurred across the globe in the recent past which has transformed the progress in the field.

The day to day healthcare that is given to the patient is known as primary care. This domain involves the broadest scope of healthcare that is concerned with patients of all socioeconomic and geographic origins and ages. It also involves patients with all manner of acute and chronic physical, mental and social health issues and the one seeking to maintain optimal health. Some examples of common chronic illnesses usually treated in primary care are hypertension, diabetes, asthma, COPD, anxiety, etc. This field also consists of many basic maternal and child health care services such as family planning services and vaccinations. Primary health care results in better health outcomes, lower spending, avoidable emergency department visits and hospital care, and reduced health disparities. This book contains some path-breaking studies in the field of primary care. It explores all the important aspects of this field in the present day scenario. The extensive content of this book provides the readers with a thorough understanding of the subject.

This book was developed from a mere concept to drafts to chapters and finally compiled together as a complete text to benefit the readers across all nations. To ensure the quality of the content we instilled two significant steps in our procedure. The first was to appoint an editorial team that would verify the data and statistics provided in the book and also select the most appropriate and valuable contributions from the plentiful contributions we received from authors worldwide. The next step was to appoint an expert of the topic as the Editor-in-Chief, who would head the project and finally make the necessary amendments and modifications to make the text reader-friendly. I was then commissioned to examine all the material to present the topics in the most comprehensible and productive format.

I would like to take this opportunity to thank all the contributing authors who were supportive enough to contribute their time and knowledge to this project. I also wish to convey my regards to my family who have been extremely supportive during the entire project.

Editor

1

A systematic review of chronic disease management interventions in primary care

Rebecca Reynolds[1], Sarah Dennis[2], Iqbal Hasan[1], Jan Slewa[1], Winnie Chen[1], David Tian[1], Sangeetha Bobba[1] and Nicholas Zwar[1,3*]

Abstract

Background: Primary and community care are key settings for the effective management of long term conditions. We aimed to evaluate the pattern of health outcomes in chronic disease management interventions for adults with physical health problems implemented in primary or community care settings.

Methods: The methods were based on our previous review published in 2006. We performed database searches for articles published from 2006 to 2014 and conducted a systematic review with narrative synthesis using the Cochrane Effective Practice and Organisation of Care taxonomy to classify interventions and outcomes. The interventions were mapped to Chronic Care Model elements. The pattern of outcomes related to interventions was summarized by frequency of statistically significant improvements in health care provision and patient outcomes.

Results: A total of 9589 journal articles were retrieved from database searches and snowballing. After screening and verification, 165 articles that detailed 157 studies were included. There were few studies with Health Care Organization (1.9% of studies) or Community Resources (0.6% of studies) as the primary intervention element. Self-Management Support interventions (45.8% of studies) most frequently resulted in improvements in patient–level outcomes. Delivery System Design interventions (22.6% of studies) showed benefits in both professional and patient-level outcomes for a narrow range of conditions. Decision Support interventions (21.3% of studies) had impact limited to professional-level outcomes, in particular use of medications. The small number of studies of Clinical Information System interventions (8.9%) showed benefits for both professional- and patient-level outcomes.

Conclusions: The published literature has expanded substantially since 2006. This review confirms that Self-Management Support is the most frequent Chronic Care Model intervention that is associated with statistically significant improvements, predominately for diabetes and hypertension.

Keywords: Chronic care, Disease management/care management, Systematic review, Endocrinology, Diabetes, Cardiovascular, Respiratory system, Musculoskeletal/connective tissue, Arthritis

Background

Chronic disease is defined by the World Health Organization (WHO) as being of long duration, generally slow in progression and not passed from person to person [1]. The Global Burden of Disease study 2013 reported a substantial (42.3%) increase in the years lived with disability (YLD) from 1990 to 2013 [2]. This was overwhelming due to non-communicable diseases, with no infectious diseases in the top 20 leading causes of YLDs globally in 2013. Chronic condition multi-morbidity is high in developed countries [3] and the prevalence of it increases with age; Australian data indicate that around 40% of people aged over 44 years have chronic disease multi-morbidity, increasing to around 50% for 65–74 year olds, and 70% for 85 years or over [4].

Addressing chronic disease is a major challenge for healthcare systems around the world, which have largely developed to deal with acute episodic care, rather than to provide organized care for people with long-term conditions [5]. A characteristic of chronic diseases is that they often require a long period of supervision, observation or care. The defining features of primary care (including

* Correspondence: nzwar@uow.edu.au
[1]UNSW, Sydney, Australia
[3]School of Medicine, University of Wollongong, Wollongong, NSW 2522, Australia
Full list of author information is available at the end of the article

continuity, coordination, and comprehensiveness) makes this setting suitable for managing chronic conditions [6]. Evidence increasingly highlights the importance of reorienting health policy and healthcare towards chronic care systems, including primary care that are proactive rather than reactive [7]. Countries with strong primary care systems tend to have better health outcomes at a lower cost [8].

The Chronic Care Model (CCM) was developed in the 1990s by Wagner et al. as a framework to improve the quality of chronic care [9]. It is an organizational approach to caring for people with chronic disease that is particularly applicable in the primary care setting. The six elements of the CCM operate within the context of the individual, community, provider organization and the health care system, see Fig. 1. The model can be used as a guide for system enhancement to provide higher-quality chronic disease management (CDM) [10–12].

Subsequent to development of the CCM there have been a number of other approaches to improving the quality and comprehensiveness of primary care including for the management of chronic diseases. These include the Patient-Centered Medical Home and The Ten Building Blocks of High-Performing Primary Care [13, 14]. Chronic disease management in primary care is an important part of both prevention and treatment of chronic conditions, but there is a need to understand which interventions are effective, for whom and in what context [6]. The literature on interventions to improve CDM in primary care, based on the CCM or otherwise, is diverse and growing. In 2006, we published a systematic review with narrative synthesis of interventions for common physical health problems managed in primary care in developed countries [15, 16]. This review classified interventions under the elements of the CCM, an approach that has subsequently been adopted by other authors [17]. In this article, we provide an updated review and narrative synthesis of the pattern of health outcomes in CDM interventions for physical health problems in the primary care setting to ensure that more recent published evidence is included and used to inform intervention development, policy and practice, as well as guide future research.

Methods

The methods for the current systematic review with narrative synthesis were based on those used in our previous review [15, 16]. The database searches for the updated review were conducted between 1 January 2006 and 31 December 2014. This systematic review was registered with PROSPERO (CRD42014009219) [18].

Literature search

Searches were run in four databases: Medline, Embase, PsycINFO and CINAHL. Inclusion and exclusion criteria for articles are described below. The database search terms are shown in Additional file 1.

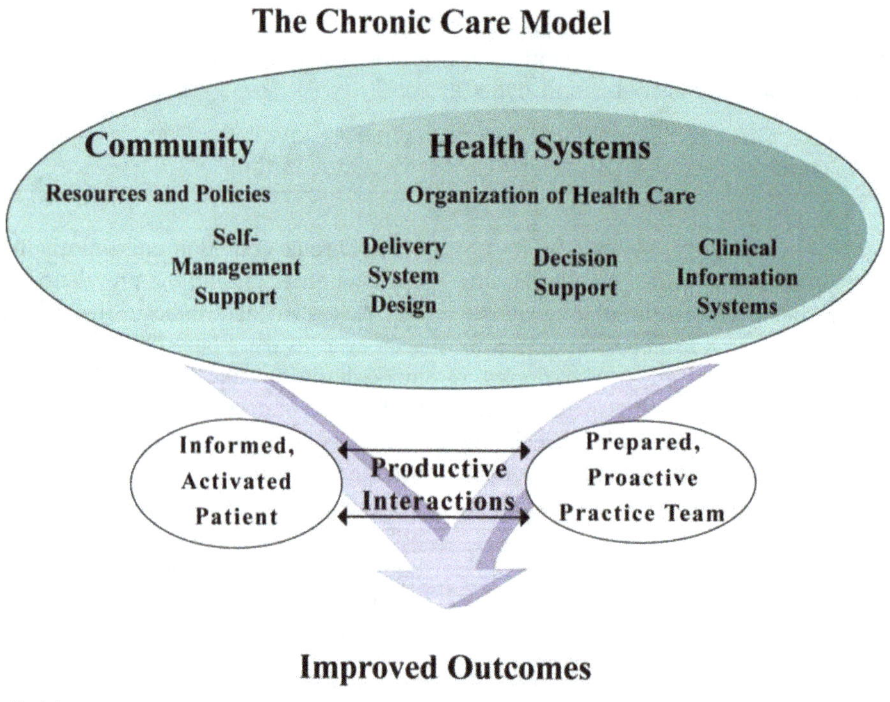

Fig. 1 Chronic Care Model

Study selection, quality assessment and data extraction

We included studies that were randomized controlled trials (RCTs), controlled clinical trials, controlled before and after and interrupted time series studies; included adults 18 years and older with the chronic physical health conditions of asthma, chronic obstructive pulmonary disease (COPD), type 2 diabetes mellitus (T2DM), heart disease (including heart failure and myocardial infarction), hypertension, lipid disorders, arthritis (osteoarthritis and rheumatoid arthritis) and osteoporosis; were delivered in a primary or community care setting (primary care, including family practice; managed care organizations; community-based but delivered by primary care professionals, including pharmacists) by non-hospital health professionals (including doctors and allied health professionals, nurses and pharmacists) in the following developed countries: Australia, Canada, Denmark, Finland, Iceland, Netherlands, New Zealand, Norway, Sweden, the UK (England, Northern Ireland, Scotland and Wales) and the USA; and the intervention could be mapped to the expanded Effective Practice and Organization of Care (EPOC) taxonomy [19]. Prior systematic reviews were not included.

Articles underwent screening of titles and abstracts; verification of full text and quality assessment used templates (see Additional file 2 and Additional file 3) developed during the previous review [15, 16]. The reference lists of included articles were used in a snowballing process to identify any missed articles. See the Preferred Reporting Items for Systematic Reviews and Meta-Analyses (PRISMA) flow diagram of this assessment process as Fig. 2 [20].

Three reviewers (RR, IH and DT) completed the title/abstract screening process and any discrepancies were reviewed by a fourth reviewer (SD), who also reviewed 20% of excluded articles. No articles were found to have been wrongly excluded. A 20% exclusion check is a validated method to assess the quality of the screening process [21].

Two reviewers (RR and IH) completed the full text verification process and any discrepancies were assessed by a third reviewer (NZ). A 20% check of excluded articles was also carried out at this full text verification stage by one reviewer (SD) and no articles were found that should not have been excluded [21]. The reference lists of all included studies were reviewed by one reviewer (NZ). A further 118 articles were identified which underwent verification and quality assessment.

All articles remaining after full text verification were quality assessed based on study design and other characteristics using the EPOC quality assessment tool [19] by four reviewers (RR, IH, DT and SD). The quality score was out of a total of 14, the included articles had a mean score of 11.1 and a median score of 11.0. Consistent with the methods of the previous review [15, 16], articles with a median score below 11.0 were excluded. The inter-rater reliability for quality scores from the four reviewers was assessed. Each reviewer assessed a 20% sample of papers scored by another reviewer. There was a 1-tailed Pearson correlation coefficient of 0.414 and significance of $p < 0.01$.

Using methods developed for the previous review [15, 16] and also used subsequently by Pasricha et al. [17], data extraction was completed by two reviewers (JS and WC). A data extraction template was developed which included the EPOC Group taxonomy for the classification of the intervention methods [19] and of up to seven categories of study outcomes based on modified methods used by Weingarten et al. 2002 [22]. We expanded the list of outcomes from the previous review [15, 16] by adding change in medication and costs.

Study interventions were coded using the EPOC taxonomy and then mapped to the elements of the CCM (NZ, SD and RR) based on published descriptions of CCM elements [11, 12], with any discrepancies addressed by NZ. Up to three CCM elements (primary, secondary and tertiary) were mapped for each study intervention. Based on the methods used in our previous review [15, 16] and by Weingarten et al. 2002 [22], we used a vote-counting approach to summarize the impact of CCM intervention elements on the primary outcome of the study (as defined by the study authors). Significant and positive (i.e. beneficial) primary and up to six additional outcomes (where present) were recorded at the $p < 0.05$ level. As in our previous review the diversity of studies, types of CCM interventions and outcomes examined prevented the use of meta-analysis to examine effect sizes. The extraction of only the primary outcome and up to six additional outcomes was a modification of the methods from our earlier review where impact of the intervention on all extracted outcomes was examined [15, 16]. Data was analyzed for descriptive statistics using Excel, SPSS (IBM Corp. Released 2013. IBM SPSS Statistics for Windows, Version 22.0. Armonk, NY: IBM Corp) and SAS/STAT® software.

Results

There were 9589 articles identified after duplicates were removed. After screening and verification 165 journal articles were included in the review, which detailed 157 original studies (some journal articles described different results from the one study design). See Fig. 2 PRISMA flow chart and Additional file 4 for a summary of the characteristics of the included studies.

The majority of the studies were of RCT design (92.9%), allocating the intervention at the patient-level (63.2%), and based in primary care (62.6%). The most common location for studies was the USA (49.0%) and

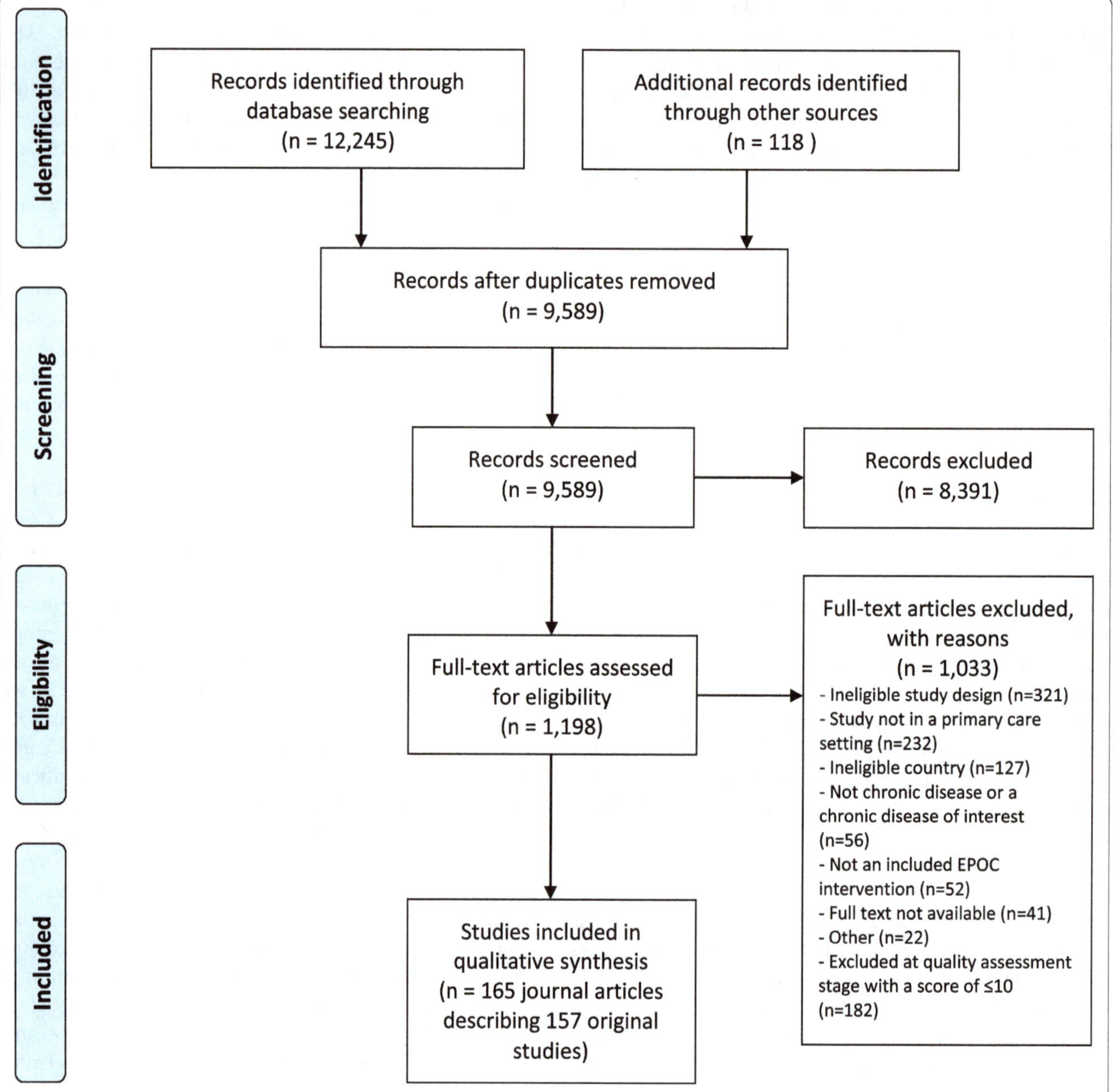

Fig. 2 Prisma flow diagram

the most common condition targeted was T2DM (43.9%). There were a total of 1,051,707 patients across 100 studies, 2961 health professionals across 14 studies and 7368 practices across 43 studies. Using mean data of participants in the control groups, the mean age was 60.7 years (SD 7.4), with 44.3% male and 23.9% in Caucasian/white populations (when ethnicity was specified). The mean duration of the studies was 14.1 (SD 11.6) months, ranging from 1 to 72 months.

Self-Management Support was the most frequent primary CCM element ($n = 71$, 45.8% of studies) followed by DS ($n = 35$, 22.6%), DSD ($n = 33$, 21.3%) and CIS ($n = 14$, 8.9%). There were relatively few studies with HCO ($n = 3$, 1.9%) or CR ($n = 1$, 0.6%) as the primary intervention element. Table 1 illustrates the CCM elements by disease; T2DM and hypertension were the most frequently studied conditions. Table 2 shows the number of CCM elements by primary outcome. Most study interventions addressed one or two CCM elements. Studies with three elements addressed in the intervention did not, in general, appear to be more effective with respect to statistically significant improvements in outcomes than studies with a smaller number of elements (Table 3).

The exception to this was where the primary element was a DSD change accompanied by SMS and DS intervention

Table 1 Types of Chronic Care Model intervention elements (primary, secondary and tertiary) by disease

Disease	Decision Support (DS)	Delivery System Design (DSD)	Clinical Information Systems (CIS)	Self Management Support (SMS)	Health Care Organization (HCO)	Community Resources (CR)	Total
Type 2 Diabetes	30	38	14	52	2	2	138
Hypertension	21	19	10	24	1	2	77
Heart disease	7	6	6	10	2		31
COPD	5	11	4	11			31
Arthritis	3	5	2	8			18
Osteoporosis	1	1	2	2			6
Asthma	4		1	4			9
Lipid disorders	3	1	1	1			6
Total	73	81	38	112	5	4	313

elements. Table 4 illustrates the proportion of studies with a significant result for professional or patient-level outcome measures (primary outcome and up to six additional outcomes) for each primary CCM intervention element overall and by disease. Self-Management Support interventions resulted in improvements in patient-level outcomes; such as physiological measures of disease, risk behavior, satisfaction and knowledge in more than half the studies analyzed. Delivery System Design interventions showed benefits in both professional and patient level outcomes but this was confined to a narrow range of conditions. Decision Support interventions tended to have impact limited to professional-level outcomes, in particular use of medications. There were small numbers of studies of Clinical Information System interventions as the primary element but the results show benefits for both professional and patient level outcomes.

Discussion

Since publication of the 2006 review [15, 16], the number of potentially eligible studies has increased considerably (9589 studies screened between 2006 and 2014 compared to 5160 studies between 1990 and 2006). This likely reflects a growing interest in how to meet the challenge of the increasing prevalence and burden of chronic disease to health systems globally. Consistent with the 2006 review [15, 16], this review showed that SMS was the most commonly tested intervention with the greatest proportion of studies demonstrating a significant result for one or more outcome measure categories for all diseases examined in the review, with the exception of lipid disorders. The effect of SMS was most often to improve physiological measures of disease in patients with T2DM and hypertension, and improve patient knowledge in T2DM and COPD. There was also some evidence of benefit on quality of life for patients with arthritis and COPD. Studies with SMS interventions as the primary element less often examined the impact of the intervention on health professional behavior.

Although the number of studies was small, CIS interventions showed benefit on both professional and patient level outcomes in particular for T2DM and hypertension. This is in contrast to our 2006 review findings and may indicate increasing sophistication of CIS interventions with computerized recall and

Table 2 Number of Chronic Care Model elements (primary only, $n = 1$; primary and secondary, $n = 2$; or primary, secondary and tertiary, $n = 3$) by primary outcome

OUTCOME CATEGORY													
	Professional-level			Patient-level									Other
Number of CCM elements	Adherence to guidelines	Change in medication	Quality of care	Adherence to treatment	Service use	PMOD	Risk behavior	Quality of life	Health status	Satisfaction	Functional status	Knowledge level	Costs
1	**2 (4)**	**5 (10)**		1 (5)	3 (9)	**11 (23)**	**4 (5)**	**7 (13)**	**6 (9)**	**1 (2)**	3 (7)	**7 (9)**	**1 (2)**
2	**12 (17)**	**12 (15)**	**1 (1)**	**7 (12)**	5 (11)	**34 (55)**	**9 (16)**	8 (18)	2 (12)	**4 (6)**	**9 (15)**	**11 (15)**	**4 (5)**
3	5 (11)	**5 (5)**		1 (5)	**4 (6)**	**20 (30)**	0 (7)	2 (12)	2 (10)	**4 (6)**	0 (3)	**3 (6)**	**4 (4)**

Numbers in cells: number of studies reporting at least one significant outcome (number of studies reporting at least one outcome for that particular category of outcome measure)
Bold font in cells is where 50% or more of studies reported a significant difference for that category of outcome
CCM Chronic Care Model, *PMOD* physiological measure of disease

Table 3 Combination of elements of Chronic Care Model and outcome measures

Single or combination CCM elements	OUTCOME CATEGORY												
	Professional-level			Patient-level									Other
	Adherence to guidelines	Change in medication	Quality of care	Adherence to treatment	Service use	PMOD	Risk behaviour	Quality of life	Health status	Satisfaction	Functional status	Knowledge level	Costs
DSD overall o Overall	**3 (5)**	**6 (7)**		1 (5)	**4 (7)**	**18(22)**	0 (4)	6 (13)	3 (8)	**4 (5)**	1 (3)	**4 (6)**	**2 (2)**
DSD						0 (1)			**1 (1)**				
DSD + CIS								**1 (1)**	0 (1)				
DSD + CIS + DS				**1 (1)**									
DSD + CIS + SMS					0 (1)	**1 (1)**		0 (1)				0 (1)	
DSD + DS		**2 (2)**				**4 (4)**			**1 (1)**				
DSD + DS + CIS	**1 (1)**					**1 (1)**			**1 (1)**				
DSD + DS + HCO	**1 (1)**									0 (1)			
DSD + DS + SMS	0 (1)	**1 (1)**			**1 (1)**	**1 (2)**	0 (1)	0 (1)				**1 (1)**	
DSD + SMS		**2 (3)**		0 (2)	**2 (3)**	**4 (5)**	0 (1)	**3 (5)**	0 (1)	**2 (2)**	**1 (2)**	**3 (3)**	
DSD + SMS + CIS	0 (1)			0 (1)	0 (1)	**1 (1)**		0 (2)	0 (1)	**1 (1)**			**1 (1)**
DSD + SMS + DS	**1 (1)**	**1 (1)**		0 (1)	**1 (1)**	**6 (7)**	0 (2)	**2 (3)**	0 (2)	**1 (1)**	0 (1)	0 (1)	**1 (1)**
DS overall	6 (13)	**8 (13)**		1 (3)	**5 (9)**	8 (22)	**2 (3)**	1 (5)	2 (9)	1 (3)	2 (10)	**1 (1)**	**1 (2)**
DS	**2 (3)**	3 (8)		**1 (2)**	**3 (6)**	3 (7)		1 (3)	**2 (2)**	0 (1)	**2 (4)**		0 (1)
DS + CIS	1 (3)	**2 (2)**				0 (3)	**1 (1)**		0 (1)		0 (1)		**1 (1)**
DS + CIS + DSD	**1 (1)**								0 (1)		0 (1)		
DS + CIS + SMS	0 (1)												
DS + DSD	0 (1)	**2 (2)**		0 (1)		**3 (4)**			0 (1)	0 (1)	0 (1)		
DS + DSD + SMS	0 (1)				**1 (1)**	1 (4)		0 (2)	0 (3)	**1 (1)**	0 (1)		
DS + HCO	**1 (1)**										0 (1)		
DS + SMS	**1 (2)**	**1 (1)**			**1 (2)**	1 (4)	**1 (2)**		0 (1)		0 (1)	**1 (1)**	
CIS overall	**4 (5)**	**2 (2)**	**1 (1)**		**1 (2)**	**5 (8)**	0 (1)			**1 (1)**	**4 (5)**		**1 (2)**
CIS + DS	**4 (4)**	**1 (1)**	**1 (1)**		**1 (1)**	1 (3)	0 (1)			**1 (1)**	**4 (4)**		**1 (1)**
CIS + DSD						**1 (1)**							
CIS + SMS	0 (1)				0 (1)	**1 (2)**					0 (1)		0 (1)
CIS + SMS + DSD		**1 (1)**				**2 (2)**							
SMS overall	**5 (7)**	**5 (6)**		6 (13)	1 (7)	**32(52)**	**11 (20)**	**10(25)**	5 (13)	**3 (5)**	**5 (5)**	**16 (23)**	**5 (5)**
SMS		**1 (1)**		0 (3)	0 (3)	8 (14)	**4 (5)**	**6 (10)**	**3 (5)**		**1 (2)**	**7 (9)**	**1 (1)**

Table 3 Combination of elements of Chronic Care Model and outcome measures *(Continued)*

Single or combination CCM elements	OUTCOME CATEGORY												
	Professional-level			Patient-level									Other
	Adherence to guidelines	Change in medication	Quality of care	Adherence to treatment	Service use	PMOD	Risk behaviour	Quality of life	Health status	Satisfaction	Functional status	Knowledge level	Costs
SMS + CIS	**1 (1)**			**2 (2)**	0 (1)	2 (5)	**1 (1)**	0 (2)	0 (1)	**1 (1)**	**1 (1)**	**1 (1)**	
SMS + CIS + DSD		**1 (1)**				**1 (1)**	0 (1)						
SMS + CR				**1 (1)**		**1 (1)**							
SMS + CR + DSD						0 (1)							
SMS + DS	**1 (1)**	**1 (1)**			0 (1)	**5 (6)**	**2 (2)**	**1 (2)**				**1 (1)**	**1 (1)**
SMS + DS + CIS	**1 (1)**	**1 (1)**				**2 (2)**		0 (1)	0 (1)				**2 (2)**
SMS + DS + DSD	0 (1)				**1 (1)**	0 (1)	0 (1)			0 (1)			
SMS + DSD	**2 (2)**	**1 (2)**		**3 (5)**	0 (1)	**9 (14)**	**4 (8)**	**3 (8)**	1 (5)	**1 (2)**	**3 (3)**	**5 (9)**	**1 (1)**
SMS + DSD + CIS						1 (1)		0 (1)	**1 (1)**	**1 (1)**		0 (1)	
SMS + DSD + CR						**1 (1)**						**1 (1)**	
SMS + DSD + DS	0 (1)			0 (2)		2 (5)	0 (2)	0 (1)				**1 (1)**	
HCO + CIS	**1 (1)**					**1 (1)**							
HCO + DSD				**1 (1)**		0 (1)							
CR + DSD		0 (1)			**1 (1)**	**1 (1)**							

Numbers in cells: number of studies reporting at least one significant outcome (number of studies reporting at least one outcome)
Bold font in cells is where 50% or more of studies reported a significant difference for that category of outcome
CCM Chronic Care Model, *CIS* clinical information systems, *COPD* chronic obstructive pulmonary disease, *CR* community resources, *DS* decision support, *DSD* delivery system design, *HCO* health care organization, *PMOD* physiological measure of disease, *SMS* self-management support

Table 4 Elements of Chronic Care Model and positive outcome measures by disease

Primary CCM element	Disease	OUTCOME CATEGORY												
		Professional			Patient									Other
		Adherence to guidelines	Change in medication	Quality of care	Adherence to treatment	Service use	PMOD	Risk behaviour	Quality of life	Health status	Satisfaction	Functional status	Knowledge level	Costs
DSD	Overall	**3 (5)**	**6 (7)**		1 (5)	**4 (7)**	**18 (22)**	0 (4)	6 (13)	3 (8)	**4 (5)**	1 (3)	**4 (6)**	**2 (2)**
	Arthritis								**1 (2)**	0 (1)		**1 (1)**		
	Asthma													
	COPD	0 (1)				1 (4)	0 (1)	0 (1)	1 (5)	0 (1)			**2 (3)**	
	Diabetes	**3 (3)**	**3 (4)**		0 (2)	**2 (2)**	**12 (14)**	0 (2)	**4 (4)**	**1 (2)**	**3 (4)**	0 (1)	**2 (2)**	**1 (1)**
	Heart disease	0 (1)			0 (2)		0 (1)	0 (1)	0 (1)	1 (3)	**1 (1)**			**1 (1)**
	Hypertension		**3 (3)**			**1 (1)**	**5 (5)**		0 (1)	1 (1)		0 (1)	0 (1)	
	Lipid disorders						**1 (1)**							
	Osteoporosis				**1 (1)**									
DS	Overall	6 (13)	**8 (13)**		1 (3)	**5 (9)**	8 (22)	**2 (3)**	1 (5)	2 (9)	1 (3)	2 (10)	**1 (1)**	**1 (2)**
	Arthritis													
	Asthma	**1 (1)**	**1 (2)**		**1 (2)**	0 (1)	0 (1)		1 (3)	**1 (1)**				
	COPD					0 (1)			0 (1)	**1 (2)**	**1 (1)**	**1 (2)**		
	Diabetes	1 (3)	**3 (4)**			**2 (3)**	4 (11)	**2 (2)**	0 (1)	0 (3)	0 (2)	0 (2)	**1 (1)**	**1 (2)**
	Heart disease	1 (3)	**2 (3)**			**1 (2)**	0 (3)	0 (1)		0 (1)		0 (2)		
	Hypertension	**2 (4)**	**2 (4)**		0 (1)	**2 (2)**	**4 (7)**			0 (2)		1 (3)		
	Lipid disorders	**1 (2)**										0 (1)		
	Osteoporosis													
CIS	Overall	**4 (5)**	**3 (3)**	**1 (1)**		**1 (2)**	**5 (8)**	0 (1)			**1 (1)**	**4 (5)**		**1 (2)**
	Arthritis													
	Asthma	**1 (1)**		**1 (1)**								**1 (1)**		
	COPD													
	Diabetes	**2 (3)**				**1 (1)**	**2 (3)**				**1 (1)**	**2 (3)**		**1 (1)**
	Heart disease		**1 (1)**			0 (1)	**1 (1)**							
	Hypertension	**1 (1)**	**2 (2)**				**2 (4)**	0 (1)				**1 (1)**		0 (1)

Table 4 Elements of Chronic Care Model and positive outcome measures by disease *(Continued)*

Primary CCM element	Disease	OUTCOME CATEGORY												
		Professional			Patient									Other
		Adherence to guidelines	Change in medication	Quality of care	Adherence to treatment	Service use	PMOD	Risk behaviour	Quality of life	Health status	Satisfaction	Functional status	Knowledge level	Costs
	Lipid disorders													
	Osteoporosis													
SMS	Overall	**5 (7)**	**5 (6)**		6 (13)	1 (7)	**32 (52)**	**11 (20)**	10 (25)	5 (13)	**3 (5)**	**5 (6)**	**16 (23)**	**5 (5)**
	Arthritis	**1 (1)**					**1 (1)**		**3 (5)**			**2 (2)**	**2 (3)**	
	Asthma		**1 (1)**			0 (2)	**1 (2)**		1 (3)	**1 (2)**				
	COPD		0 (1)			**1 (2)**		**1 (1)**	**2 (4)**	**1 (1)**	**1 (2)**	**1 (1)**	**3 (5)**	
	Diabetes	**1 (1)**			**4 (8)**	0 (1)	**17 (29)**	**9 (15)**	3 (8)	2 (6)	**1 (2)**	**1 (2)**	**11 (14)**	**1 (1)**
	Heart disease		**1 (1)**			0 (2)	2 (5)		**1 (2)**	1 (3)	**1 (1)**			**1 (1)**
	Hypertension	**3 (5)**	**3 (3)**		1 (3)		**11 (15)**	1 (4)	0 (3)	0 (1)		**1 (1)**	0 (1)	**3 (3)**
	Lipid disorders													
	Osteoporosis				**1 (2)**		**1 (1)**		0 (1)	**1 (1)**				
HCO	Overall	**1 (2)**			1 (1)		1 (3)			0 (1)		0 (1)		
	Arthritis													
	Asthma													
	COPD													
	Diabetes				1 (1)		0 (1)							
	Heart disease	**1 (1)**					**1 (1)**							
	Hypertension	0 (1)					0 (1)			0 (1)		0 (1)		
	Lipid disorders													
	Osteoporosis													
CR	Overall		0 (1)			**1 (1)**	**1 (1)**							
	Arthritis													
	Asthma													
	COPD													

Table 4 Elements of Chronic Care Model and positive outcome measures by disease *(Continued)*

Primary CCM element	Disease	OUTCOME CATEGORY												
		Professional			Patient									Other
		Adherence to guidelines	Change in medication	Quality of care	Adherence to treatment	Service use	PMOD	Risk behaviour	Quality of life	Health status	Satisfaction	Functional status	Knowledge level	Costs
	Diabetes													
	Heart disease													
	Hypertension		0 (1)			**1 (1)**	**1 (1)**							
	Lipid disorders													
	Osteoporosis													

Numbers in cells: number of studies reporting at least one significant outcome (number of studies reporting at least one outcome)
Bold font in cells is where 50% or more of studies reported a significant difference for that category of outcome
CCM Chronic Care Model, *CIS* clinical information systems, *COPD* chronic obstructive pulmonary disease, *CR* community resources, *DS* decision support, *DSD* delivery system design, *HCO* health care organization, *PMOD* physiological measure of disease, *SMS* self-management support

reminder systems, feedback to clinicians and access to computerized DS tools [23]. The next most common CCM element as a primary intervention that was associated with statistically significant improvements in outcomes was DSD, which benefited physiological measures of disease control and health professional behavior in patients with T2DM diabetes and hypertension, but had limited or no impact in other conditions. The other CCM element showing worthwhile evidence of benefit was DS which had some impact on health professional behavior including changing medication and adherence to guidelines but had limited impact on patient-level measures of disease control.

In contrast to the earlier 2006 review [15, 16], this review suggested that two CCM elements were more likely to result in significant improvements in outcomes compared to one or three, whereas the previous review found that adding multiple elements to the intervention programs did not produce better outcomes. The combination of SMS and DSD interventions was the most frequent combination of elements associated with significant improvements in outcomes, followed by SMS and DS. The results for the SMS intervention on professional and patient outcomes are consistent with those from 2006. Results for DS suggest reduced impact of the interventions on health professionals' adherence to guidelines, which was unexpected. This could be explained by increasing sophistication of CIS where DS interventions are now more frequently embedded.

Comparisons to other studies

A number of other reviews have been conducted that examined the impact of interventions based on CCM elements. Using methods for categorizing and mapping interventions based on our 2006 publication, Pasricha et al. [17] examined the effectiveness of DS and CIS interventions on improving the care of people living with HIV. They found evidence of modest improvements, with greater impact on process measures compared to outcome measures. This is consistent with our findings for DS and CIS interventions.

Baptista et al. [24] conducted a systematic review of studies which evaluated interventions based on CCM elements for T2DM. That review was restricted to RCTs with at least 3 month's follow-up and assessed only primary clinical outcomes (mortality) or intermediate clinical outcomes (glycosylated haemoglobin). They identified 12 studies that met the inclusion criteria. In six of these there was evidence of improvement of clinical outcomes. Baptista et al. [24] concluded that interventions based on isolated components of CCM may not be enough to improve clinical outcomes and suggested that greater benefits could be obtained through interventions combining the CCM's six elements. In our review, studies with three or more CCM elements in the intervention were not associated with more statistically significant improvements in outcomes than studies with a smaller number of elements. The differences in findings and conclusions may be explained by the wider inclusion criteria for this review and the broader range of outcomes examined.

Strengths and limitations of this review

The strengths of this systematic review include: the use of pre-published methods [15, 16]; the large number of articles and studies summarized; and the mapping of study interventions to the CCM, a method that is becoming increasingly common [17, 24, 25]. The limitations of this review include the exclusion of studies from developing countries. The countries included in the 2006 review were chosen according to health care systems broadly comparable to Australia, and for comparison the same countries were included in this study. Widening the inclusion criteria would have increased the number of eligible studies and may have been advantageous given that health systems in low and middle income countries are similarly challenged with increasing prevalence of chronic disease. As in our previous review, the scope of chronic disease included did not include cancer or mental health problems. The study duration of included studies ranged from 1 to 72 months and therefore information on long-term impacts is limited. A further limitation was that on this occasion we did not examine the impact of CCM interventions on all the outcomes extracted, but only on the primary outcome (as defined by the study authors) and up to six additional outcomes. This may be a factor in some of the differences observed since the previous review. A strength of our approach is that it provides a high-level overview of the pattern of effectiveness of CCM interventions on a range of outcomes across a number of chronic conditions however our approach makes it difficult to drill down to the impact of individual interventions for individual conditions. and to see the effect size of an intervention on a single outcome measure. Lastly, using *P*-values to indicate which interventions likely resulted in improvements in chronic disease outcomes has drawbacks, including not separating the estimated effect size and the estimated precision of the measure.

Conclusions

This review demonstrated benefits from implementation of interventions based on CCM elements in primary care. The findings provide further evidence to support the view that self-management education should be an integral part of high-quality primary care [26]. Kadu and Stolle [27] have identified that characteristics of the health care organization and the needs and capacity of health care providers are important influences on implementing the CCM model in primary care. There remains a paucity of research on interventions which aim to address the HCO element of the CCM and its impact on process and patient outcomes. The need for further research in this area is highlighted by both our finding and reviews by Kadu and Stolle [27] and Dauvrin et al. [28] who suggested that the scope of chronic care interventions should be expanded to transform health care organizations and systems. There is also a need for research on CR interventions, particularly given the principles of health promotion to involve communities and the recognition of the importance of environmental factors on health, as emphasized by Barr et al. in their description of an expanded CCM [29].

Abbreviations

CCM: Chronic care model; CDM: Chronic disease management; CIS: Clinical information systems; COPD: Chronic obstructive pulmonary disease; CR: Community resources; DS: Decision support; DSD: Delivery system design; EPOC: Effective practice and organisation of care; PRISMA: Preferred reporting items for systematic reviews and meta-analyses; RCT: Randomized controlled trial; SD: Standard devisation; SMS: Self-management support; T2DM: Type 2 diabetes mellitus; WHO: World Health Organization; YLD: Years lived with disability

Acknowledgements

We would like to thank Professor Tom Bodenheimer for his guidance on description of the elements of the CCM; Sarah Jacob for her help with sourcing the full texts; Dr. Nicole Mealing for her statistical help; and Yu Gu for her help with the quality assessment.

Funding

Internally funded. This review did not receive any external financial or other material support.

Authors' contributions

All authors contributed to the manuscript. RR, NZ, SD and IH were primarily responsible for the conceptualization and design of the review. RR conducted the searches. NZ conducted the snowballing. JS, WC, DT and SB were primarily responsible for data extraction. RR, SD, IH and NZ lead the analysis. RR and NZ led the drafting of the manuscript. All authors contributed to the final manuscript. All authors have read and approved the final manuscript.

Consent for publication

Not applicable

Competing interests

The authors declare that they have no competing interests.

Author details

[1]UNSW, Sydney, Australia. [2]University of Sydney, Camperdown, Australia. [3]School of Medicine, University of Wollongong, Wollongong, NSW 2522, Australia.

References

1. World Health Organization. Global status report on noncommunicable diseases. 2014. http://www.who.int/nmh/publications/ncd-status-report-2014/en/. Accessed 5 Sept 2017.
2. Vos T, Barber RM, Bell B, Bertozzi-Villa A, Biryukov S, Bolliger I, et al. Global, regional, and national incidence, prevalence, and years lived with disability for 301 acute and chronic diseases and injuries in 188 countries, 1990-2013: a systematic analysis for the global burden of disease study 2013. Lancet. 2015. doi: https://doi.org/10.1016/S0140-6736(15)60692-4.
3. Dennis S. Secondary prevention of chronic health conditions in patients with multimorbidity: what can physiotherapists do? J Comorb. 2016. doi: https://doi.org/10.15256/joc.2016.6.82.
4. Australian Institute of Health and Welfare. Chronic diseases. 2015. http://www.aihw.gov.au/chronic-diseases/. Accessed 5 Apr 2016.
5. World Health Organization. Innovative care for chronic conditions: building blocks for action. 2001. http://www.who.int/chp/knowledge/publications/icccreport/en/. Accessed 5 Sept 2017.
6. Rothman AA, Wagner EH. Chronic illness management: what is the role of primary care?. Ann Intern Med. 2003. doi: https://doi.org/10.7326/0003-4819-138-3-200302040-00034.
7. Ham C. The ten characteristics of the high-performing chronic care system. Health Econ Policy Law. 2009; doi: https://doi.org/10.1017/S1744133109990120.
8. Phillips R, Starfield B. Why does a US primary care workforce crisis matter? Am Fam Physician 2003;68(8):1494-1500. http://www.aafp.org/afp/2003/1015/p1494.html.
9. Wagner EH, Austin BT, Korff MV. Organizing Care for Patients with chronic illness. Milbank Q. 1996;74(4):511.
10. Wagner EH, Austin BT, Davis C, Hindmarsh M, Schaefer J, Bonomi A. Improving chronic illness care: translating evidence into action. Health Aff. 2001; doi: https://doi.org/10.1377/hlthaff.20.6.64.
11. Bodenheimer T, Wagner EH, Grumbach K. Improving primary Care for Patients with Chronic Illness. JAMA. 2002; doi: https://doi.org/10.1001/jama.288.14.1775.
12. Bodenheimer T, Wagner EH, Grumbach K. Improving primary care for patients with chronic illness- the chronic care model, part 2. JAMA. 2002; doi: https://doi.org/10.1001/jama.288.15.1909.
13. Nutting PA, Miller WL, Crabtree BF, Jaen CR, Stewart EE, Stange KC. Initial lessons from the first national demonstration project on practice transformation to a patient-centered medical home. Ann Fam Med. 2009; doi: https://doi.org/10.1370/afm.1002.
14. Bodenheimer T, Ghorob A, Willard-Grace R, Grumbach K. The 10 building blocks of high-performing primary care. Ann Fam Med. 2014; doi: https://doi.org/10.1370/afm.1616.
15. Dennis S, Zwar N, Griffiths R, Roland M, Hasan I, Powell Davies G, et al. Chronic disease management in primary care: from evidence to policy. Med J Aust. 2008;188(8 Suppl):S53–6.
16. Zwar N, Harris M, Griffiths R, Roland M, Dennis S, Powell Davies G, et al. A systematic review of chronic disease management. Australian Primary Health Care Research Institute. 2006. http://aphcri.anu.edu.au/projects/network/systematic-review-chronic-disease-management. Accessed 5 Sept 2017.
17. Pasricha A, Deinstadt RTM, Moher D, Killoran A, Rourke SB, Kendall CE. Chronic care model decision support and clinical information systems interventions for people living with HIV: a systematic review. J Gen Intern Med. 2012; doi: https://doi.org/10.1007/s11606-012-2145-y.
18. Reynolds R, Dennis S, Hasan I, Tian D, Bobba S, Bodenheimer T, et al. An update of a systematic review of chronic disease management interventions in primary care. PROSPERO international prospective register of systematic reviews. 2014. http://www.crd.york.ac.uk/PROSPERO/display_record.asp?ID=CRD42014009219. Accessed 5 Sept 2017.
19. Cochrane Effective Practice and Organisation of Care (EPOC). EPOC resources for review authors. 2017. epoc.cochrane.org/epoc-resources-review-authors. Accessed 5 Sept 2017.
20. Moher D, Liberati A, Tetzlaff J, Altman DG. Preferred reporting items for systematic reviews and meta-analyses: the PRISMA statement. PLoS Med. 2009; doi: https://doi.org/10.1371/journal.pmed.1000097.
21. Centre for Reviews and Dissemination, University of York. Systematic reviews: CRD's guidance for undertaking reviews in health care. 2009. https://www.york.ac.uk/media/crd/Systematic_Reviews.pdf. Accessed 5 Sept 2017.
22. Weingarten SR, Henning JM, Badamgarav E, Knight K, Hasselblad V, Gano A, et al. Interventions used in disease management programmes for patients with chronic illness—which ones work? Meta-analysis of published reports.

BMJ. 2002;325(7370):925.
23. Shojania KG, Jennings A, Mayhew A, Ramsay CR, Eccles MP, Grimshaw J. The effects of on-screen, point of care computer reminders on processes and outcomes of care. Cochrane Database Syst Rev. 2009; doi: https://doi.org/10.1002/14651858.CD001096.pub2.
24. Baptista DR, Wiens A, Pontarolo R, Regis L, Reis WC, Correr CJ. The chronic care model for type 2 diabetes: a systematic review. Diabetol Metab Syndr. 2016; doi: https://doi.org/10.1186/s13098-015-0119-z.
25. Adams SG, Smith PK, Allan PF, Anzueto A, Pugh JA, Cornell JE. Systematic review of the chronic care model in chronic obstructive pulmonary disease prevention and management. Arch Intern Med. 2007; doi: https://doi.org/10.1001/archinte.167.6.551.
26. Bodenheimer T. Patient self-management of chronic disease in primary care. JAMA. 2002; doi: https://doi.org/10.1001/jama.288.19.2469.
27. Kadu MK, Stolee P. Facilitators and barriers of implementing the chronic care model in primary care: a systematic review. BMC Fam Pract. 2015; doi: https://doi.org/10.1186/s12875-014-0219-0.
28. Dauvrin M, Lorant V. Cultural competence and social relationships: a social network analysis. Int Nurs Rev. 2016; doi: https://doi.org/10.1111/inr.12327.
29. Barr V, Robinson S, Marin-Link B, Underhill L, Dotts A, Ravensdale D, Salivaras S. The expanded chronic care model: an integration of concepts and strategies from population health promotion and the chronic care model. Hosp Q. 2003;7(1):73–82.

2

Frequent attenders in late life in primary care

Franziska D. Welzel[1*], Janine Stein[1], André Hajek[3], Hans-Helmut König[3] and Steffi G. Riedel-Heller[1,2]

Abstract

Background: High utilization of health care services is a costly phenomenon commonly observed in primary care practices. However, while frequent attendance in primary care has been broadly studied across age groups, aspects of high utilization by elderly patients have not been investigated in detail. The aim of this paper is to provide a systematic review of frequent attendance in primary care among elderly people.

Methods: We searched five databases (PubMed, PsycINFO, Web of Science, PubPsych, and Cochrane Library) for published papers addressing frequent attendance in primary health care among elderly individuals. Quality of studies was assessed using established criteria for evaluating methodological quality.

Results: Ten studies met inclusion criteria and were included for detailed analysis. The average number of patients frequently utilizing primary care services varied across studies from 10% to 33% of the elderly samples and subsamples. The definition of frequent attendance across studies differed substantially. The most consistent associations between frequent attendance and old age were found for presence and severity of physical illness. Results on mental disorders and frequent attendance were heterogeneous. Only a few studies have assessed frequent attendance in association with factors such as drug use, social support or sociodemographic aspects; however results were inconsistent.

Conclusions: Severe ill health and the need for treatment serve as the main drivers of frequent attendance in older adults. As results were scarce and divergent, future studies are needed to provide more information on this topic. Since prior studies have offered only a snapshot of this service use behaviour, a longitudinal approach would be preferable in the future.

Keywords: Primary care, General practice, Elderly, Frequent attendance

Background

General practitioners (GPs) are usually the first point of contact for elderly people for a broad range of health problems. However, a small proportion of patients, visit their GPs more frequently, thereby generating a significant amount of their workload [1, 2]. In general terms, a patient who attends general health care practices on a regular basis and who exceeds a certain number of visits within a given time interval is defined as a frequent attender (FA) [3–5]. As such, FAs are patients who consume large amounts of GP resources and generate sizable expenses for health care services [6–8]. Primary care is a main base of generalist care and serves as a major access point to the first level of professional care for people of all age groups including elderly people with depression and the oldest-old [9–12]. Thus, the primary care level provides a key setting for studying high utilization by elderly patients.

Across countries and differing definitions of frequent attendance, elderly people are overrepresented among this group of primary care utilizers [13–16]. Due to increasing life expectancy and low birth rates, the proportion of people aged 65 years and over has increased in Europe over the last decade from 16.6% in 2005 to

* Correspondence: Franziska.Welzel@medizin.uni-leipzig.de
[1]Institute of Social Medicine, Occupational Health and Public Health, Medical Faculty, University of Leipzig, Philipp-Rosenthal-Straße 55, 04103 Leipzig, Germany
Full list of author information is available at the end of the article

19.2% in 2016 [17]. In an aging society, high utilization of primary health care services among the elderly will have considerable consequences in terms of expenditure and costs for health care resources [7, 18].

While several studies have linked frequent attendance of adults of all ages to chronic physical illness [19–22], mental disorders [19, 21, 22] and female gender [16, 21, 23], the increased utilization of health care services by the elderly has also been associated with depressive symptoms, migration status, lower income and lower educational levels [24–27]. As elderly people are often more vulnerable to a variety of illnesses and life stressors, it may be reasonable to assume that older FAs have different reasons for frequent attendance than their younger counterparts.

Previous studies [28, 29] have reviewed frequent attendance in general practice in all age groups; however, they did not specifically look at the frequent attendance of elderly people in detail. To date, an overview of frequent attendance by the elderly that provides information on the associations and determinants of elderly FAs in primary health care is lacking. Furthermore, an understanding of the factors associated with frequent attendance among the elderly is important for planning for and providing cost-effective and target-oriented health care. This review sets out to fill this gap by reviewing relevant literature on frequent attendance among the elderly at the primary care level.

Unfortunately, cross-national comparisons of health care related issues are challenging because of the differences in health care systems and conflicting definitions of primary care across countries. Although health care is mainly a national matter, even in the EU, there is some agreement among European countries about the importance and role of general practitioners in delivering primary health care services [30, 31]. Therefore, this review focuses on European studies.

The objectives of this review are: (1) to systematically obtain and evaluate the relevant literature on frequent attenders in primary health care among the elderly in Europe, (2) to provide an overview and information source about elderly people frequently attending primary health care practices, and (3) to discuss the potential determinants of frequent utilization of primary health care services in old age.

Methods

This review follows the PRISMA (Preferred Reporting Items for Systematic Reviews and Meta-Analyses) guidelines [32].

Search terms and search strategy

A systematic literature search in the electronic databases PubMed, PsycINFO, Web of Science, PubPsych and Cochrane Library was conducted in November 2016. No restriction regarding the year of publication was imposed. Electronic databases were searched using MeSH keywords and free-text terms as follows: (high utiliz* OR heavy use* OR (frequent AND (consult* OR attend* OR use*))) AND ("Physicians, Primary Care" OR "Physicians, Family" OR "General Practitioners" OR "Primary Health Care" OR "Family Practice") AND (old age OR elderly). For full search strategy see Additional file 1.

Selection criteria

Abstracts were screened using the following selection criteria: (i) published studies in the primary care/general practice settings, (ii) patient recruitment in primary care/general practice, (iii) study samples consisting of patients aged 65 years and older, (iv) studies focused on frequent attendance, (v) measurement of frequency by number of contacts with general practice, (vi) studies providing an explicit definition of frequent attendance, (vii) studies conducted in Europe. Criteria for exclusion were as follows: (viii) language other than English or German, (ix) literature review only, (x) no full report of primary research (e.g. conference abstract, commentaries, study protocol), (xi) single case studies, (xii) setting is not exclusively general practice, (xiii) studies assessing primarily other aspects of health care consultation than frequent attendance.

Data extraction and data synthesis

Abstracts and titles were screened and potentially relevant articles were retrieved in full-text for a more detailed analysis. Duplicates were eliminated. In addition, the bibliographies of selected articles were assessed for further relevant literature. Identified studies that were likely to be relevant were assessed in full-text according to the above described selection criteria. Data extraction was conducted using predetermined criteria based on study characteristics and main results. The following information was extracted from each included study: a) study characteristics (authors, year, country, study design and objectives), b) sampling and characteristics of participants (study base, sampling from study base, sample gender and age, control sampling, number of participating GPs), c) definition of frequent attendance including contact initiation, included and excluded contacts, data sources and d) main results for the elderly, median or mean consultation rate and odds ratio for frequent attendance, if provided. A narrative synthesis approach was applied to describe key associations of frequent attendance in old age.

Quality assessment

The methodological quality of the studies included in this review was independently evaluated by the principal author (F.W.) and co-author (J.S.) using a 13-item checklist of predefined criteria. The checklist (see Table 1) was build based on established criteria lists applied in other reviews [33–36]. As not all of the 13 criteria were applicable to all 10 studies due to differing study designs, the overall quality of a study was assessed using the number of applicable checklist items as reference value. Studies scoring in the 75th percentile or higher were rated as high quality, while studies scoring between 50% and 75% were rated as moderate quality, and studies scoring below 50% were categorized as low quality.

Results

Literature search results

The initial search strategy yielded 1743 potentially relevant articles, of which 169 studies were excluded as they were published in languages other than English or German. For 1574 articles, titles and abstracts were screened for eligibility. From these, 104 studies were identified as eligible and two additional articles were chosen from the bibliographies of other articles. Overall, 106 studies were obtained and reviewed for final inclusion. After full-text assessment, 10 studies were identified and considered for detailed analysis. The different stages of this selection process are provided in Fig. 1.

Table 1 Criteria for assessing methodical quality of studies on frequent utilization of primary health care services

Study objective and design
1. Clearly stated study objectives and hypotheses.
Study population
2. Study sample is nationally and regionally representative, study sample includes representative sample of elderly individuals.
3. Sample inclusion and/or exclusion criteria are formulated.
4. Sociodemographic characteristics of the study sample are described.
5. Participation and response rates are reported, Participation rate > 75%.
Assessment
6. Detailed description of methods, procedures and instruments is given.
7. Stratification (e.g. age, gender) was used to assess frequent attendance.
Data reporting and analysis
8. Characteristics of responders and non-responders are presented.
9. Descriptive data (mean or median, standard deviations or percentages) are provided for the most important outcome measures and for different age groups.
10. Data on frequent attendance among elderly is given.
11. Precision of estimates is given (e.g. 95% Confidence Intervals).
12. The handling of missing values is described.
Other
13. Conflicts of interest reported and identification of funding sources is possible.

Adapted from [33–36]
Each item is scored as 1 = met the quality criterion, 0 = did not meet the quality criterion or item was not reported or unclear, – not applicable

Methodological quality

The results of the methodological quality assessment of the included ten studies are displayed in Table 2, right column. Six studies (60%) were of high quality, two studies (20%) of moderate quality, and two studies (20%) of low quality. The median score per study was nine (range five to ten) for cross-sectional and cohort studies. Methodological shortcomings according to the quality assessment (items with a score below the median) were lack of representativeness of the sample, lack of stratification for assessment of frequent attendance, missing reports on sociodemographic details and insufficient report or handling of missing values.

General and methodological characteristics of the reviewed studies

Methodological characteristics of the reviewed studies and results regarding frequent attendance in elderly samples are summarized in Tables 2 and 3.

The included studies came from the following European countries: the United Kingdom, Sweden, Germany, Denmark (two studies each), as well as Italy and Slovenia (one study each).

Most of the included studies in this review applied a cross-sectional design [37–45]. One study reported the use of a longitudinal design [46]; however, the authors did not apply a specific regression model to analyse the panel data but instead used baseline data to predict subsequent frequent attendance.

The samples of the majority of the reviewed studies were based on the population of listed patients from cooperating GPs, primary health care centres or patients registered with a health insurance company [37, 38, 42–44]. In one study, the study population consisted of listed patients with the documented diagnosis of heart failure [46]. In three out of the ten studies, the study population consisted of patients attending a general practice or primary health care centre during a predefined time interval [39, 41, 45]. In one Swedish study, the study sample was based on patients registered with the Swedish National Study on Aging and Care [40]. Only half of the included studies focused solely on elderly patients [38, 40, 44–46]. Half of the studies assessed frequency of attendance in subsamples of elderly patients among other age groups [37, 39, 41–43].

Sample sizes considering elderly samples or subsamples varied substantially across studies between $n = 112$ and $n = 123,224$. Two studies did not provide detailed information on the subsamples of elderly patients [41, 42]. Seven studies included information on gender distribution

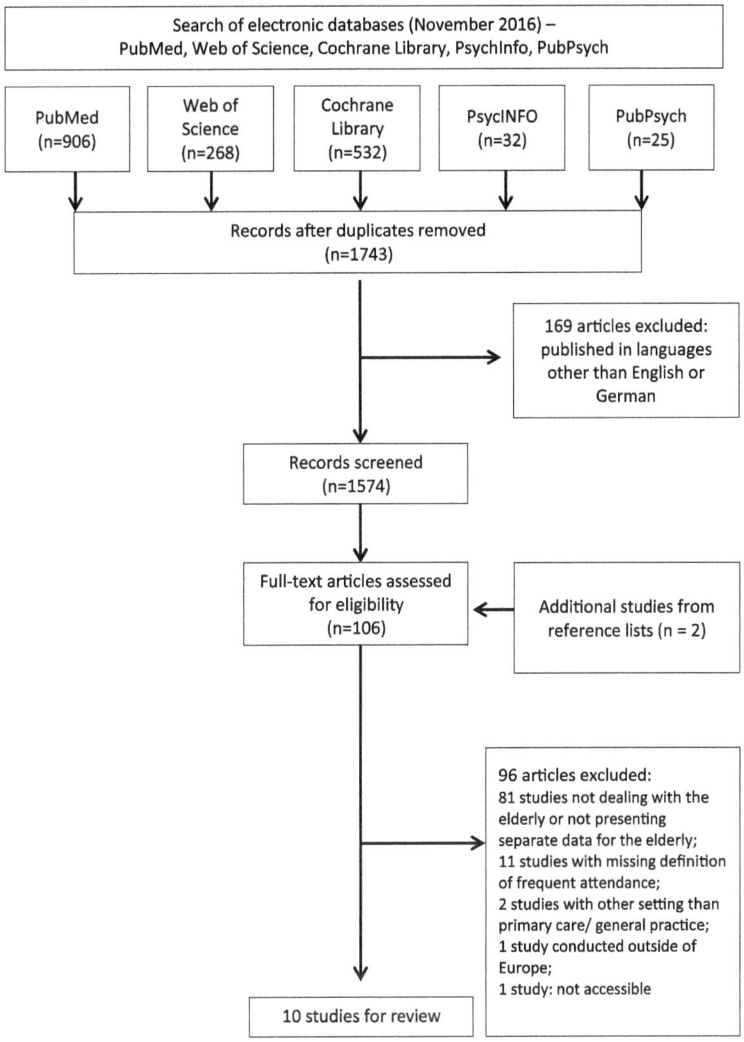

Fig. 1 PRISMA flowchart showing the different phases of the selection process

reporting a proportion of 41.4% to 68.8% female patients [37, 39–41, 44–46], with only two studies reporting a larger proportion of male patients [37, 44].

The number of participating GPs differed substantially across the included studies between $n = 7$ and $n = 320$; the number of practices varied between $n = 1$ and $n = 179$. However, three studies failed to report any information on the number of included GPs and practices [40, 42, 44], while another three studies solely reported the number of included GPs [39] or the number of included practices [38, 46].

Definition of frequent attendance

The various definitions of frequent attendance are provided in Table 3. An overview of the percentages of FAs and thresholds for frequent attendance across studies is summarized in Table 4. The percentage of elderly patients frequently utilizing primary care services varied across studies from 10% to 33%. The majority of studies considered in this review used a proportional approach to define frequent attendance and distinguished high utilizers of primary care services from other attenders. Only three studies applied an absolute number of consultations within a specified time interval as a cut-off value between FAs and non-frequent attenders (non-FAs) [39, 44, 46]. Additionally, one of these studies considered further definitions of frequent attendance [44]. In addition to the number of consultations with primary care practices within a year, the authors applied contacts with a certain number of different practices and contacts with different practices of the same medical specialty as further definitions of FAs. Four studies allocated the top 10% of most frequent primary care users into the group of FAs [37, 38, 41, 42]. Other studies used different cut-off points to define FAs: frequencies of top 25% [43], 30% [40] and 33% [45] were each employed.

Table 2 Study characteristics and study quality of the included studies

Author and year	Country	Study type	Study population	Sample			Number GP's/practices	Study quality (score)
				n (FA)/n (Controls)	Age	Sex		
Bergh and Marklund, 2003 [37]	Sweden	cross-sectional	listed patients	elderly (≥65 years): 85/126	women (≥65 years): M = 77.1 (Fa), M = 76.4 (CG) men (≥65 years): M = 77.0 (Fa), M = 74.1 (CG)	elderly (≥65 years): 46.4% female	7/1	High quality (9)
Gilleard et al., 1998 [38]	UK	cross-sectional	listed patients aged 65 years and over	95/919	range: ≥65	n/a	n/a /1	Low quality (6)
Menchetti et al., 2006 [39]	Italy	cross-sectional	attending patients aged 14 years and older	elderly (≥ 60 years): 136/470	elderly (≥ 60 years): n/a	elderly (≥ 60 years): 61% female	191/ n/a	High quality (10)
Rennemark et al., 2009 [40]	Sweden	cross-sectional	registered patients with the Swedish National Study on Aging and Care	229/511	Median = 66 range: 60–78	54.2% female	n/a	High quality (10)
Scherer et al., 2008 [46]	Germany	cohort-study	listed patients with diagnosis of heart failure	48/262	M = 72.9 (SD = 9)	68.8% female (FA)/ 50.4% female (CG)	n/a /44	Moderate quality (8)
Sheehan et al., 2003 [45]	UK	cross-sectional	attending patients aged 65 years and over	53/87	M = 76.8 (SD = 7.3) range: ≥ 65	57.9% female	14/2 (centres)	Moderate quality (9)
Svab and Zaletel-Kragelj, 1993 [43]	Slovenia	cross-sectional	listed patients	elderly (>65): 34/78	elderly (>65): n/a	elderly (>65): n/a	8/1 (primary care centre)	Low quality (5)
van den Bussche et al., 2016 [44]	Germany	cross-sectional	registered patients with a health insurance company	23,590 (19.1%)/99,634 (80.9%)	FA: M = 73, SD = 6.4 CG: M = 71.7, SD = 6.1	46.3% female (FA)/ 41.4% female (CG)	n/a	High quality (9)
Vedsted et al., 2001 [42]	Denmark	cross-sectional	listed patients aged 20 years and over	elderly (>65): n/a	elderly (>65): n/a	elderly (>65): n/a	n/a	High quality (9)
Vedsted et al., 2004 [41]	Denmark	cross-sectional	attending patients aged 20 years and over	elderly (≥65 years):6718/n/a	elderly (≥65 years): n/a	elderly (≥65 years): 57.8% female (FA)	320/179	High quality (10)

FA Frequent attender, *GP* General Practitioner, *M* Mean, *SD* Standard deviation, *CG* Control group; n/a = no information provided; – = not applicable

Table 3 Results on frequent attendance among the elderly at the primary care level across reviewed studies

Author and year	FA definition	Included contacts	Excluded contacts	Data sources	Main results
Bergh and Marklund, 2003 [37]	10% most frequent attenders in 12 months/ by sex and age group	face-to-face visits to GP		medical records	Elderly (≥ 65 years): • Most diagnostic groups and medical prescriptions more frequent among FAs than non-FAs for both sexes Most common diseases: • Women: diseases of circulatory and musculoskeletal system, similar for FAs and non-FAs • Men: circulatory & endocrine diagnoses (FAs), circulatory and musculoskeletal problems (non-FAs)
Gilleard et al., 1998 [38]	Very High Attenders: 10% most frequent attenders in 12 months (> 15 contacts in 12 months)	face-to-face visits to GP, visits to the practice nurse	home visits, out-of-hour visits	computerized records, interviews, questionnaires	Elderly (≥ 65 years): • 10% FAs responsible for 33% of all visits • Frequent attendance not associated with psychiatric morbidity, self-reported depression, use of hypnotic or antipsychotic medication • Use of antidepressants: 9.5% of FAs received prescriptions for antidepressants compared to 2.8% of low average attenders (chi-square = 13.6, df 3, $p < 0.01$)
Menchetti et al., 2006 [39]	> 1 contact to GP per month in 6 months	n/a	n/a	registered data, questionnaires, clinical judgments of GPs	Elderly (≥ 60 years): • Frequent attendance associated with moderate or severe physical illness (aOR = 2.89, 95% CI: 1.63–5.11), depression (aOR = 1.92, 95% CI: 1.10–3.35) and unexplained somatic symptoms (aOR = 1.99, 95% CI: 1.05–3.77) • Depression increased risk of being an FA fivefold and was a risk factor for frequent attendance independent of other clinical predictors
Rennemark et al., 2009 [40]	30% most frequent attenders in 12 months (≥3 contacts in 12 months)	n/a	n/a	questionnaires, cognitive tests, medical records	Elderly (≥ 60 years): • Number of GP visits positively correlated with age (0.53, $p < 0.001$), and comorbidity (0.93, $p < 0.001$), and negatively correlated with functional ability (–0.18, $p < 0.001$), education level (–0.12, p < 0.01) and internal locus of control (–0.12, p < 0.01) Results from logistic regression analyses: • Physical comorbidity as main factor determining frequent attendance (OR = 8.17, 95% CI: 5.54–12.04) • Sense of coherence (OR = 1.03, 95% CI: 1.00–1.06) and locus of control (OR = 1.14, 95% CI: 1.02–1.27) significantly related to frequent attendance • Education level and social anchorage not associated with frequent attendance
Scherer et al., 2008 [46]	> 17 contacts in 9 months	n/a	n/a	questionnaires, telephone interviews	Elderly: • Frequent attendance associated with female sex, living alone, severity of heart failure, psychological distress and quality of life • In multivariate analysis physical problems (OR = 1.1, 95% CI: 1.0–1.1, p < 0.001) and living alone (OR = 2.4, 95% CI: 1.1–5.1) independently related to frequent attendance

Table 3 Results on frequent attendance among the elderly at the primary care level across reviewed studies *(Continued)*

Author and year	FA definition	Included contacts	Excluded contacts	Data sources	Main results
Sheehan et al., 2003 [45]	top third of attenders in 9 months	medical contacts with GP at primary care centre or at home	consultations with practice nurse	patient interview, GP records, GP assessment of patients tendency to somatise	Elderly (≥ 65 years): • Frequent attendance related to depression (OR = 2.24, 95% CI: 1.11–4.50, $p < 0.05$), high rates of physical disorder (OR = 1.78, 95% CI:1.16–2.71, p < 0.05), somatic symptom reporting (OR = 1.83, 95% CI:1.13–2.97, p < 0.05), and low social support (OR = 1.73, 95% CI:1.01–2.94, p < 0.05) • In multivariate regression only low social support and somatic symptoms significantly related to frequent attendance
Svab and Zaletel-Kragelj, 1993 [43]	25% most frequent attenders in 12 months/ by age group	face-to-face visits with GP, contacts for administrative purposes	telephone contacts	medical records and registered data	Elderly (>65): • Probability for superficial (administrative) contacts larger for FAs compared to non-FAs (median percentage of superficial contacts among all contacts: FAs = 27.1%/non-FAs = 0.5%, $p = 0.05$) • Non-significant trend: larger probability of referral to specialists for FAs compared to non-FAs (median index-value for referral to a specialist: FAs = 8.0/non-FAs = 0.4).
van den Bussche et al., 2016 [44]	A: ≥ 50 contacts with physician practices in 12 months B: contacts with ≥10 different practices in 12 months C: contacts with ≥3 different practices of the same medical specialty in 12 months	visits to the practice, home, nursing home visits, telephone contacts, contacts with practice staff	appointments by phone and administrative contacts	insurance claims data/ registered data	Elderly (≥65): • Type A attendance associated with higher age, dependency on nursing care, multi-morbidity, and high impact somatic diseases • Types B and C attendance associated with younger age, less dependency on nursing care, and presence of mental diseases • Number of chronic conditions reduced the risk of being Type C FA
Vedsted et al., 2001 [42]	daytime: 10% most frequent attenders (≥ 12 contacts) in 12 months/ by sex and age group out-of-hours: 10% most frequent attenders (≥ 4 contacts) in 12 months	daytime: face-to-face visits with GP out-of-hours: telephone advice, surgery consultations, home visits	telephone contacts during daytime and administrative and routine consultations	electronic records	Elderly (≥ 65 years): • Frequent attendance during daytime strongly related to the risk of being an out-of-hours FA: OR and 95% CI of daytime users to be an FA in out-of-hours service compared to non-attenders: men with 10% most daytime contacts: OR = 72.5 (CI: 48.7–107.9) women with 10% most daytime contacts: OR = 40.7 (CI: 28.2–58.8)
Vedsted et al., 2004 [41]	10% most frequent attenders (≥ 12 contacts) in 12 months/ by sex and age group	face-to-face visits to GP, home visits during daytime	telephone contacts, administrative and routine consultations (e.g. driver's licenses)	electronic records	Elderly (≥ 65 years): • Prevalence ratio for using one or more drugs only slightly higher among FAs compared to the 50%-group with the fewest contacts • Prevalence for polypharmacy (drugs from 5 or more drug groups) 6.7 times (men) and 4.2 times (women) higher among FAs compared to the 50%-group with the fewest contacts

n/a **No information provided,** *FA* **Frequent attender,** *fa* **Frequent attendance,** *GP* **General practitioner,** *OR* **Odds ratio,** *aOR* **Adjusted Odds ratio,** *CI* **Confidence interval,** *df* **Degrees of freedom,** *p* ***p*-value**

Table 4 Overview of frequent attendance in elderly samples or sub-samples across included studies

Author and year	Percentage of FAs	Threshold for frequent attendance
Bergh and Marklund, 2003	10%	n/a
Gilleard et al., 1998	10%	> 15 contacts in 12 months
Menchetti et al., 2006	22.4%	> 1 contact per month in 6 months
Rennemark et al., 2009	30%	≥ 3 contacts in 12 months
Scherer et al., 2008	15.5%	> 17 contacts in 9 months
Sheehan et al., 2003	33.3%	≥ 11 contacts in 12 months
Svab and Zaletel-Kragelj, 1993	25%	n/a
van den Bussche et al., 2016	In total: 19% Def. A: 14.2% Def. B: 8.9% Def. C: 5.1%	Def. A: ≥ 50 contacts in 12 months
Vedsted et al., 2001	10%	≥ 12 contacts in 12 months
Vedsted et al., 2004	10%	≥ 12 contacts in 12 months

n/a = No information provided; *FA* = Frequent attender; *Def.* = Definition

While only four studies assessed attendance rates stratified by sex or age [37, 41–43], the majority of the included studies assessed attendance over a 12 month timeframe [37, 38, 40–44]. Other time intervals used to assess frequency of attendance were 6 months [39] and 9 months [45, 46].

Half of the studies exclusively considered face-to-face contacts with a GP to assess frequency of attendance [37, 41–43, 45], while two studies included patient contacts with practice staff in general [38, 44]. The remaining studies provided no information about the nature of contacts included in the assessment of frequent attendance.

To measure frequent attendance and associated factors, nine out of the ten studies used medical records or electronic registered data as data sources [37–45]. One study relied solely on patient interviews and patient questionnaires as data sources on frequency of attendance [46].

Factors associated with frequent attendance

Findings on factors associated with frequent attendance among elderly primary care patients are summarized in Table 5. Reported factors included: sociodemographic aspects, physical and mental illnesses, medical prescriptions, social support and different types of health care utilization.

Sociodemographic factors

Four studies reported on the relation between *gender* and frequent attendance at the primary care level. Analysing the relationship between gender and attendance rate, two studies found no association between gender and FA-status [39, 45]. Two studies reported female gender to be significantly associated with frequent attendance [40, 46].

Assessing *age* and frequent attendance among the elderly, no significant association was reported in two studies [45, 46]. Another study found a strong positive correlation between age and number of visits to the GP ($r = 0.53$, $p < 0.01$), however this association disappeared after logistic regression analysis [40]. One further study reported odds ratios of age and gender for the relative chance of belonging to three different types of frequent attendance [44]. They found significantly higher chances for older male and female patients (≥ 75 years) of belonging to the group of FAs consulting 50 times or more within 12 months (females: OR = 1.55, 95% CI: 1.40–1.72; males: OR = 1.38, 95% CI: 1.26–1.51) compared to somewhat younger patients (65–74 years). The authors further found that the chances of belonging to the group of FAs who contacted more than nine different practices (females: OR = 0.65, 95% CI: 0.60–0.71; males: OR = 0.79, 95% CI: 0.73–0.85) or more than two practices of the same medical specialty (females: OR = 0.60, 95% CI: 0.55–0.66; males: OR = 0.88, 95% CI: 0.81–0.95) within one year was smaller in the older age groups compared to younger patients (65–74 years) [44].

Similar to age and gender, only two studies reported results on the association between *educational level* and FA-status. One study reported a significant negative correlation ($r = -0.12$, $p < 0.01$) between educational level and number of GP visits, indicating that a higher educational level was associated with a lower number of visits to the GP. However, educational level was not found to be related to frequent attendance in logistic regression analysis [40]. Another study found no association between educational level and FA-status among the elderly [39]. One further study looked at social class with regards to high and low primary care attenders and found no significant differences between the two attendance groups [45].

Two studies reported on *living situation* and *civil status*. One study found that living alone was a significant predictor of being an FA (OR = 2.4, 95% CI: 1.2–5.1, $p = 0.02$) [46]. Another study found no association between marital status (single, married, divorced or separated) and frequent attendance [39].

Physical illness

Six out of the ten studies reported results on the association between frequent attendance at the primary care level and presence of physical diseases or multi-morbidity [37, 39, 40, 44–46]. Four studies analysed odds ratios to compare presence or severity of physical disorders among FAs and non-FAs. Three studies reported significantly

Table 5 Findings on factors associated with frequent attendance among elderly primary care patients

	Bergh and Marklund, 2003	Gilleard et al., 1998	Menchetti et al., 2006	Rennemark et al., 2009	Scherer et al., 2008	Sheehan et al., 2003	Svab and Zaletel-Kragelj, 1993	van den Bussche et al., 2016	Vedsted et al., 2001	Vedsted et al., 2004
No. or severity of somatic diseases	+		+	+	+	+		+/−		
presence of mental illness/psychological distress		0	+		+	+		+		
medical prescriptions	+	0/+								+
low social support or social anchorage				0	0	+				
sociodemographic factors:										
older age				+	0	0		+/−		
female gender			0	+	+	0				
educational level			0	−/0						
living alone					+					
lower quality of life					+					
No. of superficial contacts							+			
No. of referrals to specialists							0			
frequent attendance out-of-hours									+	

A plus sign indicates a positive association between frequent attendance and the respective factor; a minus sign indicates a negative association between frequent attendance and the respective factor; 0 indicates no association was found; blank cells mean that the factor was not studied; No. = Number

higher odds for the presence of multiple physical disorders [40, 45] or moderate to severe physical illness and unexplained somatic complaints [39] among FAs as compared to non-FAs. One study computed odds ratios for the most common medical diagnoses separately to describe the ratio of individuals among FAs and non-FAs with a certain diagnosis [37]. Most of the diagnoses (circulatory disease, musculoskeletal disease, endocrine and respiratory disease) were found more frequently among FAs as compared to non-FAs. This pattern was similar for male and female patients. However, the types of medical problems FAs and non-FAs consulted their GP for were similar [37]. Another study focusing on patients with a preceding heart failure diagnosis found significantly more physical problems and higher levels of self-rated severity of heart failure-related impairments among FAs than non-FAs, whereas perceived low severity of heart failure among the elderly patients was associated with infrequent attendance [46]. The presence of physical problems linked to the heart failure diagnosis remained associated with frequent attendance even after multivariate analysis [46]. One study reported odds ratios for multi-morbidity and dependency on nursing care for three subtypes of frequent attendance [44]. They found that number of chronic conditions and nursing care dependency was significantly associated with the group of FAs consulting physician practices 50 times or more within 12 months (type A). However, the authors showed that dependence on nursing care lowered the chance of belonging to the group of FAs who contacted either more than two practices of the same medical specialty (not including general practice or internal medicine, type C) or more than nine different physician practices within a year (type B). As for multi-morbidity, the authors reported that every additional chronic disease raised the chance of belonging to the subgroup of type A attenders by 23%, to type B attenders by 4% and lowered the chance of belonging to type C attenders by 6% [44]. In summary, six out of the ten reviewed studies reported an association between presence and severity of medical diagnoses and frequent attendance at the primary care level.

Mental illness

Four studies assessed the relationship between psychiatric morbidity [38, 39, 45] or psychological distress [46] and frequency of attendance at the primary care level. Two studies used self-assessment questionnaires to screen for depression [38] or anxiety and depressive mood [46]. Two further studies used a combination of self-assessment questionnaires and semi-structured interviews [45] or the GP's clinical judgment [39] of the presence of psychiatric disorders. In three of these four studies, significant associations were found [39, 45, 46].

One study showed that psychological distress measured with the Hospital Anxiety and Depression Scale was significantly higher among FAs [46]. Two further studies found depression significantly associated with frequent attendance [39, 45]. However, in two out of the three studies reporting a significant association between psychological distress or depression and FA-status, anxiety and depression were no longer significant after multivariate analysis [45, 46]. Only one out of these four studies found psychiatric morbidity and self-reported depression not to be associated with frequent attendance [38].

One further study calculated relative risks (RR) of becoming a frequent attender based on a single diagnosis [44]. They found that patients with the diagnosis of anxiety disorder had a risk of belonging to the group of FAs that was 2.5 points higher than belonging to the group of non-FAs. Similar results were found for the diagnoses of somatoform disorders (RR: 2.33) and depression (RR: 2.30). The relative risks of anxiety disorder and somatoform disorder were highest for the subgroup of FAs who contacted more than nine different practices during one year [44].

Medication

Medication and frequent attendance was assessed in three studies. One study showed that the prevalence of polypharmacy was 6.7 times higher among male FAs and 4.2 times higher among female FAs compared to the 50%-group of elderly patients with the fewest primary care contacts [41]. In another study, FAs were found to receive medical prescriptions for most prescribed drug groups (infection, neurological, circulatory and blood diseases) more frequently than non-FAs with odds ratios ranging from 1.3 to 5.1 for FAs and 0.5 to 1.4 for non-FAs [37]. Another study assessed the use of psychotropic drugs and attendance rates. They found no statistically significant association between the overall use of psychotropic drugs and category of attendance (low attendance, average attendance, high and very high attendance) [38]. However, they found an association between the use of antidepressant medications and the 10% most frequent attenders. Significantly more FAs (9.5%) were taking antidepressant medications than low average attenders (2.8%) (Chi-square = 13.6, $p < 0.01$) [38].

Social support and social anchorage

Three studies reported results on the association between social anchorage [40] or perceived social support [45, 46] and frequency of attendance. While one study found no association between attendance rates and self-reported social anchorage [40], two studies on social support showed contrasting results. Scherer et al. [46] found perceived social support not to be associated with frequency of attendance, whereas Sheehan et al. [45] found that FAs had significantly higher rates of perceived low social support than non-FAs. However, the number of studies on social support and elderly FAs was small and the comparability of these studies may be limited due to large differences in the measures of social support and social anchorage.

Type of health care utilization

The association between frequent attendance during regular office hours and frequent attendance during out-of-hours services at the primary care level was assessed in one study [42]. The results showed a strong risk of elderly daytime FAs to be FAs of out-of-hours services with odds ratios ranging from 40.7 (CI: 28.2–58.8) for female FAs to 72.5 (48.7–107.9) for male FAs.

Another study compared the type of health care utilization at the general practice and referral to specialists for FAs and non-FAs [43]. They found a significantly larger probability for superficial contacts (contacts for administrative purposes: e.g. repeat prescriptions) among FAs compared to non-FAs (see Table 4), whereas the difference in referral pattern was not significant.

Discussion

The objective of this paper was to systematically review existing literature on elderly FAs at the primary care level in Europe and to provide an overview and information source about older primary care patients belonging to this group of health care utilizers. While the number of studies focusing solely on elderly FAs was small, frequent attendance among elderly patients was most consistently associated with the presence and severity of physical illness. The studies included in our evaluation were found to be mostly of high to moderate quality. Lack of sample representativeness and insufficient reporting of missing values were the most common shortcomings.

General and methodological characteristics

Study Design

Cross-sectional studies on frequent attendance provide a snapshot of characteristics related to excessive health care consultations. However, previously published literature has shown that a considerably lower proportion of patients persist as FAs over a period of several years compared to the proportion of FAs identified in a shorter time slot (e.g. a calendar year) [21, 47] indicating that frequent doctor-consultations are typically a self-limiting behaviour. Furthermore, persistent FAs have been associated with more physical diseases, as well as social and psychiatric problems than short-term FAs [21]. Smits et al. [21], therefore, suggest that only the phenomenon of persistent frequent attendance should be studied in detail. Thus, while most of the reviewed studies were cross-sectional, the nature and course of a frequent health seeking behaviour may require long-term assessment to achieve a deeper understanding.

Countries of origin

While considerable variation of the task profiles of primary care providers have been found within and across European countries [48, 49], the countries included in this review seem to share similar trends in the development of GP service profiles over the last two decades. Schäfer et al. [50] reported a general increase in GPs participation in disease management across these countries, whereas several other task profiles of GPs (including GP as first contact, performance of medical technical procedures and preventive care) have declined in their frequency within the last twenty years in most countries with the exception of Sweden and Slovenia [50]. To our knowledge, frequent attendance has not been assessed with regard to differences at the primary care sector across European countries. Still, when studying frequent attendance at the primary care level it seems reasonable to assume that the context primary care is embedded within a country (e.g. dimensions of structure or service-delivery of primary care) may influence utilization behaviour.

Definition of frequent attendance

The methods used to differentiate FAs from other attenders in primary care practices varied substantially across the included studies. This resembles the results from Vedsted and Christensen [28], who could not find a widely accepted approach for the definition of frequent attendance in general practice. The way in which frequent attendance is defined may have relevant implications on the factors associated with this phenomenon [51]. The vast majority of the studies included in this review considered a proportional approach. Applying a proportion (e.g. the highest 10% or the highest 30%) of primary care patients into the group of FAs allows for comparisons across different studies, practices and regions. A proportional approach has the further advantage of allowing for stratification by sex and age. This allows researchers to compare FAs among patients with different sociodemographic characteristics, as women have been shown to consult their GP more frequently than men [14, 16, 23, 52] and older patients have been shown to consult more often than younger patients [13–16]. However, applying a certain proportion of most frequently attending patients stratified by sex or age into the group of FAs might fail to address the actual GP workload with respect to practical implications. GPs will usually have higher workloads with patients frequently attending the practice, whether or not those patients are within the 10% FAs of their specific sex and age group. Using an absolute number of consultations within a predefined time interval might, on the other hand, address all patients that occupy a certain amount of GP resources. Those patients are high utilizers of primary health care services even if they fail to fall into the group of FAs. Yet, the number of consultations applied as threshold for frequent attendance is often arbitrary chosen and differed substantially across the here included studies, thereby hampering the comparison of results on FAs across studies and countries. Still, in terms of practical implication, it may be useful to differentiate between high utilizers of primary care resources and FAs of a specific age and sex group.

Main factors associated with frequent attendance

Physical illness

Similar to the results from Vedsted and Christensen [28] a positive association between the severity of physical disorders, multi-morbidity and frequent attendance was found among the included studies. Previous literature on FAs in primary care has consistently shown that the presence of poor health and somatic diseases, particularly chronic diseases, are significantly more prevalent among FAs than non-FAs [19–22, 53]. In line with those findings, the results of this review show that frequent attendance by the elderly is strongly associated with ill health and reflects the actual and justifiable needs of older primary care patients for frequent doctor consultations. For elderly patients with serious physical illnesses, frequently utilizing primary health care services may, therefore, be necessary and a sign of a well-developed health care provision. However, the high prevalence of polypharmacy among elderly FAs found by Vedsted et al. [41] may indicate a possible avenue for optimizing health care management for this specific patient group.

Mental illness

The findings on frequency of primary care contacts and presence of psychiatric morbidity were more heterogeneous. Still, Menchetti et al. [39] and Sheehan et al. [45] consider the detection and treatment of late-life depression as an opportunity to reduce or prevent frequent attendance in the elderly. The association of mental health problems and frequent attendance is in line with previous literature assessing health care utilization among the elderly [53] and the general population [19, 21, 22, 54]. Patients with depression have been found to utilize health care services more frequently than patients without depression [55, 56]. This association of depressive symptomatology and increased health care utilization seems particularly the case for the elderly. According to Press et al. [27], depressive symptoms among elderly primary care patients were a stronger risk factor for frequent attendance than sociodemographic variables or comorbidity. As recognition of mood disorders is rather poor within the primary care context [56, 57], improving recognition rates for mental disorders might provide a starting point to approach avoidable frequent attendance. However, the assessment of depression and psychiatric morbidity varied across the here reviewed studies, including short self-assessment questionnaires, semi-structured and computer-assisted interviews, as well as GPs assessment of patient's psychiatric morbidity. As there are only a small number of studies on elderly FAs and mental illness, the findings should be interpreted with caution.

Further associations

The findings on further relationships between frequent attendance in the elderly and medical prescriptions, social support or sociodemographic factors were very limited and, therefore, do not allow valid conclusions on these issues. Future research on frequent attendance in the elderly should pay more attention to mediating aspects of this relationship beyond the mere presence of physical and mental diseases.

To sum up, while physical and psychological illnesses seem to be associated with frequent attendance in the elderly, several of the reviewed studies recommend further improvements in the health care management to deal with this health seeking behaviour. Vedsted et al. [42] suggest that an optimised care for daytime FAs may reduce their attendance both during the day and out-of-hours. Further recommendations involve improving the management of psychological illnesses in elderly patients [39, 45, 46], optimizing pharmacological therapy [41] or an improved integration of primary care and specialist care [39]. Van den Bussche et al. [44] argue that the phenomenon of frequent attendance appears to be multidimensional involving aspects of health care providers, patients and the health care system contributing to high utilization.

Strengths and limitations of this study

The strength of this review is its exclusive focus on older adults, as they seem to be overrepresented among FAs. The attendance pattern of elderly patients represents a growing source of prospective health care expenditures in aging societies. To our knowledge, a targeted review of high utilization of primary health care services among the elderly in Europe has not been done before. A further strength of this review is its evaluation of the methodical quality of the included studies based on predefined and established criteria.

Yet, the present review has some limitations. First, we excluded literature published in languages other than English or German and limited our search to published work. Hence, relevant literature may have been missed. Second, only European studies were included in this paper so that results could be compared across countries with roughly similar task profiles of GPs and health care systems. Nevertheless, there is a considerable variation in primary health care settings within and between countries. Therefore, the present study may lack generalizability, specifically to non-European countries and regions. Furthermore, during the process of reviewing, it became evident that the number of papers on primary health care utilization among older adults was small. Therefore, studies that included specific results on frequent attendance among elderly patients that encompassed other age groups were also included in this review.

Conclusions

To date, research on frequent attendance at the primary care level focusing on older adults is still unsatisfactory. Inconsistencies in the understanding of what constitutes frequent attendance hamper comparison across studies despite previous attempts in the literature to provide information on the validity of different definitions.

Still, this review indicates that severe ill health is associated with frequent attendance in the elderly and, therefore, points to a reasonable need for medical treatment as the main driver of frequent attendance in older adults. Frequent attendance is, therefore, neither right nor wrong, per se. However, it is indicative of a specific form of health seeking behaviour that should elicit stronger initiatives by health care providers so that the underlying needs of those patients can be understood.

Subsequent research is needed to shed more light on further mediating factors that contribute to frequent utilization of primary care services in the elderly. In particular, future studies should consider longitudinal approaches to study frequent attendance, carefully choose an FA definition and consider the context of primary care treatment within the health care system of their country.

Abbreviations

CI: Confidence Interval; FA: Frequent Attender; GP: General Practitioner; OR: Odds Ratio; PRISMA: Preferred Reporting Items for Systematic Reviews and Meta-Analyses; r: Correlation Coefficient; RR: Relative Risks

Acknowledgments

This study is published in affiliation with the German Federal Ministry of Education and Research (grant number: 01GY1613). We acknowledge support from the German Research Foundation (DFG) and Universität Leipzig within the program of Open Access Publishing.

Funding

Not applicable.

Author's contributions

FW, JS, and SRH conceived the study. FW performed a systematic search of the literature. FW and JS completed the data extraction and the quality assessment of the included papers. FW drafted and revised the manuscript. JS, AH, HHK, and SRH contributed to the manuscript, and have revised it critically for important intellectual content. All authors have read and approved the final version of the manuscript.

Consent for publication

Not applicable.

Competing interests

The authors declare that they have no competing interests.

Author details

[1]Institute of Social Medicine, Occupational Health and Public Health, Medical Faculty, University of Leipzig, Philipp-Rosenthal-Straße 55, 04103 Leipzig, Germany. [2]Institute of General Medicine, University of Leipzig, Leipzig, Germany. [3]Department of Health Economics and Health Services Research, University Medical Centre Hamburg-Eppendorf, Hamburg, Germany.

References

1. Neal RD, Heywood PL, Morley S, Clayden AD, Dowell AC. Frequency of patients' consulting in general practice and workload generated by frequent attenders: comparisons between practices. Br J Gen Pract. 1998;48:895–8.
2. Gill D, Dawes M, Sharpe M, Mayou R. GP frequent consulters: their prevalence, natural history, and contribution to rising workload. Br J Gen Pract. 1998;48:1856–7.
3. Heywood PL, Blackie GC, Cameron IH, Dowell AC. An assessment of the attributes of frequent attenders to general practice. Fam Pract. 1998;15:198–204.
4. Schrire S. Frequent attenders—a review. Fam Pract. 1986;3:272–5. doi:10.1093/fampra/3.4.272.
5. Browne GB, Humphrey B, Pallister R, Browne JA, Shetzer L. Prevalence and characteristics of frequent attenders in a prepaid Canadian family practice. J Fam Pract. 1982;14:63–71.
6. Morriss R, Kai J, Atha C, Avery A, Bayes S, Franklin M, et al. Persistent frequent attenders in primary care: costs, reasons for attendance, organisation of care and potential for cognitive behavioural therapeutic intervention. BMC Fam Pract. 2012;13:39. doi:10.1186/1471-2296-13-39.
7. Roos NP, Shapiro E, Tate R. Does a small minority of elderly account for a majority of health care expenditures?: a sixteen-year perspective. The Milbank Quarterly. 1989;67:347. doi:10.2307/3350220.
8. Smits FT, Brouwer HJ, Zwinderman AH, Mohrs J, Smeets HM, Bosmans JE, et al. Morbidity and doctor characteristics only partly explain the substantial healthcare expenditures of frequent attenders: a record linkage study between patient data and reimbursements data. BMC Fam Pract. 2013;14:138. doi:10.1186/1471-2296-14-138.
9. Kringos DS, Boerma WGW, Hutchinson A, van der Zee J, Groenewegen PP. The breadth of primary care: a systematic literature review of its core dimensions. BMC Health Serv Res. 2010; doi:10.1186/1472-6963-10-65.
10. Geiger K, Schneider N, Bleidorn J, Klindtworth K, Jünger S, Müller-Mundt G. Caring for frail older people in the last phase of life - the general practitioners' view. BMC Palliat Care. 2016;15:52. doi:10.1186/s12904-016-0124-5.
11. Harman JS, Veazie PJ, Lyness JM. Primary care physician office visits for depression by older Americans. J Gen Intern Med. 2006;21:926–30. doi:10.1111/j.1525-1497.2006.00497.x.
12. Macinko J, Starfield B, Shi LY. The contribution of primary care systems to health outcomes within Organization for Economic Cooperation and Development (OECD) countries, 1970-1998. Health Serv Res. 2003;38:831–65. doi:10.1111/1475-6773.00149.
13. Hauswaldt J, Hummers-Pradier E, Junius-Walker U. Health service use among patients with chronic or multiple illnesses, and frequent attenders: secondary analysis of routine primary care data from 1996 to 2006. Dtsch Arztebl Int. 2012;109:814–20. doi:10.3238/arztebl.2012.0814.
14. Smits FTM, Mohrs JJ, Beem EE, Bindels PJE, van Weert HCP. Defining frequent attendance in general practice. BMC Fam Pract. 2008;9:21. doi:10.1186/1471-2296-9-21.
15. Vedsted P, Olesen F. Frequent attenders in out-of-hours general practice care: attendance prognosis. Fam Pract. 1999;16:283–8. doi:10.1093/fampra/16.3.283.
16. Diaz E, Gimeno-Feliu L-A, Calderon-Larranaga A, Prados-Torres A. Frequent attenders in general practice and immigrant status in Norway: a nationwide cross-sectional study. Scand J Prim Health Care. 2014;32:232–40. doi:10.3109/02813432.2014.982368.
17. Eurostat. Proportion of population aged 65 and over. http://ec.europa.eu/eurostat/tgm/table.do?tab=table&init=1&language=en&pcode=tps00028&plugin=1. Accessed 18 Aug 2017.
18. Demers M. Factors explaining the increase in cost for physician care in Quebec's elderly population. Can Med Assoc J. 1996;155:1555–60.
19. Baez K, Aiarzaguena JM, Grandes G, Pedrero E, Aranguren J, Retolaza A. Understanding patient-initiated frequent attendance in primary care: a case-control study. Br J Gen Pract. 1998;48:1824–7.
20. Bergh H, Baigi A, Marklund B. Consultations for injuries by frequent attenders are found to be medically appropriate from general practitioners' perspective. Scand J Public Health. 2005;33:228–32. doi:10.1080/14034940510005761.
21. Smits FTM, Brouwer HJ, ter Riet G, van Weert HCP. Epidemiology of frequent attenders: a 3-year historic cohort study comparing attendance, morbidity and prescriptions of one-year and persistent frequent attenders. BMC Public Health. 2009;9:36. doi:10.1186/1471-2458-9-36.
22. Westhead JN. Frequent attenders in general practice: medical, psychological and social characteristics. J R Coll Gen Pract. 1985;35:337–40.
23. Scaife B, Gill P, Heywood P, Neal R. Socio-economic characteristics of adult frequent attenders in general practice: secondary analysis of data. Fam Pract. 2000;17:298–304.
24. Sole-Auro A, Guillen M, Crimmins EM. Health care usage among immigrants and native-born elderly populations in eleven European countries: results from SHARE. Eur J Health Econ. 2012;13:741–54. doi:10.1007/s10198-011-0327-x.
25. Verhagen I, Ros WJG, Steunenberg B, Laan W, de Wit NJ. Differences in health care utilisation between elderly from ethnic minorities and ethnic Dutch elderly. Int J Equity Health. 2014; doi:10.1186/s12939-014-0125-z.
26. Crespo-Cebada E, Urbanos-Garrido RM. Equity and equality in the use of GP services for elderly people: the Spanish case. Health Policy. 2012;104:193–9. doi:10.1016/j.healthpol.2011.10.007.
27. Press Y, Tandeter H, Romem P, Hazzan R, Farkash M. Depressive symptomatology as a risk factor for increased health service utilization among elderly patients in primary care. Arch Gerontol Geriatr. 2012;54:127–30. doi:10.1016/j.archger.2011.02.009.
28. Vedsted P, Christensen MB. Frequent attenders in general practice care: a literature review with special reference to methodological considerations. Public Health. 2005;119:118–37. doi:10.1016/j.puhe.2004.03.007.
29. Gill D, Sharpe M. Frequent consulters in general practice. J Psychosom Res. 1999;47:115–30. doi:10.1016/S0022-3999(98)00118-4.
30. Boerma W, Bohlken E. Profiles of general practice in Europa: an international study of variation in the tasks of general practitioners. Utrecht: NIVEL. https://www.nivel.nl/sites/default/files/bestanden/profiles-of-general-practice-in-europe.pdf
31. Kringos D, Boerma W, Bourgueil Y, Cartier T, Dedeu T, Hasvold T, et al. The strength of primary care in Europe: an international comparative study. Br J Gen Pract. 2013;63:e742–50. doi:10.3399/bjgp13X674422.
32. Moher D, Liberati A, Tetzlaff J, Altman DG. Preferred reporting items for systematic reviews and meta-analyses: the PRISMA statement. J Clin Epidemiol. 2009;62:1006–12. doi:10.1016/j.jclinepi.2009.06.005.
33. Baadjou VAE, Roussel NA, Verbunt JAMCF, Smeets RJEM, de BRA. Systematic review: risk factors for musculoskeletal disorders in musicians. Occup Med (Lond). 2016; doi:10.1093/occmed/kqw052.
34. Luppa M, Luck T, Weyerer S, Konig H-H, Brahler E, Riedel-Heller SG. Prediction of institutionalization in the elderly. A systematic review. Age Ageing. 2010;39:31–8. doi:10.1093/ageing/afp202.

35. Mols F, Vingerhoets AJJM, Coebergh JW. Van de poll-Franse LV. Quality of life among long-term breast cancer survivors: a systematic review. Eur J Cancer. 2005;41:2613–9. doi:10.1016/j.ejca.2005.05.017.
36. Stein J, Luppa M, Brahler E, Konig H-H, Riedel-Heller SG. The assessment of changes in cognitive functioning: reliable change indices for neuropsychological instruments in the elderly - a systematic review. Dement Geriatr Cogn Disord. 2010;29:275–86. doi:10.1159/000289779.
37. Bergh H, Marklund B. Characteristics of frequent attenders in different age and sex groups in primary health care. Scand J Prim Health Care. 2003;21:171–7. doi:10.1080/02813430310001149.
38. Gilleard CJ, Francis V, Brown M. Frequent attendance in primary care amongst older patients. Aging Ment Health. 1998;2:194–8. doi:10.1080/13607869856678.
39. Menchetti M, Cevenini N, de RD, Quartesan R, Berardi D. Depression and frequent attendance in elderly primary care patients. Gen Hosp Psychiatry. 2006;28:119–24. doi:10.1016/j.genhosppsych.2005.10.007.
40. Rennemark M, Holst G, Fagerstrom C, Halling A. Factors related to frequent usage of the primary healthcare services in old age: findings from the Swedish National Study on aging and care. Health Soc Care Comm. 2009;17:304–11. doi:10.1111/j.1365-2524.2008.00829.x.
41. Vedsted P, Sorensen HT, Mortensen JT. Drug prescription for adult frequent attenders in Danish general practice: a population-based study. Pharmacoepidemiol Drug Saf. 2004;13:717–24. doi:10.1002/pds.939.
42. Vedsted P, Sorensen HT, Nielsen JN, Olesen F. The association between daytime attendance and out-of-hours frequent attendance among adult patients in general practice. Br J Gen Pract. 2001;51:121–4.
43. Svab I, Zaletel-Kragelj L. Frequent attenders in general practice: a study from Slovenia. Scand J Prim Health Care. 1993;11:38–43.
44. van den Bussche H, Kaduszkiewicz H, Schaefer I, Koller D, Hansen H, Scherer M, Schoen G. Overutilization of ambulatory medical care in the elderly German population? - an empirical study based on national insurance claims data and a review of foreign studies. BMC Health Serv Res. 2016; https://doi.org/10.1186/s12913-016-1357-y.
45. Sheehan B, Bass C, Briggs R. Jacoby R. Somatization among older primary care attenders: Psychological medicine (Print). 2003;33:867–77.
46. Scherer M, Himmel W, Kochen MM, Koschack J, Ahrens D, Chenot J-F, et al. Psychosocial determinants for frequent primary health care utilisation in patients with heart failure. Psychosoc Med. 2008;5:Doc02.
47. Vrca Botica M, Kovacic L, Kujundzic Tiljak M, Katic M, Botica I, Rapic M, et al. Frequent attenders in family practice in Croatia: retrospective study. Croat Med J. 2004;45:620–4.
48. Grielen S. Unity of diversity?: task profiles of general practitioners in central and Eastern Europe. Eur J Pub Health. 2000;10:249–54. doi:10.1093/eurpub/10.4.249.
49. Boerma WG, VanderZee J, Fleming DM. Service profiles of general practitioners in Europe. Br J Gen Pract. 1997;47:481–6.
50. Schafer WLA, Boerma WGW, Spreeuwenberg P, Schellevis FG, Groenewegen PP. Two decades of change in European general practice service profiles: conditions associated with the developments in 28 countries between 1993 and 2012. Scand J Prim Health Care. 2016;34:97–110. doi:10.3109/02813432.2015.1132887.
51. Luciano JV, Fernandez A, Pinto-Meza A, Lujan L, Bellon JA, Garcia-Campayo J, et al. Frequent attendance in primary care: comparison and implications of different definitions. Br J Gen Pract. 2010;60:49–55. doi:10.3399/bjgp10X483139.
52. Howe A, Parry G, Pickvance D, Hockley B. Defining frequent attendance: evidence for routine age and sex correction in studies from primary care settings. Br J Gen Pract. 2002;52:561–2.
53. Harris T, Cook DG, Victor CR, Beighton C, Dewilde S, Carey IM. Linking survey data with computerised records to predict consulting by older people. Br J Gen Pract. 2004;54:928–31.
54. Andersson SO, Mattsson B, Lynoe N. Patients frequently consulting general practitioners at a primary health care centre in Sweden - a comparative study. Scand J Soc Med. 1995;23:251–7.
55. Herrman H, Patrick DL, Diehr P, Martin ML, Fleck M, Simon GE, Buesching DP. Longitudinal investigation of depression outcomes in primary care in six countries: the LIDO study. Functional status, health service use and treatment of people with depressive symptoms. Psychol Med. 2002; doi:10.1017/S003329170200586X.
56. Wittchen H-U, Pittrow D. Prevalence, recognition and management of depression in primary care in Germany: the depression 2000 study. Hum Psychopharmacol. 2002;17(Suppl 1):S1–11. doi:10.1002/hup.398.
57. Cameron IM, Lawton K, Reid IC. Appropriateness of antidepressant prescribing: an observational study in a Scottish primary-care setting. Br J Gen Pract. 2009;59:644–9. doi:10.3399/bjgp09X454061.

3

Primary care multidisciplinary teams in practice

Brandi Leach[1*], Perri Morgan[1], Justine Strand de Oliveira[2], Sharon Hull[1], Truls Østbye[1] and Christine Everett[1]

Abstract

Background: Current recommendations for strengthening the US healthcare system consider restructuring primary care into multidisciplinary teams as vital to improving quality and efficiency. Yet, approaches to the selection of team designs remain unclear. This project describes current primary care team designs, primary care professionals' perceptions of ideal team designs, and perceived facilitating factors and barriers to implementing ideal team-based care.

Methods: Qualitative study of 44 health care professionals at 6 primary care practices in North Carolina using focus group discussions and surveys. Data was analyzed using framework content analysis.

Results: Practices used a variety of multidisciplinary team designs with the specific design being influenced by the social and policy context in which practices were embedded. Practices overwhelmingly located barriers to adopting ideal multidisciplinary teams as being outside of their individual practices and outside of their control. Participants viewed internal organizational contexts as the major facilitators of multidisciplinary primary care teams. The majority of practices described their ideal team design as including a social worker to meet the needs of socially complex patients.

Conclusions: Primary care multidisciplinary team designs vary across practices, shaped in part by contextual factors perceived as barriers outside of the practices' control. Facilitating factors within practices provide a culture of support to team members, but they are insufficient to overcome the perceived barriers. The common desire to add social workers to care teams reflects practices' struggles to meet the complex demands of patients and external agencies. Government or organizational policies should avoid one-size-fits-all approaches to multidisciplinary care teams, and instead allow primary care practices to adapt to their specific contextual circumstances.

Keywords: Primary care, Patient care team, Qualitative research

Background

Robust primary care is known to be key to an efficient and effective health system [1, 2]. Compared to other economically developed nations, the US healthcare system places more focus on secondary and tertiary care than primary care. As a result, the US is top in healthcare spending, but at or near the bottom in health equity and quality outcomes [3]. While many policy makers, health delivery organizations, and funders would like to see a shift to more primary care delivery, a variety of factors, such as doctor shortages and an aging population with multiple chronic illnesses make strengthening a traditional primary care model increasingly difficult [4].

Current recommendations for strengthening the US healthcare system consider restructuring primary care into multidisciplinary teams as vital to improving quality and efficiency [5]. Primary care doctors alone are often unable to provide all needed care due to time constraints [6]. It is estimated that up to 47% of chronic care and 77% of preventive care could be delegated to other team members, potentially offsetting some demand for doctor services while improving access to care [7–9]. Evidence also suggests that well-organized multidisciplinary teams increase patient satisfaction [10, 11] and reduce doctor and staff burnout [12–14].

The recommendations, however, do little to recommend how to design these teams because there is a lack of information on the range of team designs being used

* Correspondence: Brandi.Leach@Duke.edu
Prior Presentation: This research was previously presented as a poster at AcademyHealth's Annual Research Meeting, June 25-27th 2017, New Orleans, LA.
[1]Department of Community and Family Medicine, Duke University School of Medicine, Durham, NC, USA
Full list of author information is available at the end of the article

[15]. Current approaches to distributing care among team members vary, resulting in a wide spectrum of team models [16, 17]. Team designs have expanded existing members' roles and added new members [15, 17–20]. For example, some practices have expanded the role of medical assistants (MAs) to include responsibility for preventive care management, patient education, and/or health coaching, and have demonstrated improvements in preventive service delivery and patient outcomes [21–24]. Other practices have included new members on the primary care team, such as physician assistants (PAs), nurse practitioners (NPs), pharmacists or behavioral health providers, to ensure access to needed services [25–28]. Many have reported encouraging results, suggesting that primary care practices have a range of team models from which to select.

Research offers some guiding principles for effective multidisciplinary care teams, including evidence from initial implementation. This work highlights the importance of factors such as physical spaces that facilitate interaction [29], cognitive factors that promote a sense of shared purpose and goals among team members [30, 31], effective communication [29, 30, 32], and leadership structures reflective of team goals and activities [29, 30]. Furthermore, this literature suggests that implementation of multidisciplinary teams should be undertaken with a flexible mindset that is sensitive to the needs of team members, as it may create unintended tensions, especially regarding role confusion [29].

Health systems outside the US have had varying degrees of success incorporating multidisciplinary teams into the delivery of primary care. For example, the uptake of multidisciplinary teams in Canada has been hampered by differences in funding and remuneration for primary care services across provinces, with some provinces adopting funding models that either explicitly or implicitly prioritize doctor-administered services [33, 34]. In contrast, the National Health Service in the UK embraced innovations conducive to multidisciplinary teams, such as funding support for non-doctor team members [35], a pay-for-performance system that encouraged the use of lower cost non-doctor personnel [36], and electronic health records that assist with care coordination [35], and as such has seen greater adoption of multidisciplinary teams than has occurred in the US.

The capacity of US primary care practices to create multidisciplinary primary care teams is complicated by a variety of issues. Firstly, due to a lack of healthcare workforce planning, the availability of healthcare professionals varies widely by geographic area [37, 38]. Also, reimbursement for services delivered can complicate team formation. Since the US has different payment structures for different populations [39], finding ways to consistently pay for the services of all team members can be challenging. A final complicating factor is that the US healthcare system is undergoing payment reform to value-based care, where quality of care delivered is factored into payment, but this reform has an uncertain future [40]. This uncertainty impedes efforts to identify and implement effective team designs. For example, in line with value-based payment reform efforts, many primary care practices are transitioning to patient-centered medical homes (PCMH). PCMH practices are characterized by assigned primary care providers for patients to facilitate continuity of care, coordinated care, enhanced access, and team-based care [41]. However the transition to a PCMH practice requires extensive administrative and financial resources that practices may be reluctant to commit without firm government backing for continued reform efforts.

As US primary care practices increasingly adopt team-based approaches to care, one issue that remains unclear is which models are being selected for implementation and which factors are influencing that selection. Primary care practices associated with large academic centers may have financial and workforce resources not available in rural areas [42–44]. The regulatory environment, reimbursement practices or organizational goals could influence and constrain the role of team members [16, 45, 46]. Additional factors related to payment or organizational policy could also be influencing the selection of team models.

The goal of this project was to understand approaches to the selection of primary care multidisciplinary team models in North Carolina (NC). The specific aims were: 1) to describe a range of primary care multidisciplinary teams being used in diverse communities in NC; 2) to describe how providers envision primary care practices' ideal team designs; and 3) to identify perceived contextual facilitating factors and barriers to implementing those ideal teams.

Methods

Study design

This is a qualitative study using focus group discussions with additional data collected via questionnaires. Focus group discussions were conducted with 44 participants from six primary care practices in NC. Two survey instruments collected additional data on [1]: individual participants' professional background and demographics, and [2] the characteristics of the practice and its patient population.

Participants and recruitment

We used purposive sampling to select primary care practices, with the final sample size based on achievement of theme saturation. Practices were selected to represent a variety of geographic locations, population health characteristics, healthcare workforce characteristics, patient populations, and organizational structures. Primary care practices in NC with at least five people (clinical and administrative workers combined) were eligible for inclusion in our study. We used primary care practice information from the Duke Primary Care Research Consortium and the NC Medical Society Foundation's Community Practitioner Program to recruit our sample. Practices were recruited by contacting practice managers via phone or email. Within each practice, with the assistance of practice personnel, we recruited 6–10 people from each practice to participate in the study. This included a mix of clinical and non-clinical personnel at each clinic, including doctors, physician assistants (PAs), nurse practitioners (NPs), clinical pharmacists, nurses, medical assistants (MAs), social workers, practice managers, or administrative staff.

Interview structure

Focus group discussions occurred at the practices. To minimize potential concerns about discomfort to speak freely arising from staff hierarchies, we divided participants into two groups with doctors, PAs, NPs, pharmacists, and managers separate from nurses, medical assistants, social workers, and administrative staff. Focus groups were led by one of three study team members (CE, PM, or BL). The focus groups lasted approximately 45 min and were audio-recorded and transcribed. We used a set of key questions to guide the focus groups (Table 1) that allowed for follow-up questions to pursue emerging themes.

Analysis

We evaluated the qualitative data using a framework content analysis approach [47]. Framework content analysis incorporates open, thematic coding into a theoretically-grounded analytic framework. Our initial framework (Fig. 1) was based on the Integrated (Health Care) Team Effectiveness Model (ITEM) [48]. This model posits that healthcare team structure is influenced not only by organizational context, but also by the larger social and policy context. Social factors influencing selection of team design may include geographic location (i.e., rural vs. urban), availability of workforce in different professions, and reimbursement policies. [46, 49, 50]

Table 1 Key questions from the focus group discussion guide

Question
If a patient asked you, "What is the most important thing you do in this practice?" what would you tell them?
How is your practice organized to deliver care?
How did that practice structure come about?
If you could create the ideal structure, what would it be?
Do you have organized or designated teams as part of this practice?

Organizational factors such as goals, provider payment practices, and availability of resources might also impact the selection of team design [16, 45]. Finally, team structure is defined by the patient population served, the type and number of team members, and the roles of each member [48]. Based on the ITEM framework, our initial thematic coding categories captured the social and policy context, organizational context, and team structures. These were refined during the analysis to include categories addressing facilitators, barriers, and aspirations (see Table 2 for examples of comments coded under each category).

Our analysis occurred in stages, beginning with an initial review of transcripts for familiarization and identification of key themes. This was followed by a secondary review to refine and adjust themes, and a systematic application of the refined themes to the full transcript data. The final stages reorganized and synthesized themed content for analysis and interpretation.

Qualitative analysis was led by two team members (CE and BL) who coded the transcripts independently before comparing and discussing their results and achieving consensus on any identified discrepancies in coding. The full study team provided feedback on preliminary results midway through data collection and after initial thematic coding and analysis. The full study team includes two doctors, three PA researchers, and one sociologist.

Results

Our final sample included 44 healthcare professionals from 6 primary care practices in NC. Most participants were female (82%) and employed full-time at their clinic (90%). They had an average age of 45 years and had worked at the same clinic for an average of 8 years (Table 3). The practices in our sample encompassed a range of organizational structures situated within different contexts (Table 4). Five of the six practices employed between 1 and 2 doctors, as well as an additional 2 to 6 NPs or PAs. The sixth practice was associated with a large academic medical center and employed over 30 full and part-time doctors, including residents. Across the US, approximately 41% of primary care doctors in 2012 worked in practices with 1–2 doctors, a further 42% were in practices with 3–10 doctors, and 16% were in practices with 11 or more doctors [51].

Team designs

The primary care practices used a variety of team designs, ranging from provider-nurse dyads (doctor, PA, or NP teamed with a nurse or medical assistant) to large multi-professional teams (Fig. 2). Most practices initially found it difficult to describe how their current team structures, staffing and workflow pattern came about, expressing a sentiment similar to that of one practice

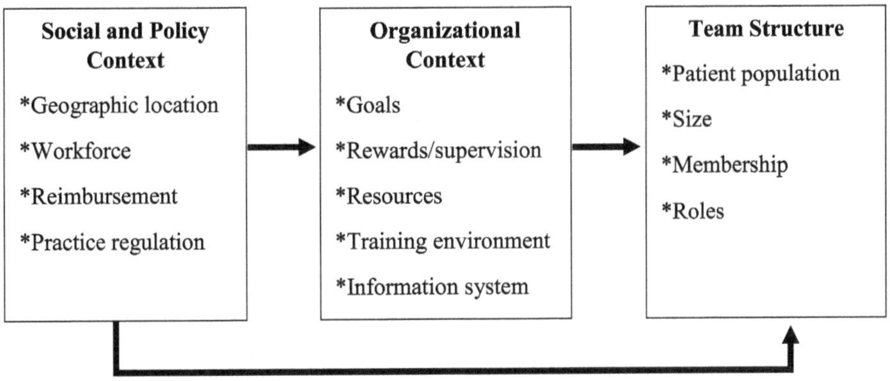
Social and Policy Context
*Geographic location
*Workforce
*Reimbursement
*Practice regulation
Organizational Context
*Goals
*Rewards/supervision
*Resources
*Training environment
*Information system
Team Structure
*Patient population
*Size
*Membership
*Roles

Note line: Based on the Integrated (Health Care) Team Effectiveness Model (ITEM) (Lemieux-Charles and McGuire 2006)

Fig. 1 Conceptual model of primary care team design used for initial analytic framework

owner who said, *"it just sort of happened that way."* When pressed, participants generally articulated that their current team structures were not the result of an explicit plan, but rather the result of various internal and external forces. Respondents from one suburban practice, for example, focused on hiring people with complementary skill sets and then developed their team structures around the individual strengths and preferences of their employees. As the practice owner described:

> *"Each one of us individual provider[s], we provide..., cutting edge, really, medicine, but we're different, ... what she's an expert on, I might not know much about. And vice versa."*

In contrast, respondents from rural practices cited difficulties in hiring and retaining doctors due to workforce availability and resource limitations, leading them to rely on NP/PAs to provide a large portion of primary care services. One rural practice manager spoke of the difficulty of retaining *any* providers beyond the initial two-year contract period for which the providers receive educational loan forgiveness, given that experienced providers could make higher salaries elsewhere:

> *"We get a lot of new NPs and PAs but as soon as they're trained they get snapped up by another provider ... And we start all over again."*

Practices facing resource limitations reported hiring staff to conform with insurance reimbursement practices that limit which provider types are eligible for incentive-based payments or can bill for specific services. For example, under the Medicaid program (government insurance for poor and disabled people) there are fewer restrictions on NPs to qualify for payments under the EHR incentive program than for PAs, which can make NPs a more economically desirable option [52]. These practices also used clinical staff (e.g. MAs) in expanded roles. Clinical staff generally appeared to value the additional responsibilities, but they also understood the underlying reasons for their expanded roles. As one MA from a rural practice stated:

Table 2 Final thematic coding categories, with examples

Theme	Example
Team Design	
Structure	*It's a free for all sister!*
Development	*We're at a cross, it seems like, between hierarchy and collaboration. And trying to find middle ground.*
Aspirations	*I think certainly reducing some of the bureaucracy or the logistical complications of getting patients the care that in our medical decision-making they need to have.*
Organizational Context	
Barriers	*Financing. And space. Money and space. Cause right now, like we, if we had the money for a social worker, I wouldn't have anywhere to put them.*
Facilitators	*Critical for me to have professional, capable, nursing staff and ancillary people to help me to make each patient visit the most efficient I possibly can.*
Culture	*You know, there's two wars going on. Some providers are like, "I don't want to see anymore [patients]." And then the administration is like, "But we gotta make money."*
Values	*We really do try to put the patients first.*
Social & Policy Context	
Structure	*We have a lot of blueberry fields... so we have a lot of, they're migrants, they go to Florida in Spring, they come here for the summer, they go to Michigan for the winter then turn right back around.*
Barriers	*You're focused on getting a patient in and out and taking care of it in a, in a highly effective way ... but all of a sudden it doesn't matter cause they can't afford it, or you know they're living on the street or something like that.*
Facilitators	*There's the Practice Transformation Network, you probably are familiar with that, is also driving some of our change. It's not necessarily the impetus, but it's helping give us some structure.*

Table 3 Participant characteristics, $N = 44$

Participant characteristics	
Age, in years [Mean/(SD)]	45/(11.1)
Time in current profession, in years [Mean/(SD)]	14/(9.0)
Time at current clinic, in years [Mean/(SD)]	8/(7.1)
Percent female	82%
Percent employed full-time	90%
Number of each Professional Type Participating	
Doctors	9
Nurse practitioners/Physician assistants	8
Pharmacists	1
Social workers	1
Nurses	5
Medical assistants	11
Administrative managers	4
Administrative staff	5

> *"With my paramedic background,...they brought me in cause I had the experience of the IVs and stuff, so basically I'm working as a ... LPN, RN, but I get paid for MA."*

In contrast, practices without significant resource limitations were able to emphasize non-financial factors when developing their teams. The approach described by members of a primary care practice associated with an academic medical center exemplified adaptive team development, with the practice adding new members or methods of coordination based on feedback from providers, staff and patients, the changing needs of the organization, or research findings. These decisions were not divorced from financial considerations, but in comparison to rural health practices and those working in higher poverty areas, this practice was able to develop its teams with more emphasis on meeting organizational goals, such as population health goals.

Aspirations

Participants' descriptions of ideal team designs frequently involved addressing gaps in important services. For example, four of the six practices cited the need for a social worker or care coordinator to manage complex patients. The specific reason for wanting a social worker/care coordinator varied by context with practices differentially emphasizing medical complexity, social complexity, or mental health needs based on contextual factors such as the characteristics of their patient population and availability of community resources. One nurse from a low-resource suburban practice captured the diversity of needs with her comment:

> *"I think adding that mental health piece, because resources are so scarce, um, and maybe adding like some sort of case management services for our really complicated patients."*

Organizational context

Focus group participants identified numerous internal organizational aspects that affected the development and functioning of multidisciplinary teams. In general, organizational contexts were seen as facilitating multidisciplinary teams. Facilitating aspects of the organizational context included technological resources such as electronic communication and electronic health record (EHR) systems (*"Being able to leave messages for them in the EHR, that's helpful. That was a big step up from the paper charts."* – administrative staff, rural practice); the skills and/or quality of their co-workers; organizational processes such as care team huddles [53], quality improvement initiatives, and staff training; and supportive and collaborative cultures within their

Table 4 Characteristics of clinics and their social context, $N = 6$

Clinic characteristics	Mean	SD	Min	Max
Median income of county[a]	$49,365	$10,322	$34,949	$67,309
Median income of city/town[a]	*	*	$19,719	$91,579
County health ranking (out of 100)[b]	35	33	96	1
County population size[a]	252,396	357,463	35,663	1,024,198
Estimated percent of patients with private insurance[c]	52%	27%	25%	91%
# practices that are patient-centered medical homes[d]	4			
# practices using electronic health records	5			

*Information not available due to small population size

[a]Source: US Census Bureau. Quick Facts, American Community Survey, 2015. http://www.census.gov/quickfacts. Accessed 2/14/17

[b]Note: County health rankings measure the health of counties in every US state using a population health model that includes policies and programs, health factors, and health outcomes. NC rankings are based out of 100 with 1 being the "healthiest" county. Source: Robert Wood Johnson Foundation, County Health Rankings & Roadmaps. 2016. http://www.countyhealthrankings.org/rankings/data/nc. Accessed 2/14/17

[c]Self-reported by practice managers. N = 4, 2 practices did not report insurance estimates

[d]For a description of patient-centered medical homes, please see: Devers KJ, Burton RA, Berenson RA. Will the patient-centered medical home transform the delivery of health care? 2011

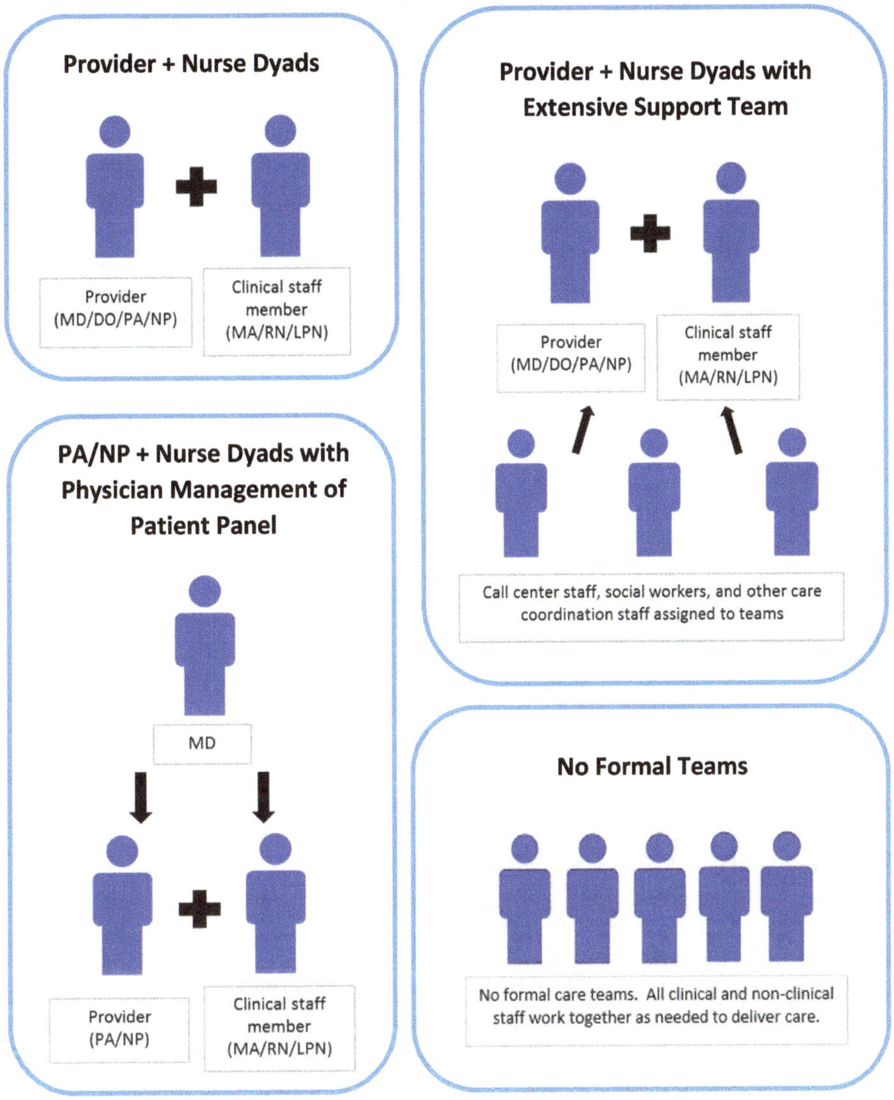

Fig. 2 Team designs used by participating clinics, $N = 6$

practices (*"We're a united front."* – administrative staff, suburban practice).

Different organizational contexts, such as practice size and ownership structure, were associated with different perceived facilitating factors. For example, one independently-owned suburban practice described their freedom as a private practice to make organizational decisions and adopt innovative practices as facilitating their implementation of multidisciplinary teams. The practice owner described their freedom to act this way:

> *"We're not really a part of any big corporate anything. … Before we make decisions…we try to really take into account everyone's, how it will impact workflows on everyone."*

Members of the practice associated with the academic medical center, in contrast, cited the extensive resources available to them as part of a large medical organization, including having a call center to help organize and triage incoming calls, and the ready availability of specialists who could be included on care teams, as facilitating the functioning of multidisciplinary teams.

Sometimes staff and providers would express differing views on whether something was a facilitating factor or a barrier, as in one practice without an EHR system. The owner of the practice resisted EHR implementation because of concerns over cost and additional time requirements that might limit the number of patients providers could see; whereas, the staff believed an EHR system would facilitate communication and improve their workflow.

Although perceived facilitating factors varied by organizational context, we found similarities that spanned contextual differences. Of particular note, members from every practice described their co-workers as essential for implementing multidisciplinary teams, with some emphasizing the skills and credentials of their co-workers and others highlighting their co-workers' supportive, collaborative behavior. Among practices that mentioned using daily or weekly huddles, there was general agreement that huddles enhanced team functioning. As one nurse from a rural practice described it:

> *"What has helped us a lot is a morning huddle... We'll have a better work flow ... That helps us to talk to each other and find out ... what we're looking forward to during the day."*

Social and policy context

With only a few exceptions, the external social and policy context was viewed as a barrier to implementing well-functioning multidisciplinary teams in primary care practices by our focus group participants. The most commonly cited social and policy barriers to well-functioning multidisciplinary teams were socially complex patients, financial constraints, and policies of external agencies and parent organizations. The specific barriers cited varied by the practice's context. For example, the perceived barriers mentioned by members of the practice associated with an academic medical center were largely related to factors controlled by their parent organization. These included the physical space of the practice which impeded team coordination, a belief among providers that the parent organization undervalued primary care, and hiring and staffing decisions. As expressed by one doctor:

> *"The fact that the staff don't actually work for us, they work for [Parent Organization], you know it's very... we're not the final ones who say what they do. It's just kind of an odd, it's an odd setup."*

In contrast, participants at privately owned practices described onerous insurance and government mandated requirements as impeding their delivery of quality team-based care:

"The amount of things that we're required to do, increasing amount of things we're required to do. Checking boxes to the point you feel like you're not delivering care almost." – PA, suburban practice

> *"We pay our employee and ... half of their time's spent on the phone with the insurance company. So that's a major barrier."* – Doctor, owner, suburban practice

Providers and staff at rural practices were likely to cite workforce availability as a barrier to implementing multidisciplinary teams, and participants at practices with high poverty patient populations reported financial barriers. One practice manager at a rural clinic with a high-poverty patient population expressed the view that delivering *"outstanding professional medical care"* often came into conflict with their financial circumstances. He stated that their practice's goal was to recruit both doctors and PAs, because *"for the level of care and some of the complexity of our patients we'd love to have another [doctor] on staff,"* but the practice's rural location and limited financial resources made it difficult to attract and retain doctors.

There were several government policies identified by study participants as facilitating their adoption of multidisciplinary teams. These included Medicaid payments for social workers, an improved state regulatory environment for clinical pharmacists, and the Centers for Medicare & Medicaid Services' (CMS) Practice Transformation Networks which provide guidance and support to primary care practices transitioning to PCMHs or other quality-based patient-centered care approaches [54].

Discussion

The six primary care practices in our study adopted an array of care team designs. Our research suggests that multidisciplinary team designs are influenced by the social and policy context in which practices are embedded, including factors such as the availability of financial and workforce resources, reimbursement practices, and patient complexity. Financial and workforce constraints appear to play a large role in determining multidisciplinary team designs for resource restricted practices. Within our study, workforce availability was especially important for multidisciplinary team design in rural practices, where a restricted doctor supply contributed to decisions to hire more NPs and PAs. Reimbursement practices influenced the types of professionals included on care teams as well as their roles. Limited resource practices used extended roles for MAs and other clinical staff in order to improve economic efficiency. Patient complexity also shaped care team design by influencing desired team members, such as a desire for social workers in practices with socially complex patients.

Primary care practices overwhelmingly located barriers to adopting their ideal multidisciplinary teams within the external social and policy context, and outside of their individual practices and outside of their control. In our study, these included parent organizations that controlled staffing decisions and undervalued primary care, complex patient populations requiring additional care coordination, and reimbursement policies that limited staffing choices. Their frustration with these external factors and their apparent inability to influence them were evident in the interviews.

Appropriate reimbursement policies for primary care services have been found by other researchers to be a key component in the success or failure of incorporating multidisciplinary team approaches to care outside the US [33, 35, 36]. Citing the examples of Canada [33, 35] and Australia [36], these researchers argue that even when there is political support for multidisciplinary teams, reimbursement models that continue to prioritize doctor-led services or offer poor or inconsistent funding streams for non-doctor team members hinder the uptake of multidisciplinary teams in practice. Funding models that offer more flexibility in service reimbursement, such as that found in the UK, may contribute to greater adoption of multidisciplinary teams in primary care [35].

In contrast to the perceived barriers, practice members viewed internal organizational contexts as the major facilitators of multidisciplinary primary care teams. These included factors facilitating communication (e.g. electronic communication and EHR systems, huddles), workforce characteristics (e.g. having skilled co-workers, availability of specialists), and practice cultures supportive of teamwork. External factors may also contribute to the adoption of multidisciplinary teams by providing financing for desired team members or offering guidance on practice transformation, but these were mentioned less often by our study sample.

Research on the effect of organizational factors on adoption of multidisciplinary teams in primary care highlights several important factors identified by our study. Most notably, this includes the importance of communication and team climate. Communication is argued to be both an important precursor to successful team implementation [30, 31] and an indicator of team functioning [29]. Research from England on the importance of team climate and culture has found conflicting results about its impact on patient outcomes [55, 56], but other research suggests that a positive team culture is necessary for team members' satisfaction with their working environment [30, 57].

Despite differences, one consistent message from primary care practices is the desire for social workers and/or care coordinators on their teams. This finding echoes that of previous research which finds that care coordinators and social workers perform valued functions on care teams [58, 59]. Social workers offer an avenue for managing patient care plans, coordinating community resources, and providing clinical behavioral interventions [59]. As noted by the participants in our study, the main barrier to including social workers or care coordinators in multidisciplinary teams was a lack of funding.

Strengths and limitations

A key strength of our interview-based approach is that it allows for the emergence of themes not previously identified by the researchers. This is important when studying emerging and developing areas such as team-based care. Our research is limited in that it only sampled practices from within a single state, although it captured a diverse set of contexts within that state and we achieved thematic saturation within our interviews. A larger sample would have permitted a more robust assessment of the effect of contextual factors on multidisciplinary care team functioning and design.

The composition of the study team presents a potential for bias in that all of the team members visiting practice sites were affiliated with a PA education program. This had the potential to affect comments made by participants regarding PAs. Although unable to eliminate this potential source of bias from within the interviews, the inclusion of several non-PA researchers on the larger study team ameliorated the potential for bias during the analysis.

Future research should seek to deepen our understanding of the range of multidisciplinary team models, and factors facilitating or impeding the establishment and ideal functioning of those models. This is needed to better inform practice transformation efforts and assist primary care practices with identifying a team model that will meet their specific needs and context.

Conclusions

The successful implementation of multidisciplinary primary care teams is influenced not only by organizational context, but by the larger social and policy context. *External* factors are often perceived as barriers to implementing multidisciplinary teams, while facilitating factors largely originate from *within* clinics. And although the participants in this study tackled the challenges of team-based primary care with energy and creativity, the internal resources of most practices are not sufficient to overcome all of the externally-imposed barriers. Solutions could include flexible payment policies that allow for a variety of care team designs, supporting innovations in care delivery. Government or organizational policies should avoid one-size-fits-all approaches to multidisciplinary care teams, and instead allow primary care practices to adapt to their specific local and contextual circumstances.

Abbreviations

CMS: Centers for Medicare and Medicaid Services; EHR: Electronic health records; LPN: Licensed practical nurse; MA: Medical assistant; NC: North Carolina; NP: Nurse practitioner; PA: Physician assistant; PCMH: Patient-centered medical home; RN: Registered nurse

Funding

This research was supported by a grant from the American Academy of Family Physicians Foundation's Joint Grant Award Program [#G1401JG]. Additional information on our data is available upon request from the corresponding author.

Authors contributions

CE developed the initial research design, conducted interviews, was a primary analyst of the data, and was a major contributor in writing the manuscript. BL conducted interviews, was a primary analyst of the data, and was the primary author of the manuscript. PM consulted on the research design, conducted interviews, contributed to the data analysis, and was a major contributor in writing the manuscript. JSD consulted on the research design, assisted with interviews, and assisted with data analysis and with writing the manuscript. TØ and SH consulted on the research design, and assisted with data analysis and with writing the manuscript. All authors read and approved the final manuscript.

Consent for publication

Not applicable.

Competing interests

The authors declare that they have no competing interests.

Author details

[1]Department of Community and Family Medicine, Duke University School of Medicine, Durham, NC, USA. [2]Barts and The London School of Medicine and Dentistry, Queen Mary University of London, London, UK.

References

1. Starfield B. Is primary care essential? Lancet. 1994;344:1129–33.
2. Starfield B, Shi L, Macinko J. Contribution of primary care to health systems and health. The milbank quarterly. 2005;83:457–502.
3. Davis K, Stremikis K, Squires D, Schoen C. Mirror, mirror on the wall. CommonWealth Fund: How the performance of the US Health care system compares internationally New York; 2014.
4. Institute of Medicine. Primary care: America's health in a new era. Washington, D.C.: National Academy Press; 1996.
5. Center for Workforce Studies (AAMC). Physician Shortages to Worsen Without Increases in Residency Training. AAMC 2010 June.
6. Ostbye T, Yarnall K, Krause K, Pollak K, Gradison M, Michener JI. There time for management of patients with chronic diseases in primary care? Ann Fam Med. 2005;3:209–14.
7. Altschuler J, Margolius D, Bodenheimer T, Grumbach K. Estimating a reasonable patient panel size for primary care physicians with team-based task delegation. The. Ann Fam Med. 2012;10:396–400.
8. Shipman S, Sinsky C. Expanding primary care capacity by reducing waste and improving the efficiency of care. Health Aff. 2013;32:1990–7.
9. Green L, Savin S, Lu Y. Primary care physician shortages could be eliminated through use of teams, nonphysicians, and electronic communication. Health Aff, 11–19 2013;32:11–19.
10. Day J, Scammon DL, Kim J, et al. Quality, satisfaction, and financial efficiency associated with elements of primary care practice transformation: preliminary findings. The. Ann Fam Med. 2013;11:S50–S9.
11. Gilfillan RJ, Tomcavage J, Rosenthal MB, et al. Value and the medical home: effects of transformed primary care. Am J Manag Care. 2010;16:607–14.
12. Willard-Grace R, Hessler D, Rogers E, Dubé K, Bodenheimer T, Grumbach K. Team structure and culture are associated with lower burnout in primary care. J. American Board Family Med. 2014;27:229–38.
13. Helfrich CD, Dolan ED, Simonetti J, et al. Elements of team-based care in a patient-centered medical home are associated with lower burnout among VA primary care employees. J Gen Intern Med. 2014;29:659–66.
14. Buttigieg SC, West MA, Dawson JF. Well-structured teams and the buffering of hospital employees from stress. Health Serv Manag Res. 2011;24:203–12.
15. Wagner EH, Flinter M, Hsu C, et al. Effective team-based primary care: observations from innovative practices. BMC Fam Pract. 2017;18:13.
16. Everett C, Thorpe C, Carayon P, Palta M, Gilchrist V, Smith M. Division of Primary Care Services Between Physicians, Physician Assistants, and Nurse Practitioners for Older Patients With Diabetes. MCCR (Medical Care Research and Review) 2013;online.
17. Goldberg D, Beeson T, Kuzel A, Love LE, Carver MA. Critical element of primary care practice transformation. Population Health Manage. 2013;16
18. Bodenheimer T, Laing B. The teamlet model of primary care. Ann Fam Med. 2007;5:457–61.
19. Jackson G, Powers B, Chatterjee R, et al. Patient-centered medical home a systematic review. Ann Intern Med. 2013;158:169–78.
20. Ladden M, Bodenheimer T, Fishman N, et al. The emerging primary care workforce: preliminary observations from the primary care team: learning from [the] effective ambulatory practices project. Acad Med. 2013;88:1830–4.
21. Hoffman R, Steel S, Yee Eea A. System-based intervention to improve colorectal cancer screening uptake. Am J Manag Care. 2011;17:49–55.
22. Loo T, Davis R, Lipsitz L, et al. Electronic medical record reminders and panel management to improve primary care of elderly patients. Arch Intern Med. 2011;171:1552–8.
23. Gensichen J, von Korff M, Peitz M, et al. Case Management for Depression by health care assistants in small primary care practices: a cluster randomized trial. Ann Intern Med. 2009;151:369–78.
24. Ivey S, Tseng W, Kurtovich E, et al. Evaluating a culturally and linguistically competent health coach intervention for Chinese-American patients with diabetes. Diabetes. Spectrum. 2012;25:93–102.
25. Bogden PE, Abbott RD, Williamson P, Onopa JK, Koontz LM. Comparing standard care with a physician and pharmacist team approach for uncontrolled hypertension. JGIM. 1998;13
26. Sandhoff B, Kuca S, Rasmussen J, Merenich J. Collaborative cardiac care service: a multi-disciplinary approach to caring for patients with coronary artery diesease. Perm J. 2008;12:4–11.
27. Mauer B. Behavioral health/primary care integration and the person-centered healthcare home.
28. Dow AW, Bohannon A, Garland S. The effects of expanding primary care access for the uninsured: implications for the health care workforce under health reform. Acad Med. 2013;88:1855–61.
29. Harris MF, Advocat J, Crabtree BF, et al. Interprofessional teamwork innovations for primary health care practices and practitioners: evidence from a comparison of reform in three countries. J Multidiscip Healthcare. 2016;9:35.
30. Fiscella K, Mauksch L, Bodenheimer T, Salas E. Improving care Teams' functioning: recommendations from team science. The Joint Commission Journal on Quality and Patient Safety. 2017;
31. Mickan SM, Rodger SA. Effective health care teams: a model of six characteristics developed from shared perceptions. J Interprofessional Care. 2005;19:358–70.
32. Mickan S, Rodger S. The organisational context for teamwork: Comparing health care and business literature.] 2000;23:179–92.
33. Wranik WD, Haydt SM, Katz A, et al. Funding and remuneration of interdisciplinary primary care teams in Canada: a conceptual framework and application. BMC Health Serv Res. 2017;17:351.
34. Misfeldt R, Suter E, Mallinson S, Boakye O, Wong S. Exploring context and the factors shaping team-based primary healthcare policies in three Canadian provinces: a comparative analysis. Healthcare Policy. 2017;13:74–93.
35. Majeed A, Bindman AB. Commentary: what can primary care in the United States learn from the United Kingdom? BMJ. 2003;326:799.
36. Freund T, Everett C, Griffiths P, Hudon C, Naccarella L, Laurant M. Skill mix, roles and remuneration in the primary care workforce: who are the healthcare professionals in the primary care teams across the world? Int J Nurs Stud. 2015;52:727–43.
37. Goodell S, Dower C, O'Neil E. Primary care workforce in the United States. Robert Wood Johnson Foundation Policy Brief No. 2011;22:2015.
38. Spero JC, Fraher E. Running the numbers: the maldistribution of health care providers is rural and underserved areas in North Carolina. N C Med J. 2014;75:74–9.
39. Bodenheimer T, Grumbach K. Paying for Healthcare. Understanding health policy. 4th ed: McGraw Hill Professional; 2012:4–13.
40. Obama B. United States health care reform: progress to date and next steps. JAMA. 2016;316:525–32.
41. Devers KJ, Burton RA, Berenson RA. Will the patient-centered medical home transform the delivery of health care? 2011.
42. Chan L, Har L, Goodman D. Geographic access to health Care for Rural Medicare Beneficiaries. J Rural Health. 2006;22:140–6.
43. Cordes S. The changing rural environment and the relationship between health services and rural development. HSR. Health Serv Res. 1989;23
44. Rittenhouse D, Casalino L, Shortell S, et al. Small and Medium-size Physician Practices Use Few Patient-centered Medical Home Processes Health Affairs, 30, no8 (2011): 2011;30:1575–84.
45. Chaix-Couturier C, Durand-Zaleski I, Jolly D, Durieux P. Effects of financial

incentives on medical practice: results from a systematic review of the literature and methodological issues. Int J Qual Health Care. 2000;12:133–42.
46. Spetz J, Parente S, Town R, Bazarko D. Scope-of-practice Laws for nurse practitioners limit cost savings that can be achieved in retail clinics. Health Aff. 2013;32:1977–84.
47. Pope C, Ziebland S, Mays N. Qualitative research in health care: Analysing qualitative data. BMJ (British Medical Journal). 2000;320:114–6.
48. Lemieux-Charles L, McGuire W. What do we know about health care team effectiveness? A review of the literature. Med Care Res Rev. 2006;63:263–300.
49. Guagliardo M. Spatial accessibility of primary care: concepts, methods and challenges. Int J Health Geogr. 2004;3
50. Elwood T. Patchwork of scope-of-practice regulations prevent allied health professionals from fully participating in patient care. Health Aff. 2013;32:1985–9.
51. Hing E, Hsiao C-J. Which states are physician assistants or nurse practitioners more likely to work in primary care? Journal of the American Academy of Physician Assistants. 2015;28:46–53.
52. Regulations and Guidance: EHR Incentive Programs - Eligibility. (Accessed October 16, 2017, at https://www.cms.gov/Regulations-and-Guidance/Legislation/EHRIncentivePrograms/Eligibility.html.)
53. Fogarty CT, Schultz S. Team huddles: the role of the primary care educator. Clin Teach. 2010;7:157–60.
54. Transforming Clinical Practice Initiative. Centers for Medicare and Medicaid Services. (Accessed April 20, 2017, at https://innovation.cms.gov/initiatives/Transforming-Clinical-Practices/.)
55. Hann M, Bower P, Campbell S, Marshall M, Reeves D. The association between culture, climate and quality of care in primary health care teams. Fam Pract. 2007:323–30.
56. Bower P, Campbell S, Bojke C, Sibbald B. Team structure, team climate and the quality of care in primary care: an observational study. Quality and Safety in Health Care. 2003;12:273–9.
57. Mickan SM. Evaluating the effectiveness of health care teams. Aust Health Rev. 2005;29:211–7.
58. Gimm G, Want J, Hough D, Polk T, Rodan M, Nichols LM. Medical home implementation in small primary care practices: provider perspectives. The Journal of the American Board of Family Medicine. 2016;29:767–74.
59. Fraser M, Lombardi B, Wu S, LdS Z, Richman E, Fraher E. Social work in integrated primary care: a systematic review. University of North Carolina, Chapel Hill: Carolina health workforce research center, the Cecil G. Sheps center for Health Serv Res. 2016;

4

Preschool children in out-of-hours primary care – a questionnaire-based cross-sectional study of factors related to the medical relevance of health problems

Grete Moth[1,2*], Linda Huibers[1,2], Astrid Ovesen[1,2], Morten Bondo Christensen[1,2] and Peter Vedsted[1,2]

Abstract

Background: Out-of-hours primary care (OOH-PC) is intended to provide medical care services for health problems that cannot wait until normal office hours. Children under five years of age represent about 19% of all OOH-PC contacts in Denmark, and the frequency of calls assessed as *severe* by health professionals is markedly lower for children than for other age groups. Several studies have questioned the appropriateness of the parents' use of OOH-PC. We aimed to identify factors associated with calls from parents of pre-school children concerning perceived non-severe health problems that were ranked by the triaging GPs as more appropriate for GP office hours (defined as 'medically irrelevant').

Methods: We used data from a cross-sectional study performed in the Central Denmark Region for a 1-year period during 2010–2011. GPs in the OOH-PC assessed random contacts, and a questionnaire was subsequently sent to registered patients. Associations between different factors and the medical irrelevance of contacts were estimated with a generalised linear model to calculate the prevalence ratio (PR).

Results: Among all included 522 telephone consultations and 1226 face-to-face consultations, we identified 71 (13.6%) telephone consultations and 95 (7.8%) face-to-face consultations that were both assessed as *non-severe* by the parents and *more appropriate for GP office hours* by the GPs. For telephone consultations, contacts at other times than 4–8 pm on weekdays were statistically significantly associated with medical irrelevance. Additionally, symptoms of longer duration than 24 h were statistically significantly associated medical irrelevance.

Conclusions: A large part of the calls to the Danish OOH-PC concern children. The results indicate that some of these calls are made for other than strictly medical reasons. To achieve more effective use of available resources, it might seem relevant to aim at directing more contacts directly to daytime care. However, future studies to enhance our knowledge on parents' motivation and behaviour would be recommendable.

Keywords: Denmark, General practice, Out-of-hours, Appropriateness, Severity, Reason for encounter

* Correspondence: moth@ph.au.dk
[1]Research Unit for General Practice, Department of Public Health, Aarhus University, Bartholins Alle 2, 8000 Aarhus, Denmark
[2]Section for General Medical Practice, Department of Public Health, Aarhus University, Bartholins Alle 2, 8000 Aarhus, Denmark

Background

Out-of-hours primary care (OOH-PC) in Denmark is organised in large cooperatives consisting of general practitioners (GPs) as in many other western countries [1–3]. The OOH-PC is intended for urgent medical problems that cannot wait until normal office hours. Nevertheless, several studies have shown that 50–77% of calls are assessed as *inappropriate* or *non-urgent* by health professionals and could have been directed to a GP in daytime or managed as self-care [4–6]. Consequently, the workload at the OOH-PC is high, and the demands are significant [7].

Studies across countries have shown that young children account for 5–19% of the OOH-PC contacts [8–10]. The proportion of calls assessed as severe is lower for children than for other age group [11]. According to a Danish study, 46% of parents who contacted OOH-PC did not consider their child's condition to be truly serious or urgent [12]. Furthermore, a Dutch study showed that about half of patients thought that OOH-PC was intended for all health-related problems, including non-urgent issues [4].

Therefore, it is relevant to analyse the medical relevance of contacts concerning children as this could provide an understanding of the OOH-PC use for this group. Our aim was to examine contacts for 0–5-year-old children at the OOH-PC regarding reasons for encounter (RFE), symptom duration, time of contact, urbanisation and severity of health problem as assessed by parents and the OOH-PC GP on duty. Furthermore, for contacts considered as non-severe by parents, we explored factors that were associated with being assessed as more suitable for own GP within office hours by the triaging GPs in order to gain knowledge on how to identify the potentially avoidable contacts.

Methods

Design

We conducted a cross-sectional study based on secondary analyses of data from a survey on RFE and disease patterns in the Danish OOH-PC (the LV-KOS cohort study) in the Central Denmark Region [8]. During the 1-year study period (1 June 2010 — 31 May 2011), data on OOH-PC contacts were generated on the basis of GP registrations of contacts and patient questionnaires. A total of 385 of all 700 GPs in the region participated in the survey at least once (55.0%), and a GP collected data for 96% of all telephone calls in each shift. In total, 21,457 random contacts were registered: 7810 telephone calls, 6973 face-to-face consultations and 6674 home visits.

Setting

The OOH-PC provides care for the 1.25 million inhabitants in the region and registers 670,000 calls annually. In the Danish OOH-PC services, patients must call the OOH-PC call centres, which are managed by fully licensed GPs. Nearly 60% of calls are terminated as telephone consultations (medical advice or direct admission to the hospital) and 40% as telephone referrals (referral to subsequent face-to-face consultation (clinic visit or home visit)).

Data collection

At the start of each shift at the OOH-PC, one GP from each type of consultation (phone, clinic, home visit) could sign up electronically in the study as they logged on to the computerized patient administration system. Participating GPs received an electronic pop-up questionnaire after terminating every tenth telephone call, every third clinic consultation and every home visit. The questions focused on a range of characteristics of the contact, such as the RFE (stated in text), and duration of symptoms. Moreover, a question concerned whether the patient ought to have attended own GP within office hours (either before or after the OOH-PC contact) instead of contacting the OOH-PC.

Two to three days after the registered OOH-PC contact, the patients received a postal questionnaire, including a question about their assessment of the severity of the health problem prompting a call. Patients registered with more than one contact in the study received only one questionnaire (after the first contact). Moreover, contacting patients with permanent address outside the region did not receive a questionnaire. Data on age, date, time and type of contact were collected from the electronic patient administration system.

Data management

Focusing on children aged 0–5 years and their parents' decision to call the OOH-PC, we categorised the children into two age groups: <3 years and 3–5 years. Contacts were categorised into two groups: telephone consultations and face-to-face consultations (clinic visits, home visits).

RFEs stated in text in the patient records were obtained and manually coded using the International Classification of Primary Care, 2nd Edition (ICPC-2) [13] by a specifically trained medical student, who was supervised by the researchers. The four most frequently applied RFE diagnoses were identified, and all additional RFEs (143 in total) formed a group of "other RFEs". Duration of symptoms was categorised into four groups: <5 h, 5–12 h, >12–24 h and >24 h. Based on the contact pattern in OOH-PC, which showed a peak during the first opening hours, the time of contact was categorised into three groups: weekday evenings (4–8 pm), weekday nights (8 pm-8 am), and weekends and holidays. Geographical location was based on the postcode of the patient's home address and categorised according to number of citizens in the postcode area: rural (≤5000) and urban (>5000).

The patient-assessed severity was dichotomised into "potentially severe" (combining *"Severe and life-threatening"* and *"Severe but not life-threatening"*) and "not severe" (combining *"Not severe, but I needed to talk to a doctor"* and *"Not ill, but I had some questions"*).

Analysis

We compared respondents and non-respondents among the parents on the basis of relevant variables available in this study (age groups, type of contact, symptom duration, geographical location and GP-assessed medical relevance for the OOH-PC). Baseline characteristics of the included contacts were presented for telephone consultations and face-to-face consultations together with the proportion of contacts that the participating OOH-PC GPs considered to be more appropriate for the daytime GP. Next, we identified the subgroup of calls that the OOH-PC GPs considered more appropriate for the daytime GP and that were also assessed as non-severe by the parents. This subgroup is henceforth referred to as "medically irrelevant contacts" in this paper. In a generalised linear model (GLM), we examined, for each consultation type, the association between being categorised in this subgroup and age, duration of symptoms, time of contact and geographical location; these associations were presented as estimates of prevalence ratios (PR) and 95% confidence intervals (95% CI). In this analysis, answers of "don't know" to assessment of severity were excluded as were RFEs with too few observations. Analyses were performed by Stata 14 statistical software.

Results

During the study period, 3857 contacts regarding children aged 0–5 years were registered. Of these, 292 were excluded, primarily because they were registered with more than one contact. Of the remaining 2923 contacts, completed patient questionnaires were returned for 1748 contacts (59.8%), which were included in the analyses (522 telephone consultations and 1226 face-to-face consultations). Respondents and non-respondents did not differ significantly, except for the GP-assessment of appropriateness. The GPs found that 18% of the contacts from respondents compared with 24% from non-respondents could have been more appropriately targeted to the daytime GP than to the OOH-PC ($P < 0.001$) (Table 1).

More contacts concerned children aged 0–2 years than children aged 3–5 years; this was found for both types of consultations (Table 2). The duration of symptoms was most often under five hours for telephone consultations (31.8%) and over 24 h for face-to-face consultations (31.6%). In total, 60.7% of telephone consultations and 40.6% of face-to-face consultations were assessed as non-severe by the parents.

According to the GPs, 17.6% of telephone consultations and 18.4% of face-to-face contacts were found to be more appropriate for the daytime GP (Table 2). Contacts at 4–8 p.m. on weekdays (24.6% of telephone consultations and 22.7% of face-to-face consultations) and contacts with symptom duration >24 h (26.9% and

Table 1 Comparison of characteristics between respondents and non-respondents

		Respondents (*n*=) (%)	Non-respondents (*n*=) (%)	*P*-value
Age	0–2 years	1216 (69.6)	829 (70.5)	0.568
	3–5 years	532 (30.4)	346 (29.5)	
Type of contact	Telephone consultation	522 (29.9)	357 (30.4)	0.764
	Face-to-face consultation	1.226 (70.1)	818 (69.6)	
Symptom duration	<5 h	439 (25.1)	278 (23.7)	0.069
	5–12 h	396 (22.7)	271 (23.1)	
	12–24 h	376 (21.5)	233 (19.8)	
	>24 h	517 (29.6)	365 (31.1)	
	Missing	20 (1.1)	28 (2.4)	
Geographical location	Urban	727 (41.6)	524 (44.6)	0.220
	Rural (<5000 inhab. Per zip code)	923 52.8)	582 (49.5)	
	Missing	98 (5.6)	69 (5.9)	
More appropriate for the daytime GP according to the OOH-PC GP	No	1.309 (74.9)	803 (68.3)	<0.001
	Yes	317 (18.1)	284 (24.1)	
	Don't know	122 (7.0)	88 (7.5)	

Table 2 Characteristics of OOH-PC contacts for preschool children and proportions considered by GPs to be more appropriately targeted to the daytime GP ($N = 1748$)

		Telephone consultations		Face-to-face contacts	
		n (%)	Appropriate for daytime GP (%)	*n* (%)	Appropriate for daytime GP (%)
All calls		522 (100.0)	17.6	1226 (100.0)	18.4
Age	0–2 years	354 (67.8)	18.4	862 (70.3)	17.8
	3–5 years	168 (32.2)	16.1	364 (29.7)	19.8
Reason for encounter[a]	Fever	167 (32.0)	12.0	464 (37.9)	17.2
	Cough	56 (10.7)	16.1	224 (18.3)	18.8
	Earache	41 (7.9)	9.8	77 (6.3)	19.5
	Vomiting	34 (6.5)	8.8	65 (5.3)	15.4
	Other RFE	285 (54.6)	22.8	595 (48.5)	19.5
Duration of symptoms	<5 h	166 (31.8)	13.3	273 (22.3)	13.2
	5–12 h	126 (24.1)	15.9	270 (22.0)	17.9
	12–24 h	86 (16.5)	15.1	290 (23.7)	15.5
	>24 h	130 (24.9)	26.9	387 (31.6)	24.6
	Missing	14 (2.7)	–	6 (0.5)	–
Time of contact	Weekdays 4–8 p.m.	110 (21.1)	24.6	216 (17.6)	22.7
	Weekday nights (8 pm - 8 am)	172 (33.0)	17.4	299 (24.4)	18.7
	Weekends and holidays	240 (46.0)	14.6	711 (58.0)	16.9
Geographical location	Urban	222 (42.5)	17.1	505 (41.2)	17.8
	Rural (<5000 inhab. Per postal code)	279 (53.5)	18.3	644 (52.5)	18.3
	Missing	21 (4.0)	–	77 (6.3)	–
Parent-assessed severity	Potentially severe	203 (38.9)	9.4	721 (58.8)	15.3
	Not severe	317 (60.7)	23.0	498 (40.6)	22.9
	Missing	2 (0.4)	–	7 (0.6)	–

[a]The five most frequent RFEs; numbers add up to more than the total as several RFEs were stated for some cases

24.6%, respectively) were most often assessed to be more relevant for daytime care than OOH-PC.

Table 3 depicts the parent-assessed problem severity in relation to the GP-assessed appropriateness of contacts for OOH-PC. For telephone consultations that were considered more appropriate for daytime care by the GPs, 79.4% of the consultations were assessed as non-severe by the parents. For face-to-face consultations, the corresponding figure was 50.7%. It should be noted that the agreement between GP-assessed appropriateness of contact and parent-assessed severity of health problem generally was low.

Table 3 Distribution of parent-assessed severity and GP-assessed appropriateness of OOH-PC contacts

		More appropriately targeted to the daytime GP			
	Parent-assessed severity	Yes (*n*=) (%)	No (*n*=) (%)	Don't know (*n*=) (%)	All
Telephone consultations	Not severe	73 (79.4)	221 (56.5)	23 (59.0)	317 (60.7)
	Potentially severe	19 (20.6)	169 (43.2)	15 (38.5)	203 (38.9)
	Don't know	0	1 (0.3)	1 (2.5)	2 (0.4)
	All	92 (100)	391 (100)	39 (100)	522 (100)
Face-to-face consultations	Not severe	114 (50.7)	346 (37.7)	68 (45.8)	498 (40.6)
	Potentially severe	110 (48.9)	566 (61.7)	45 (54.2)	721 (58.8)
	Don't know	1 (0.44)	6 (0.6)	0	7 (0.6)
	All	225 (100)	918 (100)	83 (100)	1.226 (100)

Table 4 Factors associated with medically irrelevant contacts (problems considered non-severe by parents and more appropriate for the daytime GP by triaging GPs)

Characteristics	Telephone consultations ($n = 71$[a])			Face-to-face contacts (n=95[a])		
	Prevalence	Adj. prevalence ratio[b] (95% CI)	p-value	Prevalence	Adj. prevalence ratio[b] (95% CI)	p-value
Age						
< 3 years	0.15	1 (reference)		0.09	1 (reference)	
3–5 years	0.13	0.99 (0.61–1.62)	0.982	0.11	1.41 (0.96–2.06)	0.077
Duration of symptoms						
< 5 h	0.13	1 (reference)		0.06	1 (reference)	
5–12 h	0.13	0.94 (0.50–1.75)	0.834	0.10	1.86 (0.95–3.62)	0.069
> 12–24 h	0.14	1.30 (0.67–2.49)	0.437	0.09	1.91 (0.99–3.69)	0.055
> 24 h	0.17	1.50 (0.86–2.61)	0.150	0.12	2.65 (1.45–4.86)	0.002
Time of contact						
4–8 pm on weekdays	0.22	1 (reference)		0.11	1 (reference)	
8 pm-8 am on weekdays	0.13	0.57 (0.34–0.95)	0.033	0.07	0.70 (0.40–1.22)	0.205
Weekends and holidays	0.11	0.40 (0.23–0.68)	0.001	0.10	0.69 (0.44–1.61)	0.112
Geographical location						
Urban	0.14	1 (reference)		0.09	1 (reference)	
Rural	0.15	1.11 (0.12–0.34)	0.639	0.09	1.11 (0.76–1.61)	0.588

[a]Two and 19 in telephone consultations and face-to-face consultations, respectively, excluded from analysis due to missing responses
[b]Adjusted for age groups, duration of symptoms and time of contact

Table 4 shows the 166 medically irrelevant contacts (assessed by the GPs to be inappropriately directed to OOH-PC and by the parents concern be non-severe problems). For telephone consultations, these contacts were statistically significantly more often seen on weekday evenings compared to weekday nights (adj. PR: 0.57 (95% CI: 0.34–0.95)) and weekends and holidays (adj. PR: 0.40 (95% CI: 0.23–0.68)). For face-to-face contacts, a similar trend (although not statistically significant) was seen. There was a tendency that longer symptom duration was associated with assessment as medically irrelevant for OOH-PC. Age of child and geographical location were not significantly associated with assessment as medically irrelevant for OOH-PC.

Discussion

Main results

In 60% of telephone consultations and 40% of face-to-face consultations, parents considered the health problem as non-severe. In one fifth of these, the GPs also considered the problem as unappropriate for OOH-PC. For telephone consultations, we found that contacts during 4–8 p.m. on weekdays was significantly associated with assessment as medically irrelevant for OOH-PC, that is, considered to be more appropriately directed to daytime care by GPs *and* health problem was considered non-severe by parents. In face-to-face consultations, symptom duration of more than 12 h was significantly associated with medical irrelevance for OOH-PC.

Strengths and limitations

Data originated from a large study on contacts to the OOH-PC service (LV-KOS), which ensured high statistical precision. Furthermore, the participating GPs and the random inclusion of contacts have been demonstrated to be highly representative of all contacts to OOH-PC [8]. As patient contacts were randomly recruited through electronic pop-up questionnaires and the participation rate among GPs was high, the risk of selection bias was limited. Respondents and non-respondents did not differ significantly on the included variables, except that the GPs rated the medical relevance for OOH-PC somewhat lower for non-respondents. As a larger share of the medically irrelevant contacts are likely to be perceived as non-severe by parents, we may have underestimated the number of contacts with low parent-assessed severity; if this is the case, our results represent conservative estimates of the investigated association.

The short time period between contacting OOH-PC and receiving the questionnaire reduced the risk of recall bias in the parents. Still, we cannot entirely rule out the possibility of recall bias as the parents assessed the severity of the health problem several days after the contact. Their child may have recovered, and this may have affected their response and their assessment of the treatment received. This might result in an underestimation of the severity in retrospect among parents and an overestimation of the proportion of contacts assessed as non-severe.

The share of contacts assessed as unappropriate for OOH-PC was similar for the two contact types. This may be surprising as the children seen in face-to-face consultations had already been triaged by a GP by telephone. However, the basis for the GP assessment of the medical appropriateness for OOH-PC varies by type of contact as the triaging GP only had information from the telephone interview and needed a safety margin. Therefore, some of these cases may have been referred to a face-to-face consultation even though they turned out to be medically irrelevant for OOH-PC. Moreover, according to the Danish clinical guidelines, all children below the age of six months with fever should be seen in a face-to-face consultation.

It would have been relevant to include RFEs in the regression analyses in a study focusing on medical relevance. However, due to the large diversity in RFEs, the statistical precision would be reduced by including RFEs in the multivariate analyses.

Comparison with existing literature

Young children are more often sick than older children or adults [14, 15]. Therefore, this patient group is more frequently seen in OOH-PC; this group accounts for about one fifth of all calls [8, 16]. In accordance with other studies of children aged less than 5 years, we found fever, earache, coughing, breathing difficulties and vomiting the most common RFEs [12, 15, 17].

Our finding that many calls from parents to OOH-PC concern health problems in children which are often considered medically inappropriate for OOH-PC by the GPs is in line with results from other studies in similar settings [4–6, 18]. In a Norwegian survey on the urgency of calls to OOH-PC, 84.4% of calls regarding children below ten years of age were considered to concern non-urgent health problems [6]. Similarly, 44.9% of all contacts regarding children below two years of age and 55.8% contacts regarding children above two years of age to the emergency department of a paediatric department in Belgium were considered to concern non-urgent health problems [18]. In addition, a study showed that the rate of telephone consultations was almost four times as high for Danish children than for Dutch children [3]. The organisation of health care in general, including OOH primary care, is rather similar in the two countries [1]. Therefore, this difference could indicate that more contacts in Denmark concern health issues that are considered medically irrelevant for OOH-PC. Yet, previous studies indicate similar patterns of patient behaviour in the two countries [4].

We found several factors to be related to medical irrelevance for OOH-PC. The parents' motives for contacting the OOH-PC have been investigated in several studies. Frequently mentioned motives were feelings of worry or fear, inadequateness to take care of their sick child, lack of control of their child's condition and need for medical information or symptom relief [12, 15, 19]. To increase the quality of care and the efficiency in OOH-PC, it may be best for parents to wait and present their child's health problem to the GP in the daytime. Moreover, the GP often knows the family beforehand and is more able to estimate the condition of the child using the already established relation with the parents. However, several studies indicate that this may not be possible in all cases as the psychosocial context of a child's illness and the feeling of worry are likely to overrule other more rational reflections on the most relevant behaviour and the best use of resources [20–22].

Decisions on calling for medical advice are influenced by an array of various elements. Besides the actual medical problem, the parents' knowledge and degree of feeling secure in managing their child's illness are the main drivers for the decision-making [12]. Moreover, sociodemographic factors have been found to be associated with patient behaviour [23, 24]. These would have been relevant to include in the analyses of present study, but such information was not available. Future studies focusing on children in the OOH-PC should be designed to address the potential association between parent behaviour and sociodemographic factors.

Generalisability and implications for research and practice

As parents frequently worry when their child is ill, it is relevant to aim directly at this issue in future studies to gain more knowledge and to identify potential ways of redirecting calls to daytime care. This may especially be relevant if calls are related to structural factors, such as perceived inaccessibility to own GP in the daytime, which has been shown to be associated with increased use of acute care services [25, 26]. The finding that most of the telephone consultations that were considered medically irrelevant for OOH-PC were seen during the first opening hours of the OOH-PC services on weekdays supports that this could be an important structural issue. As parents considered their child's condition as non-severe in many cases, it would be relevant to examine more closely their motives for contacting the OOH-PC anyway. More insight in the reasons for contacting OOH-PC could provide input for better patient education and GP training. It would be particularly relevant to address the different elements that influence the motives for different help-seeking behaviour, such as individual sociodemographic factors and former experience with help-seeking. These components could be supplemented by exploring organizational factors related to the structure of the health care services, such as the accessibility to a GP within office hours.

Conclusions

In this study of contacts concerning health issues in young children under six years of age to OOH-PC in Denmark, we found that fever, cough and ear pain were the most common RFEs. Parents assessed 60.7% of telephone consultations and 40.6% of face-to-face consultations to concern non-severe problems. GPs assessed that about 18% of contacts concerning children should have been directed to the daytime GP. Of these GP-assessed inappropriate contacts, parents considered the health problems as non-severe in 80% of the telephone consultations and in 50% of the face-to-face consultations. Contacts in the early evening on weekdays and contacts involving longer symptom duration (>24 h) were associated with medical irrelevance for OOH-PC. The results show varying perspectives between parents and GPs and confirm the challenge of defining the appropriate use of OOH-PC. Future studies focusing on parents' motives and behaviour would be recommendable to establish more evidence on factors related to medical relevance of calls to OOH-PC in order to identify avoidable contacts.

Abbreviations

CI: Confidence interval; GP: General practitioner; ICPC-2: International Classification of Primary Care, 2nd Edition (ICPC-2); LV-KOS: Danish survey (and cohort) on contact and disease patterns in out-of-hours primary care; OOH-PC: Out-of-hours primary care; PR: Prevalence ratio; RFE: Reason for encounter

Acknowledgements

The authors would like to thank all the GPs who participated in this study.

Funding

This project was supported by the County of Aarhus, the Central Denmark Region, the Danish General Practice Fund and the Danish foundation Trygfonden. The financial support provided by these organisations partly covered the salaries of the researchers, the logistic expenses of the study (e.g. printing and postage of questionnaires), and the remuneration fees for participating GPs. The funding bodies were not involved in any part of the study nor in the writing of the manuscript.

Authors' contributions

GM designed the study and contributed substantially to the acquisition, analysis and interpretation of data. GM made the first draft and the subsequent revisions of the manuscript and approved the final version. LH contributed substantially to defining the aim of the article and interpreting the data and participated actively in the writing and critical revision of the manuscript. Furthermore, LH approved the final version of the manuscript. AO contributed substantially to the literature search related to the study, participated in the writing and revision of the manuscript and approved the final version of the manuscript. MBC contributed substantially to the design of the LV-KOS study, participated in the writing and revision of the manuscript and approved the final version of the manuscript. PV contributed substantially to the design of the study and the interpretation of data and participated in the writing and critical revision of the manuscript and approved the final version of the manuscript. All authors read and approved the final manuscript.

Consent for publication

Not applicable.

Competing interests

The authors declare that they have no competing interests.

References

1. Grol R, Giesen P, van Uden C. After-hours care in the United Kingdom, Denmark, and the Netherlands: new models. Health Aff (Millwood). 2006; 25(6):1733–7.
2. Huibers L, Giesen P, Wensing M, Grol R. Out-of-hours care in western countries: assessment of different organizational models. BMC Health Serv Res. 2009;9:105-6963-9-105.
3. Huibers L, Moth G, Andersen M, van Grunsven P, Giesen P, Christensen MB, et al. Consumption in out-of-hours health care: Danes double Dutch? Scand J Prim Health Care. 2014;32(1):44–50.
4. Keizer E, Smits M, Peters Y, Huibers L, Giesen P, Wensing M. Contacts with out-of-hours primary care for nonurgent problems: patients' beliefs or deficiencies in healthcare? BMC Fam Pract. 2015;16(1):157-015-0376-9.
5. Vedovetto A, Soriani N, Merlo E, Gregori D. The burden of inappropriate emergency department pediatric visits: why Italy needs an urgent reform. Health Serv Res. 2014;49(4):1290–305.
6. Hansen EH, Zakariassen E, Hunskaar S. Sentinel monitoring of activity of out-of-hours services in Norway in 2007: an observational study. BMC Health Serv Res. 2009;9:123–6963–9-123.
7. Iliffe S, Haug U. Out of hours work in general practice. BMJ. 1991;302(6792): 1584–6.
8. Flarup L, Moth G, Christensen MB, Vestergaard M, Olesen F, Vedsted P. A feasible method to study the Danish out-of-hours primary care service. Dan Med J. 2014;61(5):A4847.
9. Huibers LA, Moth G, Bondevik GT, Kersnik J, Huber CA, Christensen MB, et al. Diagnostic scope in out-of-hours primary care services in eight European countries: an observational study. BMC Fam Pract 2011;12:30–2296–12-30.
10. Zwaanswijk M, Nielen MM, Hek K, Verheij RA. Factors associated with variation in urgency of primary out-of-hours contacts in the Netherlands: a cross-sectional study. BMJ Open. 2015;5(10):e008421-2015-008421.
11. Moth G, Huibers L, Christensen MB, Vedsted P. Out-of-hours primary care: a population-based study of the diagnostic scope of telephone contacts. Fam Pract. 2016;33(5):504–9.
12. Kallestrup P, Bro F. Parents' beliefs and expectations when presenting with a febrile child at an out-of-hours general practice clinic. Br J Gen Pract. 2003; 53(486):43–4.
13. WONCA. International classification of primary care. ICPC-2-R. Second ed. New York: Oxford University Press; 2005.
14. Bruijnzeels MA, Foets M, van der Wouden JC, van den Heuvel WJ, Prins A. Everyday symptoms in childhood: occurrence and general practitioner consultation rates. Br J Gen Pract. 1998;48(426):880–4.
15. Ertmann RK, Siersma V, Reventlow S, Soderstrom M. Infants' symptoms of illness assessed by parents: impact and implications. Scand J Prim Health Care. 2011;29(2):67–74.
16. Moth G, Flarup L, Christensen M, Olesen F, Vedsted P. Reasons for encounter and disease patterns in the Danish out-of-hours primary care service. LV-KOS (in Danish). 1st ed. Aarhus: The Research Unit for General Practice, Aarhus University; 2012.
17. Kai J. What worries parents when their preschool children are acutely ill, and why: a qualitative study. BMJ. 1996;313(7063):983–6.
18. Benahmed N, Laokri S, Zhang WH, Verhaeghe N, Trybou J, Cohen L, et al. Determinants of nonurgent use of the emergency department for pediatric patients in 12 hospitals in Belgium. Eur J Pediatr. 2012;171(12):1829–37.
19. Shipman C, Dale J. Using and providing out-of-hours services: can patients and GPs agree? Health Soc Care Community. 1999;7(4):266–75.
20. Richtsmeier AJ, Hatcher JW. Parental anxiety and minor illness. J Dev Behav Pediatr. 1994;15(1):14–9.

21. Hopton J, Hogg R, McKee I. Patients' accounts of calling the doctor out of hours: qualitative study in one general practice. BMJ. 1996;313(7063):991–4.
22. Bernthal EM, Lathlean J, Gobbi M, Simpson RG. Mothers' decision-making during times of stress as a lone parent: a qualitative study. J R Army Med Corps. 2015;161(Suppl 1):i26–33.
23. Buja A, Toffanin R, Rigon S, Lion C, Sandona P, Carraro D, et al. What determines frequent attendance at out-of-hours primary care services? Eur J Pub Health. 2015;25(4):563–8.
24. Jansen T, Zwaanswijk M, Hek K, de Bakker D. To what extent does sociodemographic composition of the neighbourhood explain regional differences in demand of primary out-of-hours care: a multilevel study. BMC Fam Pract 2015;16:54–015–0275-0.
25. Smits M, Peters Y, Broers S, Keizer E, Wensing M, Giesen P. Association between general practice characteristics and use of out-of-hours GP cooperatives. BMC Fam Pract 2015;16:52–015–0266-1.
26. Zhou Y, Abel G, Warren F, Roland M, Campbell J, Lyratzopoulos G. Do difficulties in accessing in-hours primary care predict higher use of out-of-hours GP services? Evidence from an English National Patient Survey. Emerg Med J. 2015;32(5):373–8.

5

Patient-perceived barriers and facilitators to the implementation of a medication review in primary care

Mirella Carolin Uhl[1*], Christiane Muth[1], Ferdinand Michael Gerlach[1], Goentje-Gesine Schoch[2] and Beate Sigrid Müller[1]

Abstract

Background: Although polypharmacy can cause adverse health outcomes, patients often know little about their medication. A regularly conducted medication review (MR) can help provide an overview of a patient's medication, and benefit patients by enhancing their knowledge of their drugs. As little is known about patient attitudes towards MRs in primary care, the objective of this study was to gain insight into patient-perceived barriers and facilitators to the implementation of an MR.

Methods: We conducted a qualitative study with a convenience sample of 31 patients (age ≥ 60 years, ≥3 chronic diseases, taking ≥5 drugs/d); in Hesse, Germany, in February 2016. We conducted two focus groups and, in order to ensure the participation of elderly patients with reduced mobility, 16 telephone interviews. Both relied on a semi-structured interview guide dealing with the following subjects: patients' experience of polypharmacy, general design of MRs, potential barriers and facilitators to implementation etc. Interviews were audio-recorded, transcribed verbatim, and analysed by two researchers using thematic analysis.

Results: Patients' average age was 74 years (range 62–88 years). We identified barriers and facilitators for four main topics regarding the implementation of MRs in primary care: patient participation, GP-led MRs, pharmacist-led MRs, and the involvement of healthcare assistants in MRs. Barriers to patient participation concerned patient autonomy, while facilitators involved patient awareness of medication-related problems. Barriers to GP-led MRs concerned GP's lack of resources while facilitators related to the trusting relationship between patient and GP. Pharmacist-led MRs might be hindered by a lack of patients' confidence in pharmacists' expertise, but facilitated by pharmacies' digital records of the patients' medications. Regarding the involvement of healthcare assistants in MRs, a potential barrier was patients' uncertainty regarding the extent of their training. Patients could, however, imagine GPs delegating some aspects of MRs to them.

Conclusions: Our study suggests that patients regard MRs as beneficial and expect indications for their medicines to be checked, and possible interactions to be identified. To foster the implementation of MRs in primary care, it is important to consider barriers and facilitators to the four identified topics.

Keywords: Multimorbidity, Multiple chronic conditions, Polypharmacy, Patients, Primary health care

* Correspondence: mirellauhl@hotmail.com
[1]Institute of General Practice, Goethe University Frankfurt, Theodor-Stern-Kai 7, 60590 Frankfurt am Main, Germany
Full list of author information is available at the end of the article

Background

The prevalence of multimorbidity rises with age and already affects more than 60% of patients above the age of 50 [1–3]. Multimorbidity is defined as the simultaneous occurrence of several acute or chronic illnesses and medical conditions in one person [4]. Increasing life expectancy can be expected to lead to a significant increase in its prevalence [5]. Multimorbidity is often associated with polypharmacy. No universally accepted definition of polypharmacy exists, but the term is generally used to describe patients taking five or more medicines per day [6, 7]. The number of patients taking five or more medicines increases with age, and the number prescribed 10 or more nearly doubles between the ages of 65 and 80 [8]. Additionally, about 24% of elderly patients are prescribed at least one potentially inappropriate medication [9]. As falls and hospital admissions often result from drug-disease interactions and adverse drug reactions, polypharmacy is a risk factor for adverse health outcomes [10–13]. Additionally, patients with polypharmacy often know too little about their drugs and have difficulties with treatment compliance [14].

A regular medication review (MR) defined as "a structured, critical examination of a patient's medicines with the objective of reaching an agreement with the patient about treatment, optimising the impact of medicines, minimising the number of medication-related problems and reducing waste" can curb inappropriate polypharmacy [15]. MRs are also a first essential step towards gaining a comprehensive overview of a patient's current medication [16]. Although evidence on the effect of MRs on hard clinical outcomes is lacking [17], a reduction in drug-related problems and the number of prescribed drugs has been demonstrated [18–20]. General practitioners (GPs) play a key role in MRs because of their generalist perspective and role in the coordination and continuity of care [21]. However, the workload of GPs hinders the use of MRs [22]. Pharmacists have also been involved in MRs, but their acceptance by patients varies considerably. High implementation rates for their recommendations (up to 86%) have been observed when the relationship between GPs and pharmacists has existed for some time [23, 24].

Although successful MRs require the active participation of patients, studies on patients' attitudes to MRs are scarce [25]. Patients expect MRs to provide them with detailed information on their current medication, e.g. on necessity, and hope they will lead to simplified medication regimens. Not all patients feel the need to undergo an MR [26, 27], but those that have done see benefits in the enhancement of their knowledge about their medication, and the chance to ask about new drugs [15, 25, 28, 29]. Overall, little is known about patient-perceived barriers and facilitators to MRs in general practice.

Structured MRs are not regularly conducted in primary care in Germany. We therefore developed and tested a complex intervention involving GPs and their healthcare assistants (HCAs)[1] to optimise and prioritise multiple medications in older patients with multimorbidity in primary care. The intervention included an MR and was generally feasible for health care professionals and patients during the pilot study [22]. After conducting the main study (publication in progress), to facilitate routine implementation of MRs in general practice, we have now conducted a qualitative barrier analysis to obtain patient perspectives on hindering and facilitating factors.

Methods

Design and setting

The study was conducted in primary care, where most prescriptions are managed. To include patients with reduced mobility and to support patient interaction, we investigated patients' perspectives using two different approaches, namely 1) telephone interviews and 2) focus groups. Both relied on a semi-structured interview guide. The telephone interviews were conducted first.

Participants

From January to February 2016, we recruited a convenience sample of patients from 17 general practices in the city and region of Frankfurt am Main. GPs from these practices belonged to "Forschungsnetzwerk Allgemeinmedizin Frankfurt" (ForN, Frankfurt research network of general practices) [30]. We asked GPs via e-mail to invite patients to participate in the study if they 1) were ≥60 years old, 2) had ≥3 chronic diseases, and 3) took ≥5 drugs per day. GPs were told about the study and its ultimate aim (to design an MR for primary care) and informed that travel expenses would be refunded for focus group participants. When a GP agreed to recruit patients, we sent him or her five consent forms and patient information sheets, with further copies available on request. Patients received written information on the study (general importance of medicines, polypharmacy as potential problem, and drug-related problems), the choice between telephone interview and focus group, and data protection regulations. After receiving written informed consent, their GP informed the study centre, the Frankfurt Institute of General Practice. The Institutional Review Board of the University Hospital Frankfurt/Main approved the study protocol in January, 2016 (No 443/15).

Data collection

Patients were called up by the Frankfurt Institute of General Practice to arrange appointments for either a telephone interview or a focus group session to be carried out in February 2016. Patients had no previous association with the Institute. A preliminary interview guide was developed by BSM (academic GP, MD) and a student assistant (during the final term of his sociology studies), and revised after discussion with CM (principal investigator, MD, MPH) on the basis of her own research and existing literature [16, 22, 31]. The semi-structured interview guide covered the following subjects: patients with polypharmacy, design of a medication review (person in charge, benefits, difficulties) and services provided by health insurers (see Additional file 1). Conversations were structured but open, enabling patients to add their own comments [32]. At the beginning of both telephone interviews and focus groups, the two female interviewers (BSM, MCU) introduced themselves as staff from the Institute, but did not provide information on personal goals or academic background in order to minimise their influence on the conversation. BSM and MCU also provided background information on the study (see Additional file 1). BSM has considerable experience in conducting interviews and focus groups, and briefed MCU (doctoral candidate) carefully in advance. To get comprehensive insights into patients' perspectives, we adapted the content of our interviews and focus groups by expanding on subjects that seemed important to them, and rewording and clarifying questions for better understanding. Subsequent interviews and focus groups were improved, based on field notes that were made when it had proven necessary to reword or clarify questions. Focus groups took place at the Institute. Patients did not receive payment but travel expenses were refunded. BSM and MCU conducted the focus groups and ensured that all important subjects were covered without interrupting the discussions. At the beginning of each focus group, BSM explained the procedure (talking and interacting with each other is encouraged, different attitudes are welcomed, others should be permitted to finish speaking). After each focus group, a short debriefing took place. Telephone interviews and focus groups were audio recorded.

Data analysis

Telephone interviews and focus groups were anonymised and transcribed verbatim using f4transkript [33] software. Transcripts were not returned to interviewees for comment, correction, or feedback on the findings.

We used thematic analysis - a form of qualitative content analysis - to analyse the transcripts [34]. It contains the following phases: 1) familiarisation with the data; 2) generate initial codes; 3) search for themes; 4) review themes; 5) define and name themes; and 6) produce the report including a selection of illustrative data and quotations [34]. To explore the diversity of patient perspectives on barriers to and facilitators of the implementation of an MR, we analysed transcripts from telephone interviews and focus groups together. There was no evidence of any relevant differences in the findings between the two types of interviews, the same topics emerged from the respective transcripts.

BSM and MCU independently coded a sample of three transcripts and then checked for agreement on the codes. Afterwards, both coded the remaining transcripts. They then discussed the codes and emerging subjects, and reached a consensus by recoding or redefining them in case of disagreement. To minimise personal bias stemming from the differing disciplinary perspectives of the coders, the transition from codes to preliminary and then to the final themes included frequent discussions with the principal investigator (CM). We used an analytic framework involving the identification of key concepts to discover core ideas, and to understand how participants viewed the topic [35]. MAXQDA 11 [36] software was used to assist with coding and analysis. MCU and BSM selected illustrative quotations. All quotations were translated into English by a native speaker. The consolidated criteria for reporting qualitative research (COREQ) (see Additional file 2) were used to report the findings of the study.

Results

Characteristics of participants and interviews

Forty-five patients were recruited by 13 general practices and 33 patients ultimately included in our study. The 12 remaining patients were not invited to participate as we noticed during our debriefings that no new topics arose in the course of interviews and focus groups. Two patients withdrew from the study (unavailable on the phone; cancelled the focus group). The final sample consisted of 16 women and 15 men. Sixteen telephone interviews (average duration 12.5 min) and two focus groups with the remaining 15 patients (average duration 1 h 12 min) were conducted. Table 1 displays the sample characteristics. Most patients reported they took six to seven medicines a day, always got them from the same pharmacy and had received a medication plan from their GP. None of the participants had previously received a structured medication review on a regular basis.

Each quotation is assigned a code: P stands for "patient", and the number indicates the individual. An ellipsis surrounded by parentheses (...) denotes omitted text.

Table 1 Sample characteristics ($n = 31$)

	Patients (male/female) (n)	Mean age (years)	Range (years)
Telephone interviews	16 (10/6)	72 (SD 7,1)	(62–82)
Focus group 1	8 (3/5)	74 (SD 6,6)	(62–82)
Focus group 2	7 (2/5)	78 (SD 6,3)	(71–88)
All participants	31 (15/16)	74 (SD 7,0)	(62–88)

Patient participation in an MR

Barriers

Some of our interviewees were sceptical about the need for MRs in general, or could understand why other patients might refuse participation. The three main reasons they gave concerned patient autonomy. The first point was satisfaction with the current medication regime and therefore reluctance to have anyone change it. The second point was an unwillingness to disclose all medicines during an MR. This unwillingness was mainly related to psychiatric treatment and over-the-counter (OTC) drugs. Patients wanted to decide for themselves when to speak about psychiatric diagnoses, and not to be forced to do so during an MR. Furthermore, OTC drugs are often not disclosed, sometimes because patients are unaware they can also lead to interactions, and sometimes because they fear having to justify what they take.

"I didn't mention it either, that I take them. I didn't think it was important because it's herbal medicine (...)." (P 4, 66 years, telephone interview).

"Well, what they're taking may not be that good, but when your sister has said, or your brother, that that's ideal, you don't want to be sort of dictated to ... to be told what you have to take, when and why." (P 9, 63 years, telephone interview).

The third point was that some patients disapproved of only having an MR at predetermined intervals. They agreed to have a review on a regular basis, e.g. once a year, but stressed that MRs should be available to them upon request, following hospitalisation, when new medicines are prescribed, or when medicines are changed. One patient, who was taking eight prescribed medicines per day, said he could not "wait half a year, or a year" (P24, 76 years, focus group 1) to talk to a doctor when he had a problem with his medication.

Facilitators

Most of our interviewed patients saw no reason to refuse an MR themselves, and regarded it as "definitely necessary that such a check is done" (P27, 76 years, focus group 2), not least because the majority of participants had already reflected upon the appropriateness of their medication and some had even undertaken measures to check it. These measures ranged from reading the patient information leaflet provided with their medicines, to preparing their own digital medication plan, or proactively asking their GP to check their medicines for potential interactions. These patients regarded a structured MR as a good opportunity to discuss their medications. Many patients could also imagine playing an active role by, for example, preparing a list of their medicines in advance, thus facilitating and shortening MRs.

During an MR, patients expected indications for their medicines to be checked, possible interactions with other drugs identified, information provided on the availability of new and better medicines, and possibilities to reduce the number of drugs they were taking to be investigated. Two main reasons for these expectations were revealed during interviews and focus groups. The first reason was medication-related somatic problems faced by the interviewees themselves, e.g. stomach bleeding or a restricted choice of headache pills when taking anticoagulants. The second reason was a more general distrust of the complex healthcare system and its various stakeholders. It was repeatedly seen as a problem that consulting several doctors (GPs and specialists) frequently led to uncoordinated prescription of multiple different medicines.

"If I could stop taking something - well I do take a lot - I should add that I really am all for stopping (...)" (P8, 77 years, telephone interview).

"Yes, especially concerning interactions. Do they agree with one another? Is it necessary that I take this kind of medicine? That's really the main priority, and how they interact with one another. Yes, I always think; as many as necessary but as few as possible." (P 12, 62 years, telephone interview).

GP-led MRs

Barriers

The main arguments against GPs conducting MRs were a perceived lack of resources (financial and time constraints) on the one hand, and a lack of pharmacological competence on the other. Patients who were concerned that GPs would not have enough time for MRs based their doubts on the experience that the practice was always crowded. They feared a lack of time might prevent GPs from discussing patients' medicines in the necessary detail. One patient questioned whether GPs would receive appropriate financial compensation. A few patients also doubted whether GPs had the necessary pharmaceutical expertise for an MR. However, such patients were never referring to their own GPs, and most of them were actually in favour of GP-led MRs.

"Well I reckon you're opening a can of worms - it's definitely necessary that such a check is done - because I can't imagine that all the things we swallow, that all those things agree with one another, but I don't know if the GP has the ability or the time to do the research on it." (P 27, 76 years, focus group 2).

Facilitators

The main facilitators to GP-led MRs were firstly his or her perceived pharmaceutical competence, and secondly the trusting relationship between patient and GP.

GPs were generally mentioned explicitly as the first point of contact in the event of medication-related problems. Most patients expected their GPs to have more medication-related experience and knowledge than pharmacists. They therefore concluded that GPs were best suited to conducting an MR.

"(...) when I get a new or a different medicine, I can read the description as often as I want, I still only understand 10% of it. Simple! I need someone that knows about it and who says, yes, that works or that doesn't work. And if it's not the GP, who sees me regularly and has known me for years, who is it going to be?" (P 21, 67 years, focus group 1).

"In that case I'd prefer the doctor. I don't want to criticise the pharmacist. (...) I can just imagine the doctor knows more about side effects (...)." (P 13, 65 years, telephone interview).

Most of our interviewees reported having confidence in their GPs and regarded the trusting relationship with him or her as a good basis for a successful MR. They had often consulted the same GP for a long time. One participant also mentioned that his GP visited him at home as he was physically disabled. (Pharmacists in Germany do not currently perform home visits on a regular basis,) So he perceived he had "not many options" (P8, 77 years, telephone interview) other than a GP-led MR for practical reasons.

Pharmacist-led MRs

Barriers

The main barrier to a pharmacist leading the MR was a lack of confidence in their pharmacological expertise. This mistrust was specifically described as resulting from personal experience when buying medicines in a pharmacy. When obtaining medicines, patients expected to be asked about illnesses and the other medications they were taking to ensure there was no danger of interactions. However, several patients reported that this had not always been the case. One 76-year-old patient, for instance, described reading the patient information leaflet after buying eye drops and discovering that his coronary heart disease was contra-indicated. Another 64-year-old patient said it upsets him for safety reasons that when buying aspirin, he was never asked whether he was taking anticoagulants. In consequence, he now mentions that he is taking anticoagulants when obtaining a medication from a pharmacy.

As a result, very few patients discussed problems with prescribed medicines with pharmacists but only consulted them when obtaining OTC drugs.

Facilitators

Few patients saw any benefit in MRs being conducted by pharmacists. However, one patient mentioned that it was an advantage that some pharmacies already have digital records of the medicines taken by regular customers.

"That means that when I go to the pharmacy, all the medications I'm being prescribed are entered into a computer programme so that it's possible to see, like I said, when I received what medication and in what dosage (...) Then they can see exactly what has been prescribed to date." (P9, 63 years, telephone interview).

Involvement of HCAs in MRs

Barriers

Several patients were unsure whether HCAs should be involved in MRs, generally because they were unsure whether HCAs received the necessary training.

"The problem is really to what extent the assistants can or are allowed to discuss such things. I don't know what their training entails and whether they are competent enough for it (...) But if the doctor says Mrs. Whatever is capable enough then of course I would speak to her about it." (P 2, 64 years, telephone interview).

Facilitators

Most patients found it acceptable that GPs should delegate parts of MRs to an HCA. They expected HCAs' support to reduce the doctor's workload and to facilitate the MR. As examples of such supportive tasks, participants said they could imagine HCAs calling up patients to make a list of their medications, or entering the medicines into a computer programme prior to the MR appointment.

Discussion

Main findings

Our study identified barriers and facilitators for four main topics regarding the implementation of MRs in primary care. These four topics comprised patient participation, GP-led MRs, pharmacist-led MRs, and involvement of HCAs in MRs.

Barriers to patient participation related to patient autonomy and included reluctance to change current drug regime, unwillingness to disclose psychiatric and OTC drugs, as well as disapproval of excessive rigidity in the intervals between MRs. However, as the majority of patients had already reflected upon the appropriateness of their medications, their awareness of medication-related problems was a facilitator. During an MR, patients expected indications for their medicines to be checked, possible interactions with other drugs identified, information provided on the availability of new and better medicines, and possibilities to reduce the number of drugs they were taking to be investigated. Barriers to GP-led MRs concerned GP's lack of resources, whereas facilitators related to the trusting relationship between patient and GP. Respondents had differing views on the pharmaceutical competence of GPs. Although most had confidence in their doctor's skill, some doubted he or she had sufficient pharmaceutical knowledge. Pharmacist-led MRs may be hindered by patients' mistrust of pharmacists' expertise, but could be facilitated by pharmacies' digital records of a patient's medicines. With regard to the involvement of HCAs in an MR, a potential barrier was that some patients doubted whether their training and competence were sufficient. However, most patients were happy with the idea that GPs would delegate some aspects of MRs to an HCA and thus facilitate their implementation.

Findings in relation to the literature

Our findings are supported in the literature [15, 27, 28, 37] insofar as our patients' attitudes towards MRs were mostly positive. Unlike as in some other studies, none of our patients viewed MRs negatively or as unnecessary due to the workload of existing medical appointments [26, 38]. Fears and suspicions that the purpose of MRs was to save money by stopping or changing medicines were mentioned by Petty et al. [27, 39]. Some of our patients also feared a change in a drug regimen they were satisfied with, but did not voice fears that the aim was to cut costs. Others found that additional drugs, such as herbal treatments, had only been documented by approximately 60% of GPs [40], and that some patients withheld information on these drugs from their doctor [41, 42]. Our interviewees also mentioned this problem. As inappropriate use can lead to potentially hazardous drug interactions, structured MRs should explicitly ask about additional drugs [43]. However, our findings suggest that patients need to be informed about the importance of disclosing additional drugs, as some of our interviewees perceived for instance herbal medicines as not important and never mentioned them to their GPs. Patients should not be forced to reveal all their medicines, but motivated to do so in a supportive manner.

Reports by patients that they had no opportunity to discuss medication-related questions and problems with a health professional can be found in the literature [15, 41]. These patients want to be properly informed about their medications, including possible side effects, and to receive detailed instructions on taking them [27, 44]. Such patients would undoubtedly appreciate the opportunity to discuss these issues in an MR [27, 45], and to have their questions answered [29], just like our interviewees. The wish to cease taking medications that are no longer necessary and to reduce the number of drugs being taken was a point mentioned in both telephone interviews and focus groups. Other authors have reported similar finding [46].

The majority of our patients had reflected upon the appropriateness of their medicines, and a few had even asked their GP to check their current medicines. However, in other studies, GPs' lack of time and patients' fears of wasting it were barriers to seeking help [47]. This may explain why many of our interviewees had not asked their GPs to review their medicines. Nonetheless, the inclusion of MRs in routine primary care would be welcomed by patients who are aware of potential problems and willing to do something about it, e.g. by seeking advice from journals, or on the internet [48, 49]. Our participants also undertook measures to check their medicines by, for instance, reading patient information leaflets. Our patients were able to imagine being actively involved in MRs. This could well be a facilitator, as patients would then be more likely to provide information on their actual drug use (including OTC drugs), adverse drug events, and practical and management problems [25].

Our interviewees welcomed the idea of GPs conducting MRs in preference to pharmacists. Other authors have also reported that patients welcomed MRs conducted by GPs [15, 27, 50]. However, considering the lack of research into patients' views on MRs, it cannot be ruled out that many patients would be happy for pharmacists to perform them. Patients that had undergone an MR with a pharmacist spoke positively about it, and viewed the pharmacist as an expert on medicines [51]. Indeed, some of our interviewees could imagine that a pharmacist would conduct their MR.

Strengths and limitations

One strength of our study is that some of our elderly patients expressed their opinions in telephone interviews and some in focus groups. Their average age was 74, and ranged from 62 to 88 years, enabling us to cover a wide spectrum of patients. Furthermore, our sample was balanced with respect to gender. As a result of our inclusion criteria, we selected patients who had most likely experienced medication-related problems, and could contribute to the discussion.

The study has several limitations. As we recruited patients in general practice, where patients generally have confidence in their GPs, our participants may have overemphasized the role of the GP in MRs. Furthermore, as we work at an institute of general practice, we may also have tended to overstate the role of GPs. To prevent this, we thoroughly discussed codes during the analysis. Studies inviting patients to community pharmacies might find slightly different attitudes. Although we conducted test interviews, our interview guide was not systematically pilot tested. Furthermore, patients could choose between telephone interview and focus group. The choice enabled us to lower the threshold for participation because housebound people could participate in a telephone interview. A similar study, by contrast, excluded housebound patients [27].

Patients participated voluntarily, so it is likely that they had a greater interest in MRs than the average patient. Furthermore, in the "project background" section of our interview guide, we state that taking many different medicines can cause problems. This may have encouraged patients to speak in more detail about their medication-related problems, as they felt confident that their problems were of interest to others. In general, participants' statements have to be rated as assumptions – none had experienced a structured MR so far. Limitations usually associated with focus groups such as difficulties surrounding mutual self-disclosure on uncomfortable subjects may apply to our study as well [52]. However, in anticipation of this limitation we also conducted telephone interviews, which created a more personal atmosphere. Additionally, we used circular questions, inviting our interviewees to refer to other patients' viewpoints, e.g. relatives or friends who had different experiences and problems [53]. Nevertheless, such viewpoints remain speculative.

Conclusion

Our study suggests that patients regard MRs as beneficial and expect indications for their medicines to be checked, and possible interactions with other drugs to be identified. To foster the use of MRs in primary care, it is important to consider potential barriers and facilitators for the four different topics we identified. These topics comprised patient participation, GP-led MRs, pharmacist-led-MRs, and the involvement of HCAs.

These findings will be used to support the further implementation of our complex intervention on "PRIoritising MUltimedication in Multimorbidity in general practices (PRIMUM)" [22] to facilitate MRs in primary care. Furthermore, our findings may help in the design of MRs. According to our study, invitations should describe possible effects (e.g. reduction in number and complexity of medicines), and explicitly invite patients to consult their GPs. The structured MRs should also include questions on additional drugs, such as OTC medicines. Although our patients thought differently, we could envisage cooperation between GPs and pharmacists. Further research is needed here to identify and address possible obstacles from the point of view of all stakeholders. Our patients considered MRs to be necessary, but as resources in primary care are limited, further research should focus on precise inclusion criteria for the target group.

We confirm all patient/personal identifiers have been removed or disguised so that the patient/person(s) described are not identifiable and cannot be identified on the basis of the manuscript.

Endnotes

[1]HCAs are medical assistants in the practice who receive less training than nurse practitioners and U.S. physician assistants and are comparable to certified medical assistants in the USA. They mainly perform administrative work and simple tasks such as weighing patients [54, 55]. HCAs have already been repeatedly and successfully involved in primary care-based, chronic care interventions in Germany. Under GP supervision, they have followed evidence-based protocols and algorithms with fixed interview questions, and provided telephone monitoring to check, for example, adherence to medication in patients with major depression, chronic heart failure, and osteoarthritis [56–58]

Abbreviations

ForN: Forschungsnetzwerk Allgemeinmedizin Frankfurt; GP: General Practitioner; HCA: Health care assistant; MR: Medication review; OTC: Over-the-counter; PRIMUM: PRIoritising MUltimedication in Multimorbidity in general practices; TK: Techniker Krankenkasse

Acknowledgements

The authors would like to express their thanks to all participating patients and general practices. We also thank Birgit Kemperdick for her project management skills, Corina Güthlin and Jennifer Engler for their comments on a former version of the manuscript, Jonas Biedermann for his assistance regarding the interview guide, and Phillip Elliott and Dagmar Dornbierer for the English-review of this paper.

Funding

The study was funded by the German Statutory Health Insurance Company "Techniker Krankenkasse (TK)".

Authors' contributions

MCU contributed towards data-collection and analysis, wrote the first draft of the manuscript, and critically edited revisions to it. CM contributed towards the study concept and design, supervised the study, contributed towards data analysis and writing the initial manuscript, and commented on successive drafts. FMG contributed towards the study concept and design, and commented on the manuscript and successive drafts to it. GGS contributed towards the study concept and design. BSM contributed towards the study concept and design, as well as to data-collection and analysis, and contributed towards writing the manuscript, and commenting on successive drafts. All authors read and approved the final manuscript.

Consent for publication

Not applicable.

Competing interests

CM and BSM received grants from the German Statutory Health Insurance Company "Techniker Krankenkasse (TK)" for the study. However, the "TK" had no involvement in study design; collection, analysis and interpretation of data; writing of the study report; and in the decision to submit the article for publication. The other authors declare no conflict of interest.

Author details

[1]Institute of General Practice, Goethe University Frankfurt, Theodor-Stern-Kai 7, 60590 Frankfurt am Main, Germany. [2]Scientific Institute for Benefit and Efficiency in Health Care (WINEG), Techniker Krankenkasse (TK), Bramfelder Straße 140, 22305 Hamburg, Germany.

References

1. Glynn LG, Valderas JM, Healy P, Burke E, Newell J, Gillespie P, Murphy AW. The prevalence of multimorbidity in primary care and its effect on health care utilization and cost. Fam Pract. 2011;28:516–23.
2. Violan C, Foguet-Boreu Q, Flores-Mateo G, Salisbury C, Blom J, Freitag M, et al. Prevalence, determinants and patterns of multimorbidity in primary care: a systematic review of observational studies. PLoS One. 2014;9: e102149.
3. Fortin M, Bravo G, Hudon C, Vanasse A, Lapointe L. Prevalence of multimorbidity among adults seen in family practice. Ann Fam Med. 2005;3:223–8.
4. van Den Akker M, Buntinx F, Knottnerus JA. Comorbidity or multimorbidity: what's in a name? A review of literature. Eur J Gen Pract. 2009;2:65–70.
5. Pötzsch O, Rößger F. Bevölkerung Deutschlands bis 2060–13. koordinierte Bevölkerungsvorausberechnung. 2015. https://www.destatis.de/DE/PresseService/Presse/Pressekonferenzen/2015/bevoelkerung/Pressebroschuere_Bevoelk2060.pdf?__blob=publicationFile. Accessed 24 Mar 2016.
6. Maher RL, Hanlon J, Hajjar ER. Clinical consequences of polypharmacy in elderly. Expert Opin Drug Saf. 2013;13:57–65.
7. Wehling M, Burkhardt H. Arzneitherapie für Ältere. 2nd ed. Berlin, Heidelberg: Springer-Verlag Berlin Heidelberg; 2011.
8. Fillit HM, Futterman R, Orland BI, Chim T, Susnow L, Picariello GP, et al. Polypharmacy management in Medicare managed care: changes in prescribing by primary care physicians resulting from a program promoting medication reviews. Am J Manag Care. 1999;5:587–94.
9. Voigt K, Gottschall M, Köberlein-Neu J, Schübel J, Quint N, Bergmann A. Why do family doctors prescribe potentially inappropriate medication to elderly patients? BMC Fam Pract. 2016;17:93.
10. Fried TR, O'Leary J, Towle V, Goldstein MK, Trentalange M, Martin DK. Health outcomes associated with polypharmacy in community-dwelling older adults: a systematic review. J Am Geriatr Soc. 2014;62:2261–72.
11. Chan M, Nicklason F, Vial JH. Adverse drug events as a cause of hospital admission in the elderly. Intern Med J. 2001;31:199–205.
12. Payne RA, Abel GA, Avery AJ, Mercer SW, Roland MO. Is polypharmacy always hazardous? A retrospective cohort analysis using linked electronic health records from primary and secondary care. Br J Clin Pharmacol. 2014; 77:1073–82.
13. Guthrie B, Makubate B, Hernandez-Santiago V, Dreischulte T. The rising tide of polypharmacy and drug-drug interactions: population database analysis 1995-2010. BMC Med. 2015;13:74.
14. Nathan A, Goodyer L, Lovejoy A, Rashid A. Brown bag' medication reviews as a means of optimizing patients' use of medication and of identifying potential clinical problems. Fam Pract. 1999;16:278–82.
15. Shaw J, Seal R, Pilling M. Room for review: a guide to medication review : the agenda for patients, practitioners and managers. London: Task Force on Medicines Partnership; 2002.
16. Bergert FW, Braun M, Ehrenthal K, Feßler J, Gross J, Hüttner U, et al. Recommendations for treating adult and geriatric patients on Multimedication. Int J Clin Pharmacol Ther. 2014;52:1–64.
17. Patterson SM, Cadogan CA, Kerse N, Cardwell CR, Bradley MC, Ryan C, Hughes C. Interventions to improve the appropriate use of polypharmacy for older people. Cochrane Database Syst Rev. 2014;(10):CD008165. https://doi.org/10.1002/14651858.CD008165.pub3.
18. Chau SH, APD J, van de Ven PM, Hoogland P, PJM E, Hugtenburg JG. Clinical medication reviews in elderly patients with polypharmacy: a cross-sectional study on drug-related problems in the Netherlands. Int J Clin Pharm. 2016;38:46–53.
19. Fiss T, Meinke-Franze C, van den Berg N, Hoffmann W. Effects of a three party healthcare network on the incidence levels of drug related problems. Int J Clin Pharm. 2013;35:763–71.
20. Huiskes VJ, Burger DM, van den Ende CH, van den Bemt BJ. Effectiveness of medication review: a systematic review and meta-analysis of randomized controlled trials. BMC Fam Pract. 2017;18:5.
21. Haggerty JL, Reid RJ, Freeman GK, Starfield BH, Adair CE, McKendry R. Continuity of care: a multidisciplinary review. BMJ. 2003;327:1219–21.
22. Muth C, Harder S, Uhlmann L, Rochon J, Fullerton B, Guthlin C, et al. Pilot study to test the feasibility of a trial design and complex intervention on PRIoritising MUltimedication in multimorbidity in general practices (PRIMUMpilot). BMJ Open. 2016;6:e011613.
23. Zermansky AG, Petty DR, Raynor DK, Lowe CJ, Freemantle N, Vail A. Clinical medication review by a pharmacist of patients on repeat prescriptions in general practice: a randomised controlled trial. Health Technol Assess. 2002; 6:1–86.
24. Bryant LJM, Coster G, Gamble GD, McCormick RN. The general practitioner-pharmacist collaboration (GPPC) study: a randomised controlled trial of clinical medication reviews in community pharmacy. Int J Pharm Pract. 2011;19:94–105.
25. Willeboordse F, Hugtenburg JG, Schellevis FG, Elders PJM. Patient participation in medication reviews is desirable but not evidence-based: a systematic literature review. Br J Clin Pharmacol. 2014;78:1201–16.
26. Lee CY, George J, Elliott RA, Stewart K. Exploring stakeholder perspectives on medication review services for older residents in retirement villages. Int J Pharm Pract. 2012;20:249–58.
27. Petty DR, Knapp P, Raynor DK, House AO. Patients' views of a pharmacist-run medication review clinic in general practice. Br J Gen Pract. 2003;53:607–13.
28. Jameson JP, VanNoord GR. Pharmacotherapy consultation on polypharmacy patients in ambulatory care. Ann Pharmacother. 2001;35:835–40.
29. Sheridan J, Butler R, Brandt T, Harrison J, Jensen M, Shaw J. Patients' and pharmacists' perceptions of a pilot medicines use review service in Auckland, New Zealand. J Pharm Health Serv Res. 2012;3:35–40.
30. Allgemeinmedizin If, Frankfurt. ForN - Forschungsnetzwerk Allgemeinmedizin Frankfurt. 2016. http://www.allgemeinmedizin.uni-frankfurt.de/forschung4/forn.html. Accessed 4 May 2016.
31. Muth C, van Den Akker M, Blom JW, Mallen CD, Rochon J, Schellevis FG, et al. The Ariadne principles: how to handle multimorbidity in primary care consultations. BMC Med. 2014;12:223.
32. Mayring P. Einführung in die qualitative Sozialforschung: Eine Anleitung zu qualitativem Denken. 5th ed. Beltz: Weinheim; 2002.
33. dr. dresing & pehl GmbH. f4transkript - Audiodateien schneller abtippen. 2016. https://www.audiotranskription.de/f4.htm. Accessed 9 May 2016.
34. Braun V, Clarke V. Using thematic analysis in psychology. Qual Res Psychol. 2006;3:77–101.
35. Krueger RA, Casey MA. Focus groups: a practical guide for applied research. 5th ed. Thousand Oaks: SAGE; 2015.
36. VERBI Software. Consult. Sozialforschung. GmbH. MAXQDA 11. 1995-2016. http://www.maxqda.de/produkte/maxqda11/. Accessed 9 May 2016.
37. Swain LD. A pharmacist's contribution to an ambulatory neurology clinic. Consult Pharm. 2012;27:49–57.
38. Bissell P, Blenkinsopp A, Short D, Mason L. Patients' experiences of a community pharmacy-led medicines management service. Health Soc Care Community. 2008;16:363–9.
39. Petty DR, Zermansky AG, Raynor DK, Vail A, Lowe CJ, Freemantle N, Buttress AD. "no thank you": why elderly patients declined to participate in a research study. Pharm World Sci. 2001;23:22–7.
40. Jaski ME, Schwartzberg JG, Guttman RA, Noorani M. Medication review and documentation in physician office practice. Eff Clin Pract. 2000;3:31–4.
41. Moen J, Bohm A, Tillenius T, Antonov K, Nilsson JLG, Ring L. "I don't know how many of these medicines are necessary." - a focus group study among elderly users of multiple medicines. Patient Educ Couns. 2009;74:135–41.
42. Serper M, McCarthy DM, Patzer RE, King JP, Bailey SC, Smith SG, et al. What patients think doctors know: beliefs about provider knowledge as barriers to safe medication use. Patient Educ Couns. 2013;93:306–11.
43. Fendrick AM, Pan DE, Johnson GE. OTC analgesics and drug interactions: clinical implications. Osteopath Med Prim Care. 2008;2:2.
44. Tarn DM, Paterniti DA, Williams BR, Cipri CS, Wenger NS. Which providers should communicate which critical information about a new medication? Patient, pharmacist, and physician perspectives. J Am Geriatr Soc. 2009;57:462–9.
45. White L, Klinner C, Carter S. Consumer perspectives of the Australian home medicines review program: benefits and barriers. Res Social Adm Pharm. 2012;8:4–16.
46. Reeve E, To J, Hendrix I, Shakib S, Roberts MS, Wiese MD. Patient barriers to and enablers of deprescribing: a systematic review. Drugs Aging. 2013;30:793–807.
47. Cromme SK, Whitaker KL, Winstanley K, Renzi C, Smith CF, Wardle J. Worrying about wasting GP time as a barrier to help-seeking: a community-based, qualitative study. Br J Gen Pract. 2016;66:82.
48. Bezreh T, Laws MB, Taubin T, Rifkin DE, Wilson IB. Challenges to physician-patient communication about medication use: a window into the skeptical patient's world. Patient Prefer Adherence. 2012;6:11–8.
49. Löffler C, Kaduszkiewicz H, Stolzenbach C-O, Streich W, Fuchs A, van den Bussche H, et al. Coping with multimorbidity in old age–a qualitative study. BMC Fam Pract. 2012;13:45.
50. Salter C, Holland R, Harvey I, Henwood K. "I haven't even phoned my doctor yet." the advice giving role of the pharmacist during consultations for

medication review with patients aged 80 or more: qualitative discourse analysis. BMJ. 2007;334:1101.
51. Latif A, Pollock K, Boardman HF. Medicines use reviews: a potential resource or lost opportunity for general practice? BMC Fam Pract. 2013;14:57.
52. Morgan DL. Focus groups. Annu Rev Sociol. 1996;22:129–52.
53. Evans N, Whitcombe S. Using circular questions as a tool in qualitative research. Nurse Res. 2016;23:26–9.
54. Bosley S, Dale J. Healthcare assistants in general practice: practical and conceptual issues of skill-mix change. Br J Gen Pract. 2008;58:118–24.
55. Gensichen J, Jaeger C, Peitz M, Torge M, Guthlin C, Mergenthal K, et al. Health care assistants in primary care depression management: role perception, burdening factors, and disease conception. Ann Fam Med. 2009; 7:513–9.
56. Rosemann T, Korner T, Wensing M, Gensichen J, Muth C, Joos S, Szecsenyi J. Rationale, design and conduct of a comprehensive evaluation of a primary care based intervention to improve the quality of life of osteoarthritis patients. The PraxArt-project: a cluster randomized controlled trial ISRCTN87252339. BMC Public Health. 2005;5:77.
57. Peters-Klimm F, Muller-Tasch T, Schellberg D, Gensichen J, Muth C, Herzog W, Szecsenyi J. Rationale, design and conduct of a randomised controlled trial evaluating a primary care-based complex intervention to improve the quality of life of heart failure patients: HICMan (Heidelberg integrated case management). BMC Cardiovasc Disord. 2007;7:25.
58. Gensichen J, von Korff M, Peitz M, Muth C, Beyer M, Guthlin C, et al. Case management for depression by health care assistants in small primary care practices: a cluster randomized trial. Ann Intern Med. 2009;151:369–78.

6

What gives rise to clinician gut feeling, its influence on management decisions and its prognostic value for children with RTI in primary care

Sophie Turnbull[1,10*], Patricia J. Lucas[2], Niamh M. Redmond[3], Hannah Christensen[4], Hannah Thornton[1], Christie Cabral[1], Peter S. Blair[5], Brendan C. Delaney[6], Matthew Thompson[7], Paul Little[8], Tim J. Peters[9] and Alastair D. Hay[1]

Abstract

Background: The objectives were to identify 1) the clinician and child characteristics associated with; 2) clinical management decisions following from, and; 3) the prognostic value of; a clinician's 'gut feeling something is wrong' for children presenting to primary care with acute cough and respiratory tract infection (RTI).

Methods: Multicentre prospective cohort study where 518 primary care clinicians across 244 general practices in England assessed 8394 children aged ≥3 months and < 16 years for acute cough and RTI. The main outcome measures were: Self-reported clinician 'gut feeling'; clinician management decisions (antibiotic prescribing, referral for acute admission); and child's prognosis (reconsultation with evidence of illness deterioration, hospital admission in the 30 days following recruitment).

Results: Clinician years since qualification, parent reported symptoms (illness severity score ≥ 7/10, severe fever < 24 h, low energy, shortness of breath) and clinical examination findings (crackles/ crepitations on chest auscultation, recession, pallor, bronchial breathing, wheeze, temperature ≥ 37.8 °C, tachypnoea and inflamed pharynx) independently contributed towards a clinician 'gut feeling that something was wrong'. 'Gut feeling' was independently associated with increased antibiotic prescribing and referral for secondary care assessment. After adjustment for other associated factors, gut feeling was not associated with reconsultations or hospital admissions.

Conclusions: Clinicians were more likely to report a gut feeling something is wrong, when they were more experienced or when children were more unwell. Gut feeling is independently and strongly associated with antibiotic prescribing and referral to secondary care, but not with two indicators of poor child health.

Keywords: Child, Respiratory tract infections, Primary health care, Prognosis, Emotions, Decision making, Paediatric, Cough

* Correspondence: Sophie.turnbull@bristol.ac.uk
[1]Centre for Academic Primary Care, Population Health Sciences, Bristol Medical School, University of Bristol, Canynge Hall, 39 Whatley Road, Bristol BS8 2PS, UK
[10]Centre for Academic Primary Care, School of Social and Community Medicine, University of Bristol, Bristol BS8 2PS, UK
Full list of author information is available at the end of the article

Background

Acute cough with respiratory tract infection (RTI) in children is the most common problem managed by health services internationally [1, 2]. While the majority of childhood RTIs are self-limiting, a small number result in serious illness and hospitalisation [3]. Clinicians report that uncertainty regarding both the diagnosis and prognosis of some children with RTIs are important drivers of antibiotic prescribing, [4–6] contributing to over-prescribing [7] and antimicrobial resistance [8]. Knowing the prognosis of children presenting to primary care with acute RTIs can be challenging as clinicians cannot always be certain where in the illness trajectory the child has presented, and whether red flag symptoms and signs are absent or are yet to develop. In cases where there is uncertainty, clinical intuition or 'gut feeling' is thought to play a part in management decisions.

The current literature offers two definitions of clinician gut feeling. Both propose it arises when the clinician feels uncertain or has a low 'feeling of rightness', [9, 10] and both have been shown to influence management decisions [11]. In some studies, a comparison has been made between a sense of reassurance versus a feeling that 'something is wrong' which defines a broad set of cases where clinicians are worried [11]. In others, authors define a gut feeling as a sense of dissonance between intuitive and analytic reasoning; a gut feeling something is wrong despite a lack of clinical markers [9]. The latter definition draws on theories of clinical reasoning distinguishing between "intuitive" processing, which is rapid and unconscious and "analytic" processing that involves slow deliberative reasoning [12–14].

In primary care, gut feeling has been described as an incorporation of clinician knowledge, experience and information about the patient [9]. In the case of childhood RTI, clinicians report using immediately apparent symptoms and signs (the child's energy, pallor and breathing) to distinguish severe from non-severe cases, using pattern recognition and drawing on past experience [5]. A recent study in children with any acute illness, found that: general appearance, breathing pattern, weight loss, history of convulsions and parental concern that the illness was different from any previously experienced predicted the feeling something was wrong when clinical impression was of non-serious illness [15]. This evidence goes some way to characterising the factors influencing clinical gut feeling, but does not identify the specific clinical features associated with particular illnesses, or provide objective assessments of illness severity.

Despite qualitative studies indicating the importance of clinician intuition for primary care doctors and in nursing, [16] there is a paucity of quantitative evidence regarding the prognostic value of gut feelings and whether primary care clinicians utilise them in their decision making. A systematic review suggested that gut feeling in itself should be viewed as a 'diagnostic red flag' and that it had greater diagnostic value than the majority of illness specific symptoms and signs [17]. Another study indicated that in situations where there was uncertainty after clinical assessment, gut feeling was highly predictive of serious infective illness [15].

We used a large prospective cohort study of children presenting to primary care with acute cough and RTI to address three objectives regarding 'gut feeling that something is wrong' (from here on 'gut feeling'): (i) to describe the clinician and child characteristics that drive clinician to have a gut feeling that something is wrong; (ii) to investigate if gut feeling influences management decisions; and (iii) to evaluate the prognostic value of gut feeling in relation to primary care reconsultations with evidence of illness deterioration, and hospital admissions.

Methods

Design and setting

The 'TARGET' study [18] was a multicentre, prospective cohort study that recruited children presenting to general practices with acute cough and RTI, between July 2011 and May 2013. Practices were recruited and trained by four University hubs (Bristol, London, Oxford and Southampton). The primary aim of the study was to develop a clinical rule that could help clinicians improve their use of antibiotics by using baseline clinical characteristics to predict the children that would be hospitalised in the next 30 days [3]. Here we present findings from secondary analysis of this dataset, which are reported following the Strengthening the Reporting of Observational Studies in Epidemiology (STROBE) recommendations [19].

Participants

Clinicians (General Practitioners: GPs and 'prescribing' Nurse Practitioners: NPs), were eligible to recruit to the study if they were working in participating primary care practices and reported that they prescribed antibiotics in ≤30% children with RTIs (to reduce the possibility of confounding by indication). Clinicians were asked to specify a priori their preferred recruitment strategy (for example, consecutive or first eligible on the day). Children were eligible if aged ≥3 months to < 16 years and presenting with an acute (≤28 days) cough and other symptoms of an RTI. Children with an infected exacerbation of asthma and those severely unwell (for example, requiring same day hospital assessment or admission) were included. Children were excluded if: presenting with a non-infective exacerbation of asthma; immunocompromised; previously recruited or recently participated in other research; or temporarily registered at the GP practice.

Data collection

Clinician characteristics

Clinician characteristics included the clinician type (GP or NP), number of years qualified and evidence of further medical/ health qualifications (Diploma in Child Health (DCH) or Membership of the Royal College of General Practitioners (MRCGP)).

Child characteristics

At the baseline consultation the recruiting clinician used a structured case report form (CRF) to record socio-demographic information, parent-reported symptoms (including severity of symptoms in the past 24 h) and physical examination findings. A parent and clinician reported illness severity score was collected, scored 0-10 (see Fig. 1. Case report form). Information about the child's past medical history was collected from the primary care medical record. The 2010 Indices of Multiple Deprivation (IMD) provided a measure of neighbourhood deprivation linked to the child's home postcode [20].

Gut feeling

At the end of their clinical evaluation, the clinician was also asked to respond 'yes' or 'no' to the statement "my gut feeling is 'something is wrong'" with the child. A definition was provided in the clinician instruction booklet that gut feeling in this context "represents clinicians gut feeling that the child's illness may be more serious than is superficially apparent". This question was located at the end of the CRF, following the socio-demographic, symptoms and physical examination findings, but prior to the reporting of management decisions.

Management decisions

Clinicians were asked to record if the child was referred for a secondary care assessment and if they prescribed antibiotics.

Prognostic value

Two indicators of poor child health were collected from the primary care medical record by trained notes reviewers at least 3 months after study entry (to allow sufficient time for the hospital discharge information to reach the medical record): primary care re-consultations for the same RTI with evidence of symptom deterioration; and hospital admissions for RTI in the 30 days following recruitment (using hospital discharge summaries). The 30 days threshold for hospitalisation was selected for two reasons. First, the rationale for the primary aim of the TARGET study [3] (from which the 'gut feeling' paper derives its data) was that clinicians report they prescribe antibiotics 'just in case' children are subsequently admitted to hospital with their RTI, and we sought to use an inclusive definition. Second, our previous [21] and more recent [22] research has shown the symptoms of acute cough and RTI take 25 days for most (90%) of children to resolve. A hospitalisation outcome with a ≤ 7 day cut off was also used as a sensitivity analysis to ensure that there was not a temporal association between the prognostic value of gut feeling and the hospitalisation outcome. We calculated the Kappa statistic to assess inter-rater reliability of the two reviewers that independently assessed the primary care medical record for these two health outcomes.

Statistical analysis

Treatment of variables

Parent-reported symptom severity (mild, moderate, severe) in the 24 h prior to consultation was transformed into a binary outcome with a threshold dependent on overall prevalence: to either 'severe/not severe' (where > 5% of children reported as being severe or 'moderate or severe/not moderate or severe' (where < 5% of children reported being severe). This pragmatic cut-off was chosen prior to analysis to avoid severity variables with very low prevalence. We used accepted clinical cut offs (temperature > 37.8 °C, [23] capillary refill time (CRT) ≥3 s, [24, 25] oxygen saturation ≤ 95% [26]) or 25th percentile or 75th percentile thresholds to dichotomise continuous data, and we used age-adjusted thresholds for heart and respiratory rates [27]. Given the large number of variables being tested, continuous outcomes were initially categorised to help interpret and contextualise the final model, a sensitivity analysis was then conducted to assess the distribution of these continuous variables if included in the model.

Determinants of gut feeling

We first used univariable multilevel random effects logistic regression (accounting for between-clinician differences) to assess associations between clinician profile and children's baseline characteristics, with gut feeling. Modelling was conducted using a multivariable multilevel random effects logistic regression model (accounting for clustering at the clinician level) and variable selection using the backward stepwise method with a 5% model entry threshold. For the 'determinant' analyses, the outcome variable was the clinician's gut feeling and (given the large number of variables investigated) model retention was set at the 1% level. A more liberal threshold was employed for the univariable stage than for the multivariable stage because the former was used as a selection filter for the latter and we did not want to miss any potential associations of interest, whereas for the final selection of variables it was necessary to be more

CASE REPORT FORM — TARGET

ID
Today's date ☐☐/☐☐/20☐☐

Informed consent for study obtained ☐

Background information
DOB ☐☐/☐☐/☐☐☐☐
Gender ☐ Female ☐ Male
Ethnicity ☐☐ PTO for codes, if other ethnicity, please describe below ☐☐☐☐☐☐☐☐☐☐☐☐☐☐

Mother's age ☐☐
children in home (inc. unwell child) ☐☐
Does the mother smoke? ☐ No ☐ Yes ☐ Don't know
Mother still breast feeding child at 3 months? ☐ No ☐ Yes ☐ Don't know

Carer reported symptoms
How unwell does the parent consider the child to be? Well ☐0 ☐1 ☐2 ☐3 ☐4 ☐5 ☐6 ☐7 ☐8 ☐9 ☐10 Very unwell

Duration of illness ☐☐ days
Has illness got a lot worse recently? ☐ No ☐ Yes
If Yes, how many days ago did it start to get worse? ☐☐ days

Symptoms present	During illness? No	Yes	If yes	Last 24 hours? No	Yes	If yes	Severity in last 24 hours (tick one) Mild	Moderate	Severe
Dry cough	☐	☐		☐	☐		☐	☐	☐
Productive/ wet cough	☐	☐		☐	☐		☐	☐	☐
Barking/ croupy cough	☐	☐		☐	☐		☐	☐	☐
Blocked or runny nose	☐	☐		☐	☐		☐	☐	☐
Change in cry	☐	☐		☐	☐		☐	☐	☐
Breathing faster than normal (shortness of breath)	☐	☐		☐	☐		☐	☐	☐
Wheeze or whistling in the chest	☐	☐		☐	☐		☐	☐	☐
Fever	☐	☐		☐	☐		☐	☐	☐
Chills/ shivering	☐	☐		☐	☐		☐	☐	☐
Diarrhoea	☐	☐		☐	☐		☐	☐	☐
Vomiting (including after cough)	☐	☐		☐	☐		☐	☐	☐
Taking fewer fluids/ milk feeds	☐	☐		☐	☐		☐	☐	☐
Eating less	☐	☐		☐	☐		☐	☐	☐
Low energy/ fatigue/ lethargy	☐	☐		☐	☐		☐	☐	☐
Disturbed sleep	☐	☐		☐	☐		☐	☐	☐
Passing urine less often/ dryer nappies	☐	☐		☐	☐		☐	☐	☐
Please tick NA if the child is too young/ uncommunicative for the parent to know about the following > NA ☐									
Chest/ shoulder pain	☐	☐		☐	☐		☐	☐	☐
Headache	☐	☐		☐	☐		☐	☐	☐
Muscle aches all over	☐	☐		☐	☐		☐	☐	☐
Confusion/ disorientation	☐	☐		☐	☐		☐	☐	☐

Clinician examination and management

	Absent	Present
Pallor	☐	☐
Grunting	☐	☐
Nasal flaring	☐	☐
Stridor	☐	☐
Inter/ subcostal recession	☐	☐
Inflamed pharynx/ tonsils	☐	☐

	Absent	Unilateral	Bilateral
Wheeze	☐	☐	☐
Crackles/ crepitations	☐	☐	☐
Bronchial breathing	☐	☐	☐

Temperature ☐☐.☐ °C Pulse ☐☐☐ bpm
Respiratory rate ☐☐ bpm O_2 sat ☐☐☐ % ☐ Unable to take O_2 sat/no equipment
Consciousness level ☐ normal ☐ irritable ☐ drowsy
Capillary refill time ☐ 2 seconds or less ☐ 3 seconds or more
How unwell do you consider the child to be? Well ☐0 ☐1 ☐2 ☐3 ☐4 ☐5 ☐6 ☐7 ☐8 ☐9 ☐10 Very unwell

Main working respiratory tract diagnosis ☐☐☐☐☐☐☐☐☐☐☐☐☐☐
My gut feeling is 'something is wrong' ☐ No ☐ Yes
Antibiotics prescribed? ☐ No ☐ Yes, immediate ☐ Yes, delayed by ☐☐ days
Referral for acute admission today? ☐ No ☐ Yes

2011 04 08 TARGET CRF LOS centre version 1.0

Fig. 1 Case report form

conservative given both the number of variables considered and the large sample size (which could potentially result in small effects being detected statistically). Global clinician illness severity score was not included in this analysis as it was suspected that there was overlap in what this and gut feeling variables represented to the clinician. Considering prior literature indicating prognostic value of gut feeling in the absence of clinical signs of severe illness, we undertook a sensitivity analysis to explore the contribution of high illness severity score to the model.

Evidence that clustering by clinician was important in the multivariable model was explored using the Likelihood-ratio test (LRT). The accuracy of the resulting model was represented by the Area Under the Receiver Operating Characteristic (AUROC) curve.

Multiple imputation was employed as a sensitivity analysis to check whether the model was robust [28].

Management decisions and prognostic value

Univariable and multivariable multilevel logistic regression modelling was employed, using backward stepwise selection (accounting for between-clinician differences), as well as variables associated with each of those outcomes retaining variables with a p-value of < 0.05. Two models were used to investigate the associations between clinician gut feeling and the decision to: 1) prescribe antibiotics, and 2) refer the child to hospital for acute admission. Two further models were used to investigate the associations between gut feeling and: 1) reconsultation for the same RTI with evidence of deterioration, and; 2) hospitalisation for a RTI in the 30 days following recruitment. A further multivariable model was used in the sensitivity analysis exploring the association between gut feeling and the hospitalisation outcome with a ≤ 7 day cut off. To ensure the prognostic value of gut feeling did not differ with definition of gut feeling, a univariable analysis was conducted to explore the association between hospitalisation and the more focused definition described by a previous study: gut feeling when clinical impression was of non-serious illness [15]. Due to the exploratory nature of these analyses, and to ensure we did not miss any potential influences, the more liberal threshold was employed for the multivariable analysis. LRT was used to explore the influence of clustering by clinician in the multivariate models. Data were analysed using STATA version 13.1.

Results

Clinicians and children

Of the 842 clinicians agreeing to participate, 519 (62%) located at 247 general practices recruited at least one child (median 5, inter-quartile range (IQR) 2-15 children) into the study. Of the clinicians who recruited at least one child who was retained in the study, data were available about clinician type for 502 (97%) clinicians; of these 77 (15%) were NPs and 425 (85%) were GPs. Data on years since qualification were available for 498/518 (96%) of the clinicians: median of 20 years (range 1-44, IQR 13-26 years). Of the 519 clinicians, 85 (16%) reported having at least one additional qualification (DCH or MRCGP).

A total of 8613 children were recruited to the study, of whom 219 (3%) children were excluded: 181 did not meet the eligibility criteria, 32 did not have baseline data and six were withdrawn. Of the 8394 children recruited and retained, clinicians recorded their gut feeling for 8377 (99.8%) - all analyses that follow use these 8377 children. Participant flow through the study is available in Fig. 2. Oxygen saturation was removed from all analysis as these data were missing for 50% of children due to a lack of available paediatric oxygen saturation monitors. All other reported variables had < 2% missing data. Children's median age was 3 years (range 3 months-15 years, IQR, 1-6 years) and 1390 (17%) were under 1 year. There were slightly more boys (52%) than girls, and of the 8333 (99.5%) for whom ethnicity data were available the majority (6540, 78%) were white (similar to UK Census 2011 data) [29]. Families' median deprivation (IMD) score was 16.7 (IQR 8.8-29.5), similar to the English median (17.2, IQR 9.8-30.2) [20]. Median clinician reported illness severity was 3 (range 0-9, IQR 2-4).

Clinicians reported a gut feeling something was wrong in 1706 (20%) cases. 3110 (37%) were prescribed an antibiotic, with 2341 (28%) given an immediate script and 769 (9%) given a delayed script. Seventy-four children were immediately referred for secondary care assessment at the recruiting consultation, of whom 13 were subsequently admitted. A further 65 children were admitted to hospital with a RTI in the subsequent 30 days. For the 78 hospitalised children the median number of days to hospitalisation was 2 days (IQR 1-12 days). The hospital discharge diagnoses were: lower respiratory tract infection (19%); bronchiolitis (18%); viral wheeze (15%); upper respiratory tract infection (13%); croup (8%); infected exacerbation of asthma (8%); tonsillitis (6%); viral illness (5%); febrile illness (3%); and pneumonia (1%). Of the 8193 children for whom data were available relating to primary care reconsultations in the 30 days following baseline, 1847 reconsulted for an RTI. Of these 354 (4%) reconsulted for the same illness with evidence of symptom deterioration, with a median of 5 days (IQR 2-11 days) to this reconsultation. The percentage inter-rater agreement (kappa) for hospitalisation and reconsultation for the same illness with evidence of deterioration were 90% (Kappa 0.80) and 84% (Kappa 0.67) respectively. There were 242/8377 (3%) children in whom the clinician reported a low illness severity score (≤ 2) whilst also reporting they a gut feeling something was wrong.

Determinants of gut feeling

Univariable analyses

Fifty-one (84%) of the 61 variables measured were associated with a gut feeling (with p-values < 0.05 (Additional file 1: Web Appendix, Table S1). Two of the three clinician characteristics were associated: those with more years since qualification and NPs reported having a gut feeling in a higher proportion of the children than GPs (27% vs. 18%), while additional qualifications were not associated. Only one of the five sociodemographic variables collected were associated: being male (55% vs 51%). There was no evidence of a difference in the children's ethnicity, age, the mother's age at the time of the child's birth, or home IMD score in the two groups.

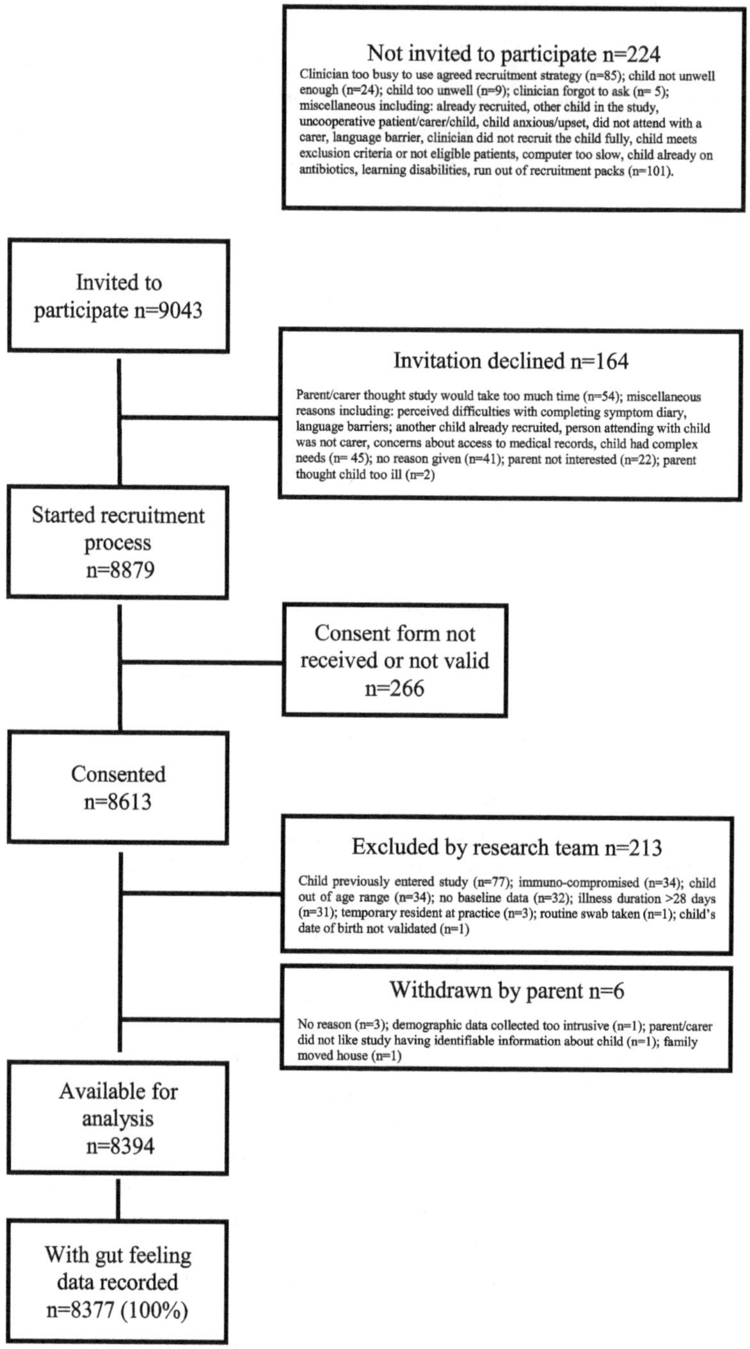

Fig. 2 Flow of participants through the study

All the four variables collected regarding the child's medical history were associated with gut feeling. The child was more likely to: have a chronic condition (21% vs 18%), a previous or current asthma diagnosis (12% vs 8%), and to have consulted for an RTI on two or more occasions in the 12 months prior to recruitment (36% vs 35%), than the children for whom the clinician did not have a gut feeling. There was evidence that 44/49 (90%) of the symptoms and signs that were recorded at baseline were associated with gut feeling. The five symptoms and signs that did not reach the 5% threshold were low illness duration prior to recruitment, barking or croupy cough, blocked or runny nose, diarrhoea and stridor (Additional file 1: Web Appendix, Table S1).

Multivariable analysis

There was strong evidence that increasing years since clinician qualification, five carer-reported symptoms and eight clinically-reported signs were independently associated with gut feeling (Table 1). The strongest was crackles and crepitations. In the multivariable model there was no evidence of association with clinician type (NP versus GP), additional clinician qualifications or any of the socio-demographic variables. There was strong evidence that clustering by clinician was important in the model (LRT of rho = 0: $p < 0.001$) when compared with the multivariable model without clustering. The AUROC curve was 0.82, 95% confidence interval (CI) 0.80-0.83. Imputing the missing data for the final model made little difference to the odds ratios, confidence intervals and *p*-values. The sensitivity analysis exploring the impact of high clinician illness score on the model resulted in few changes: high clinician illness severity score was retained, while severe fever in the last 24 h and parent reporting that that illness was worse recently dropped out of the model. There was little change to the remaining estimates, except for crackles and crepitations, where the OR fell from 14.56 (95% CI 11.71-18.12) to 9.57 (95% CI 7.64-11.99) and the AUROC increased from 0.81 (95% CI 0.80-0.83) to 0.82 (95% CI 0.83-0.85).

Management decisions and gut feeling

There was strong evidence in both the univariable and multivariable analysis that when clinicians report a gut feeling, they were more likely to prescribe antibiotics and refer for same day further secondary care assessment (Table 2, including description of the covariates retained in the multivariate model at the < 1% level). These findings were independent of clinician's impression of illness severity.

Prognostic value of gut feeling

There was no evidence to suggest that the children for whom the clinician had a gut feeling were more likely to re-consult for the same illness with evidence of illness deterioration in the 30 days following recruitment in the univariable or multivariable analysis. They were over twice as likely to be admitted to hospital for a RTI

Table 1 Determinants: Multivariable associations between parent-reported symptoms, clinician-reported observations, clinician profile and 'gut feeling'

Significant predictors	No gut feeling		Yes gut feeling		OR	95% CI	*p*-value
	n/N	%	n/N	%			
Years qualified (Categorical)							
1-9 years	646/720	89.7	74/720	10.3	Ref	Ref	< 0.001 5 d.f.*
10-14 years	1790/2213	80.9	423/2213	19.1	0.55	0.30-1.02	
15-19 years	971/1206	80.5	235/1206	19.5	1.44	0.71-2.90	
20-24 years	1219/1586	76.9	367/1586	23.1	1.28	0.57-2.87	
25-29 years	875/1159	75.5	284/1159	24.5	1.67	0.76-3.68	
30+ years	1170/1493	78.4	323/1493	21.6	1.08	0.47-2.46	
Parent reported symptoms							
High parent illness severity score (≥7/10)	1459/6650	21.9	681/1702	40.0	1.67	1.39-2.01	< 0.001
Fever in the last 24 h (severe)	363/6647	5.5	177/1700	10.4	1.66	1.23-2.26	0.001
Low energy during illness	3404/6669	51.0	1100/1704	65.6	1.65	1.36-1.99	< 0.001
Shortness of breath during illness	2115/6670	31.7	857/1704	50.3	1.50	1.25-1.81	< 0.001
Illness worse recently	4182/6663	62.8	1339/1704	78.6	1.44	1.18-1.76	< 0.001
Clinical signs							
Crackles and crepitations	695/6661	10.4	901/1704	52.9	14.56	11.71-18.12	< 0.001
Recession	164/6663	2.5	239/1704	14.0	3.31	2.29-4.79	< 0.001
Pallor	6185/6663	7.2	345/1705	20.2	3.10	2.30-4.18	< 0.001
Bronchial breath	136/6658	2.0	142/1703	8.3	2.99	1.90-4.70	< 0.001
Wheeze (recorded in consultation)	675/6663	10.1	560/1703	32.9	2.78	2.23-3.46	< 0.001
High temperature (≥37.8 °C recorded in consultation)	629/6653	9.5	415/1702	24.4	2.32	1.84-2.91	< 0.001
High respiratory rate (age related cut offs)	825/6634	12.4	414/1698	24.4	1.64	1.30-2.07	< 0.001
Inflamed pharynx	1873/6647	28.2	521/1702	30.6	1.51	1.23-1.86	< 0.001

N = 8217/8377 (98.1% of the sample) 514 clusters (clinicians)
*Degrees of freedom

Table 2 Management decisions: relationship between 'gut feeling' and subsequent clinical management

Treatment	No gut feeling		Yes gut feeling		Univariable analysis controlling for clustering			Multivariable analysis controlling for clustering and significant covariates		
	n/N	%	n/N	%	OR	95% CI	*P*-value	OR	95% CI	*P*-value
Prescribed antibiotics at baseline consultation										
Any antibiotics prescribed	1707/6671	25.6	1403/1706	82.2	20.80	17.42-24.83	< 0.001	5.85	4.67-7.32	< 0.001[±]
Referred for acute admission (during the recruiting consultation)										
Referral for acute admission	16/6671	0.2	58/1706	3.4	19.27	9.83-37.79	< 0.001	12.64	6.31-25.32	< 0.001[¥]

[±]Co-variates of any antibiotic prescription (retained at the < 1% level): illness has got worse recently, child's age (< 2 years), barking cough, fever, diarrhoea, low energy and productive cough during the illness, moderate/severe wheeze and severe fever in the last 24 h, recession, crackles and crepitations, wheeze (as reported by the clinician), bronchial breath, inflamed pharynx, high temperature, high clinician and parent illness severity scores, low illness duration and gut feeling that something is wrong
[¥]Co-variates of referral for acute admission (retained at the < 1% level): Recession, gut feeling that something is wrong and capillary refill time (CRT)

in the 30 days following recruitment. However, after adjusting for other variables associated with hospital admission, this relationship was attenuated. This was also true for the sensitivity analysis examining the 7-day hospitalisation outcome. The presence of clinician reported wheeze and/or recession in the multivariate model reduced the association with gut feeling below the < 5% threshold (Table 3, including description of covariates retained in the multivariate model). There was evidence of clinician clustering effect for re-consultation (LRT of rho = 0: $p < 0.001$) but not hospitalisation (30 days LRT of rho = 0: $p = 0.30$, 7 days LRT of rho = 0: $p = 0.43$), indicating that there was a relationship between the clinician who had seen the child and the likelihood of child reconsulting, but not being hospitalised. There was also no evidence of an association between hospitalisation and the more focused definition of gut feeling (described in previous studies) was explored at univariate level(OR 1.26, 95% CI 0.38-4.13, $p = 0.71$).

Discussion

Summary of findings

In a large, rigorously conducted, prospective cohort study, gut feeling was more commonly reported by more experienced clinicians and in children with parent-reported symptoms and physical examination signs suggesting more severe illnesses. Gut feeling was strongly associated with management decisions – both antibiotic prescribing and same-day referral for admission. Despite this, we did not find strong evidence that gut feeling was associated with indicators of poorer prognosis in the following 30 days, such as reconsulting in primary care with evidence of illness deterioration or being hospitalised for a RTI, at least not after controlling for potential confounders.

Strengths and limitations

To our knowledge, ours is the largest, prospective study to describe the determinants, management decisions and prognostic value of gut feeling for respiratory tract infections in children in routine, office-based primary

Table 3 Prognosis: relationship between 'gut feeling' and children's health outcomes

Health outcome	No gut feeling		Yes gut feeling		Univariable analysis controlling for clustering			Multivariable analysis controlling for clustering and significant covariates		
	n/N	%	n/N	%	OR	95% CI	*P*-value	OR	95% CI	*P*-value
Health outcome										
Re-consultation for the same illness with evidence of illness deterioration (≥1) in the 30 days following recruitment	271/6523	4.2	83/1670	5.0	1.30	0.99 -1.71	0.06	1.08	0.80-1.46	0.60[¥]
Admitted to hospital in the 30 days following recruitment	48/6671	0.7	30/1706	1.8	2.47	1.55-3.95	< 0.001	1.11	0.65-1.89	0.71[ǂ]
Sensitivity analysis										
Admitted to hospital in the ≤7 days post recruitment	24/6647	0.4	25/1681	1.5	4.20	2.34-7.54	< 0.001	1.62	0.83-3.14	0.16[α]

[¥]Co-variates of re-consultation for the same RTI with evidence of deterioration (retained at the < 5% level): ≥2 consultations for RTI in primary care in the year prior to baseline, low illness duration prior to baseline, previous asthma diagnosis, current asthma diagnosis, child's age at baseline (< 2 years), white ethnicity, parent reported barking cough, wheeze and taking fewer fluids during the illness, moderate/severe vomiting and fewer fluids in the 24 h prior to baseline, severe eating less in the 24 h prior to baseline, wheeze and recession (as reported by the clinician)
[ǂ]Co-variates of hospitalisation (retained at the < 5% level): child's age (< 2 years), low illness duration prior to baseline, current asthma diagnosis, moderate/severe vomiting, recession, wheeze (as reported by the clinician), high temperature (age related cut offs)
[α]Co-variates of hospitalisation ≤7 days post recruitment (retained at the < 5% level): child's age (< 2 years), low illness (< 3 days) duration prior to baseline, current asthma diagnoses, moderate/severe vomiting, recession, wheeze (as reported by the clinician), high temperature (age related cut offs)

care [2]. We included a broad range of clinician, demographic, child and clinical characteristics and the study focussed on a clinical group in whom clinicians report diagnostic and prognostic uncertainty [6]. Determinants of gut feeling were measured according to routine clinical practice using standardised reporting forms on the day of recruitment, blind to the prognostic outcomes, which were reliably measured from the primary care record. We used rigorous techniques to adjust for confounding.

We are aware of five main limitations. First, while we offered some instructions to support completion of the question "My gut feeling is 'something is wrong'", including a definition, there was no attempt to interpret it and clinicians were simply asked to report its presence/absence. While the low question refusal suggests clinicians understood the question, it is likely the presence of gut feeling means different things to different clinicians. Definitions of gut feeling overlap, and may not be clear to clinicians. Given our relatively high (20%) prevalence of gut feeling, the strong associations found with symptoms and signs (such as crepitations/crackles) and with high clinician reported illness severity score, it is likely our clinicians were using a broad definition, such as "the presence of a significant illness". Second, although focussing on an extremely common primary care presentation, [2] findings may not generalise to other illnesses or different age groups. Third, we adjusted for a wide range of potential confounders but it is possible that other unmeasured factors could be important. We are aware of another study that found 'parent concern that the illness was different to other illnesses,' weight loss and history of convulsions have been shown to be associated with gut feeling and these were not collected in our study [15]. Fourth, while our conservative model entry and exit thresholds have minimised scope for Type I error, the relative infrequency of the hospitalisation outcome, and the fact this was a secondary analysis of data collected for another purpose, [18] could have led to Type II error and us incorrectly concluding that gut feeling does not have prognostic value. The large study size mitigates against this for re-consultation. It is plausible some cases of re-consultation or hospitalisation were avoided where antibiotics were given and this may mask associations with gut feeling (so-called confounding by indication). However, there is limited evidence of the mitigating effects of antibiotics on prognostic outcome for RTI. Two studies, one with adults [30] and the other with children (in submission [31]) with RTIs found antibiotics did not reduce hospitalisation, and immediate antibiotics did not reduce reconsultations. Finally, the outcomes used to explore the prognostic value of gut feeling are indicators of poor health, but we acknowledge that other factors beyond the child's illness severity can influence these, such as parent behaviour and available services in the area.

Comparison with existing literature

Determinants of gut feeling

Previous studies have described gut feeling in primary care clinicians as being derived from a combination of patient characteristics and clinicians' knowledge and past experience [32, 33]. Like others we found that pallor or appearance, energy and breathing patterns were associated with gut feeling [5, 15].

Our results contrast with a previous study, which did not find evidence to support their hypothesis that high temperature contributed towards gut feeling, but we found high temperature and carer-reported severe fever both contributed [15]. The literature is contradictory regarding the role of clinician experience. For instance, both we and a previous qualitative study found more experienced family primary physicians were more likely to report having a gut feeling something was wrong, [17] whereas another quantitative study found that more senior doctors were less likely to report it [15]. These differences may be due to differences in participating children or definition of gut feeling; van den Bruel's study included children with any non-serious acute illness, whereas we studied children with RTI regardless of clinician-reported illness severity. In their study they conceptualised gut feeling as "intuitive feeling that something was wrong even if the clinician was unsure why" and included the 3.1% children where the clinician reported a gut feeling in addition to the illness was not severe. Our definition was broader and included 20% of the children. However, in our sample a clinician reported a gut feeling combined with a low illness severity score approximates this definition, and we found the same proportion (3%). The concept that gut feeling is more commonly reported in more experienced clinicians is supported by the learning perspective of intuition: where intuition is the consequence of unconscious drawing on an implicit knowledge base and recognition of patterns of clinical markers that is developed though experience and may be associated with previous negative or uncertain outcomes. As demonstrated by our findings, more experienced does not mean more accurate. The validity of the gut feeling as a guide to decision-making relies not only on the quantity but also the quality of the feedback. If there is good feedback during the learning process, this results in good or accurate gut feeling and associated decision-making. Conversely, poor or absent feedback results in poor intuition [34].

Management decisions and gut feeling

Our findings agree with previous studies [32] that found gut feeling can play a substantial role in treatment decisions.

Prognostic value of gut feeling

A recent systematic review suggested that gut feeling was of greater diagnostic value than the majority of symptoms and signs [17]. Two recent prospective studies reported that gut feeling in primary care was also associated with serious infectious illness in children in Belgium [15] and serious disease in adults and children in Denmark [35]. In contrast, we did not find evidence that gut feeling was associated with subsequent reconsultations with evidence of deterioration. When considered in isolation, we found gut feeling was associated with hospitalisation, however, when other clinical signs (wheeze and/or recession) were taken into account, gut feeling was no longer associated. Indeed, our recent paper identified seven other characteristics that were independently associated with hospitalisation – namely age less than 2 years, current asthma, illness duration of 3 days or less, parent-reported moderate or severe vomiting in the previous 24 h, severe fever in the previous 24 h or a body temperature of 37·8 °C or more at presentation, clinician-reported intercostal or subcostal recession, and wheeze on auscultation [3]. Use of these may reduce prognostic uncertainty and reduce reliance on gut feeling.

Clinical, teaching and research implications

Our study suggests that for children presenting to primary care with acute cough and RTI, the gut feeling that something is wrong, which appears to drive clinical decision-making in this group, are not associated with either re-consultation or hospital admission, at least not after potential confounding effects were taken into account [30, 31]. Given the high levels of uncertainty reported by clinicians looking after this group of patients, [5, 36] it is not surprising they wish to use all the tools at their disposal, including gut feeling. However, our results suggest some clinicians may over-value gut feeling in their clinical decision making in this group of patients and that they are using gut feeling as a proxy or unconscious marker of other important symptoms and signs. Gut feeling may have value in the absence of known, objectively assessed markers of risk, however, attending to objective assessment of these risks is preferable when this information is available. Future research may wish to focus on a more specific definition of gut feeling, including perhaps the sense of dissonance arising when conscious and unconscious assessment processes are in conflict.

Conclusions

Clinicians were more likely to report a gut feeling something is wrong, when they were more experienced and when children were more unwell. Gut feeling is independently and strongly associated with antibiotic prescribing and referral to secondary care, but not with two indicators of poor child health.

Abbreviations

AUROC: Area under the receiver operating Characteristic; CRF: Case report form; CRT: Capillary refill time; DCH: Diploma in child health; GPs: General practitioners; IMD: Indices of multiple deprivation; IQR: Inter-quartile range; LRT: Likelihood-ratio test; MRCGP: Membership of the royal college of general Practitioners; NPs: 'Prescribing' nurse practitioners; RTI: Respiratory tract infection; STROBE: Strengthening the reporting of observational studies in epidemiology

Acknowledgements

The National Institute for Health Research funds the Programme Grant for Applied Research TARGET Programme grant at the University of Bristol and NHS Bristol Clinical Commissioning Group.

This paper summarises independent research funded by the National Institute for Health Research (NIHR) under its Programme Grants for Applied Research Programme (Grant Reference Number RP-PG-0608-10018). HC is supported by the National Institute for Health Research Health Protection Research Unit (NIHR HPRU) in Evaluation of Interventions at the University of Bristol, in partnership with Public Health England (PHE). ADH is funded by NIHR Research Professorship (NIHR-RP-02-12-012). NMR's time is supported by the NIHR Collaboration for Leadership in Applied Health Research and Care West (CLAHRC West) at University Hospitals Bristol NHS Foundation Trust. The views expressed are those of the authors and not necessarily those of the NHS, the NIHR, and the Department of Health of Public Health England.

The authors are extremely grateful to the children, parents/carers and families who have participated in the study, all GP practices including recruiting clinicians, administrative and research contacts and all other staff whose participation made this study possible. We thank all our colleagues from the TARGET Programme, the TARGET Programme Management Group and the TARGET Programme Steering Committee (Sandra Eldridge, Nick Francis, Joe Kai, Victoria Senior, Anna Thursby-Pelham, Mireille Williams) for their time, expertise and support. We are grateful to the following individuals who have helped with the study; James Austin, Denis Baird, Tony Beard, Stephen Beckett, Issy Bray, Peter Brindle, Kate Brooks, Sue Broomfield, Joanna Cordell, Judy Cordell, Tania Crabb, Hazel Crabb-Wyke, Mike Crawford, Julie Cunningham, Christina Currie, Rachel Davies, Elizabeth Derodra, Elena Domenech, Stevo Durbaba, Lucy Feather, Caroline Footer, Emily Gale, Anna Gilbertson, Victoria Hardy, Rose Hawkins, Abigail Hay, Lisa Hird, Sandra Hollinghurst, Julie Hooper, Jonathan Hubb, Catherine Jameson, Grania Jenkins, Amy Jepps, Mari-Rose Kennedy, Michael Lawton, Mel Lewcock, Lyn Liddiard, Sandra Mulligan, Sharen O'Keefe, Lucy O'Reilly, Marilyn Peters, Aled Picton, Ilaria Pinna, Fiona Redmond, Isabel Richards, Kim Roden, Sharon Salt, Douglas Shedden, Ella Simmonds, Sue Smith, Carol Stanton, Kate Taylor, Elizabeth Thomas, Nicki Thorne, Sara Tonge, Abby Waterhouse, Eleanor Woodward. The TARGET study team acknowledges the support of the National Institute for Health Research, through the Comprehensive Clinical Research Network. To Robert Ross from the Department of Psychology at the Royal Holloway who advised on the dual process theory of clinical reasoning. Also to George Leckie, from the multi-level modelling centre at Bristol University who advised on statistical methods.

Funding

This paper reports independent research funded by the National Institute for Health Research (NIHR) under its Programme Grant for Applied Research (Grant Reference Number RP-PG-0608-10018). The views expressed are those of the author(s) and not necessarily those of the NHS, the NIHR or the Department of Health. The funder did not have a role in the design of the study, data collection, analysis, interpretation of the data or in writing the manuscript.

Authors' contributions

PLu and ST were responsible for conceiving the research question. ADH, PLu, PLi, PSB, BD, MT, and TJP conceived the original idea for the TARGET cohort study and were responsible securing funding. ADH, CC, PLu, PLi, PSB, HC, BD, NMR, MT, ST and TJP were responsible for the study design, data collection and interpretation. NMR, HC and ST were responsible for study management and co-ordination. ST, HT, NR, PSB and TJP were responsible for study analysis; ST led the analysis for this paper. ST drafted the paper. All authors have read and approved the final manuscript. ST (corresponding and guarantor author) affirms that the manuscript is an honest, accurate, and transparent account of the study being reported; that no important aspects of the study have been omitted; and that any discrepancies from the study as planned (and, if relevant, registered) have been explained.

Consent for publication

Not applicable.

Competing interests

The authors declare that they have no competing interests.

Author details

[1]Centre for Academic Primary Care, Population Health Sciences, Bristol Medical School, University of Bristol, Canynge Hall, 39 Whatley Road, Bristol BS8 2PS, UK. [2]School for Policy Studies, University of Bristol, 8 Priory Road, Bristol BS8 1TZ, UK. [3]National Institute for Health Research Collaborations for Leadership in Applied Health Research and Care West (NIHR CLAHRC West), University Hospitals Bristol NHS Foundation Trust, 9th Floor, Whitefriars, Lewins Mead, Bristol BS1 2NT, UK. [4]Population Health Sciences, Bristol Medical School, University of Bristol, Oakfield House, Oakfield Grove, Bristol BS8 2BN, UK. [5]Population Health Sciences, Bristol Medical School, University of Bristol, Level D, St Michael's Hospital, Southwell St, Bristol BS2 8EG, UK. [6]Department of Surgery and Cancer, Imperial College London, St Mary's Hospital, W2 1NY, London, UK. [7]Department of Family Medicine, University of Washington, Seattle, WA 98195-4696, USA. [8]Primary Care and Population Sciences Unit, University of Southampton, Aldermoor Health Centre, Aldermoor Close, Southampton SO16 5ST, UK. [9]School of Clinical Sciences, University of Bristol, 69 St Michael's Hill, Bristol BS2 8DZ, UK. [10]Centre for Academic Primary Care, School of Social and Community Medicine, University of Bristol, Bristol BS8 2PS, UK.

References

1. Hay AD, Heron J, Ness A. The prevalence of symptoms and consultations in pre-school children in the Avon longitudinal study of parents and children (ALSPAC): a prospective cohort study. Fam Pract. 2005;22(4):367–74.
2. Okkes IM, Oskam SK, Lamberts H. The probability of specific diagnoses for patients presenting with common symptoms to Dutch family physicians. J Fam Pract. 2002;51(1):31–6.
3. Hay AD, Redmond NM, Turnbull S, Christensen H, Thornton H, Little P, Thompson M, Delaney B, Lovering AM, Muir P, et al. Development and internal validation of a clinical rule to improve antibiotic use in children presenting to primary care with acute respiratory tract infection and cough: a prognostic cohort study. Lancet Respir Med. 2016;(11):902–10.
4. Lucas PJ, Cabral C, Hay AD, Horwood J. A systematic review of parent and clinician views and perceptions that influence prescribing decisions in relation to acute childhood infections in primary care. Scand J Prim Health Care. 2015:33(1):11-20.
5. Horwood J, Cabral C, Hay AD, Ingram J. Primary care clinician antibiotic prescribing decisions in consultations for children with RTIs: a qualitative interview study. B J Gen Pract. 2016;66(644):e207–13.
6. Cabral C, Lucas PJ, Ingram J, Hay AD, Horwood J. "It's safer to ..." parent consulting and clinician antibiotic prescribing decisions for children with respiratory tract infections: an analysis across four qualitative studies. Soc Sci Med. 2015;136-137C:156–64.
7. Washington TWH. National strategy for combating antibioticresistant bacteria. Washington: Centers for Disease Control and Prevention publisher location; 2014.
8. Costelloe C, Metcalfe C, Lovering A, Mant D, Hay AD. Effect of antibiotic prescribing in primary care on antimicrobial resistance in individual patients: systematic review and meta-analysis. BMJ. 2010;340:c2096.
9 Woolley A, Kostopoulou O. Clinical intuition in family medicine: more than first impressions. Ann Fam Med. 2013;11(1):60–6.
10 Thompson VA, Prowse Turner JA, Pennycook G. Intuition, reason, and metacognition. Cogn Psychol. 2011;63(3):107–40.
11 Stolper E, van Bokhoven M, Houben P, Van Royen P, van de Wiel M, van der Weijden T, Jan Dinant G. The diagnostic role of gut feelings in general practice. A focus group study of the concept and its determinants. BMC Fam Pract. 2009;10:17.
12. Kahneman D. A perspective on judgment and choice: mapping bounded rationality. Am Psychol. 2003;58(9):697–720.
13. Evans JS, Stanovich KE. Dual-Process Theories of Higher Cognition: Advancing the Debate. 2013;8(3):223–41.
14. Toplak ME, West RF, Stanovich KE. The cognitive reflection test as a predictor of performance on heuristics-and-biases tasks. Mem Cogn. 2011; 39(7):1275–89.
15 Van den Bruel A, Thompson M, Buntinx F, Mant D. Clinicians' gut feeling about serious infections in children: observational study. BMJ. 2012;345:e6144.
16 Hams SP. A gut feeling? Intuition and critical care nursing. Intensive Crit Care Nurs. 2000;16(5):310–8.
17 Van den Bruel A, Haj-Hassan T, Thompson M, Buntinx F, Mant D. Diagnostic value of clinical features at presentation to identify serious infection in children in developed countries: a systematic review. Lancet. 2010; 375(9717):834–45.
18 Redmond NM, Davies R, Christensen H, Blair PS, Lovering AM, Leeming JP, Muir P, Vipond B, Thornton H, Fletcher M, et al. The TARGET cohort study protocol: a prospective primary care cohort study to derive and validate a clinical prediction rule to improve the targeting of antibiotics in children with respiratory tract illnesses. BMC Health Serv Res. 2013;13:322.
19 von Elm E, Altman DG, Egger M, Pocock SJ, Gotzsche PC, Vandenbroucke JP. Strengthening The Reporting of Observational Studies in Epidemiology (STROBE) statement: guidelines for reporting observational studies. BMJ. 2007;335(7624):806–8.
20 Lad M. English Indices of Deprivation 2010. London: Department for Communities and Local Government; 2010.
21 Hay AD, Wilson A, Fahey T, Peters TJ. The duration of acute cough in pre-school children presenting to primary care: a prospective cohort study. Fam Pract. 2003;20(6):696–705.
22 Thompson M, Vodicka T, Cohen H, Blair P, Buckley T, Heneghan C, Hay A. Duration of symptoms of respiratory tract infections in children: systematic review. BMJ. 2013;347:f7027.
23 Craig JV, Lancaster GA, Williamson PR, Smyth RL. Temperature measured at the axilla compared with rectum in children and young people: systematic review. BMJ. 2000;320(7243):1174–8.
24 Strozik KS, Pieper CH, Roller J. Capillary refilling time in newborn babies: normal values. Arch Dis Child Fetal Neonatal Ed. 1997;76(3):F193–6.
25 Tibby SM, Hatherill M, Murdoch IA. Capillary refill and core-peripheral temperature gap as indicators of haemodynamic status in paediatric intensive care patients. Arch Dis Child. 1999;80(2):163–6.
26 National Collaborating Centre for Women's and Children's Health. Feverish Illness in Children: Assessment and Initial Management in Children Younger than 5 Years. London: National Collaborating Centre for Women's and Children's Health; 2013.
27 Ferguson J. Advanced paediatric life support. 3rd ed. London: BMJ Books; 2001.
28 Sterne JA, White IR, Carlin JB, Spratt M, Royston P, Kenward MG, Wood AM, Carpenter JR. Multiple imputation for missing data in epidemiological and clinical research: potential and pitfalls. BMJ. 2009;338:b2393.
29 Census statistical bulletin: Population and Household Estimates for Wales, March 2011 [http://www.ons.gov.uk/ons/rel/census/2011-census/population-and-household-estimates-for-wales/stb-2011-census-wales.html].
30 Little P, Stuart B, Smith S, Thompson MJ, Knox K, van den Bruel A, Lown M, Moore M, Mant D. Antibiotic prescription strategies and adverse outcome for uncomplicated lower respiratory tract infections: prospective cough complication cohort (3C) study. BMJ. 2017;357:j2148.

31 Redmond NM, Turnbull S, Stuart B, Thornton HV, Christensen H, Blair PS, Delaney BC, Thompson M, Peters TJ, Hay AD et al: Do antibiotics prescribed for children presenting to primary care with cough and respiratory tract infections (RTIs) modify adverse outcomes? In submission 2017.
32 Stolper E, Van de Wiel M, Van Royen P, Van Bokhoven M, Van der Weijden T, Dinant GJ. Gut feelings as a third track in general practitioners' diagnostic reasoning. J Gen Intern Med. 2011;26(2):197–203.
33 Hogarth RM. Educating intuition. Chicago, IL: University of Chicago Press; 2001.
34 Betsch T. The nature of intuition and its neglect in research on judgment and decision making. New York, NY: Psychology Press; 2008.
35 Hjertholm P, Moth G, Ingeman ML, Vedsted P. Predictive values of GPs' suspicion of serious disease: a population-based follow-up study. Br J Gen Pract. 2014;64(623):e346–53.
36 Horwood J, Cabral C, Hay AD, Ingram J. "Recognising the sick child in amongst the just unwell": health practitioner prescribing decisions in consultations for acute RTI in children. In: Society for Academic Primary Care Annual Research Meeting. Glasgow: Society for Academic Primary Care; 2012.

7

Cost-effectiveness of a multicomponent primary care program targeting frail elderly people

Franca G. H. Ruikes[1*], Eddy M. Adang[2], Willem J. J. Assendelft[1], Henk J. Schers[1], Raymond T. C. M. Koopmans[1,3] and Sytse U. Zuidema[4]

Abstract

Background: Over the last 20 years, integrated care programs for frail elderly people aimed to prevent functional dependence and reduce hospitalization and institutionalization. However, results have been inconsistent and merely modest. To date, evidence on the cost-effectiveness of these programs is scarce. We evaluated the cost-effectiveness of the CareWell program, a multicomponent integrated care program for frail elderly people.

Methods: Economic evaluation from a healthcare perspective embedded in a cluster controlled trial of 12 months in 12 general practices in (the region of) Nijmegen. Two hundred and four frail elderly from 6 general practices in the intervention group received care according to the CareWell program, consisting of multidisciplinary team meetings, proactive care planning, case management, and medication reviews; 165 frail elderly from 6 general practices in the control group received usual care. In cost-effectiveness analyses, we related costs to daily functioning (Katz-15 change score i.e. follow up score minus baseline score) and quality adjusted life years (EQ-5D-3 L).

Results: Adjusted mean costs directly related to the intervention were €456 per person. Adjusted mean total costs, i.e. intervention costs plus healthcare utilization costs, were €1583 (95% CI -4647 to 1481) higher in the intervention group than in the control group. Incremental Net Monetary Benefits did not show significant differences between groups, but on average tended to favour usual care.

Conclusions: The CareWell primary program was not cost-effective after 12 months. From a cost-effectiveness perspective, widespread implementation of the program in its current form cannot be recommended.

Keywords: Cost-benefit analysis, Frail elderly, Delivery of health care, Integrated, Activities of daily living, Primary health care

Background

Frail elderly account for a disproportionally large share of healthcare costs, spending over $70,000/year in 2011 in the United States, with particularly high expenditure on in-patient and post-acute care [1, 2]. In the Western world, the prevalence of frailty - a state of increased vulnerability to adverse outcomes through a complex interplay of physical, psychological, social and environmental factors [3] - will even increase due to population ageing, since frailty is thought to be present in 10% of people aged ≥65 years up to 25%–50% of people aged ≥85 years [4, 5]. Western countries are forced to adapt their healthcare policies addressing frail elderly in order to achieve cost reductions in health and social services and maintain financial sustainability.

Proactive integrated care programs, addressing the complex and interacting healthcare and welfare needs, are thought to have the potential to prevent adverse outcomes and lower healthcare costs [6, 7]. However, results so far have shown merely modest, inconsistent results regarding their effectiveness and efficiency [8–12]. Some studies pointed out the potential to prevent hospitalization and

* Correspondence: Franca.Ruikes@radboudumc.nl
[1]Radboud Institute for Health Sciences, Department of Primary and Community Care, Radboud university medical centre, Nijmegen, the Netherlands
Full list of author information is available at the end of the article

nursing home admissions [10, 11, 13], but accompanying increases in home care and social services use might impede overall cost savings [8, 10, 14]. Formal economic evaluations of integrated programs targeting frail elderly are scarce [15, 16]. Moreover, heterogeneity between studies regarding target population (age, low or high risk of functional decline), context (home-, primary care- or institution based), and intervention components hinder comparability and generalizability. Moreover, results of economic evaluations need to be interpreted in the light of national contexts [17].

In the Netherlands, the Dutch Ministry of Health, Welfare and Sports initiated the National Care for the Elderly Program in 2008, in which over 650 organizations in health, welfare and housing work together in eight regional networks led by academic medical centres to improve care for elderly people with complex care needs. As part of this program, we developed the CareWell primary care program that aimed to reduce functional decline, institutionalization, and hospitalization of community-dwelling frail elderly. Although effectiveness of the program could not be demonstrated [18], the program might theoretically save overall costs and, depending on the trade-off between costs and effects, might be cost-effective. Therefore, we conducted a separate economic evaluation to answer the following research questions:

- What are the differences in health care costs between participants receiving care according to the CareWell primary care program and those receiving care as usual?
- Is the CareWell primary care program cost-effective from a healthcare perspective after 12 months?

Methods

Design

This economic evaluation from a healthcare perspective was performed alongside a cluster controlled effectiveness study with a follow-up of 12 months. Design, methods and outcomes of the effectiveness study have been reported elsewhere [18].

Setting and participants

The study was conducted between September 2011 and September 2012 in 12 general practitioner (GP) practices in the region of Nijmegen, the Netherlands. After informed consent, frail elderly aged ≥70 years were included with the use of the EASY-Care TOS instrument [19]: First, GPs use prior knowledge to subdivide 'not frail' from '(possibly) frail' elders. Then, trained nurses perform a comprehensive geriatric assessment of (possible) frail elders during a home visit. Last, GPs and nurses weigh all signs into a final frailty judgment. Exclusion criteria were institutionalization, and/or critical or terminal illnesses. Details on the recruitment and informed consent procedures have been reported previously [18, 20].

Intervention

In brief, the CareWell primary care program consisted of four key components: 1) multidisciplinary team (MDT) meetings, 2) proactive care planning, 3) case management, and 4) medication reviews.

Each practice assembled a MDT consisting of a general practitioner (GP), practice nurse(s) and/or community nurse(s), an elderly care physician (ECP) [21], and a social worker with elderly care expertise. Each participant was discussed in a MDT meeting at least half-yearly, more often if needed. Meetings were planned every 4–8 weeks. Tailor-made proactive care plans, based on the individual health-related problems and goals as assessed with the EASY-Care TOS [19], were formulated for each participant on enrolment in the program and revised after discussion in a MDT meeting at least every 6 months. A case manager, either a nurse or social worker, was assigned to each participant. They were responsible for care planning and coordination, patient-support in goal setting and self-management, and caregivers support. Last, the GP and nurse conducted a yearly medication review in collaboration with a pharmacist for each participant with polypharmacy (use of ≥5 chronically prescribed drugs).

Professionals received financial reimbursement to cover time-investment and overhead costs.

Usual care

In the Netherlands, GPs provide continuous, person-centred care to community-dwelling frail elderly, facilitated by the use of high-standard electronic medical records and patient panels, defining the population under care [22, 23]. GPs often collaborate with practice and/or community nurses. Moreover, elderly care physicians, i.e. medical practitioners that are specialized as primary care experts in geriatric medicine, increasingly operate (as consultants) in the care for community-dwelling frail elderly [21]. However, the coordination between GPs, other primary and specialist care providers, and home care and community services is often perceived to be insufficient, leading to a fragmented delivery of care [24].

GPs in the usual care group were explicitly asked to decline new relevant inter professional collaborations during the intervention period. No restrictions on pre-existing collaborations between GPs and (practice) nurses were imposed.

Outcome measures

Dependence in functioning in (instrumental) activities of daily living (measured with the Katz-15 [25] change score, i.e. follow-up score minus baseline score) and health-related quality of life (measured with the EuroQol five-dimensional three-level instrument (EQ-5D-3 L) [26]) were collected at baseline and at follow-up after 12 months by structured interviews by trained nurses. The Katz-15 score ranges from 0 to 15 points with higher scores indicating more dependence in (instrumental) activities of daily living. The EQ-5D-3 L instrument is a 'preference-based' measure of health status [27], that defines health-related quality of life according to five dimensions (mobility, self-care, usual activities, pain/discomfort, and anxiety/depression) at three levels (no problems, some problems, severe problems) [26]. In line with the guidelines of the National Care for the Elderly Program, we used the modified EQ-5D + C-3 L instrument that includes cognitive functioning as an additional dimension, with a similar operationalization at three levels [28]. To date, to the best of our knowledge, there is no validated weighting formula for the EQ-5D + C-3 L. Utilities, reflecting the relative desirability of each health state, were thus calculated for the EQ-5D-3 L, without the cognitive dimension, using the Dutch tariff [29]. EQ-5D-3 L scores range from − 0.33 to 1.00, with a higher score indicating a higher health status. Quality Adjusted Life Years (QALYs) were then calculated by multiplying the utilities by the amount of time spent in a particular health state. 1 QALY represents 1 year in perfect health [29].

Healthcare utilization costs and intervention costs

We assessed intervention costs and healthcare utilization during the follow up period. [17] An overview of the healthcare cost variables, prices per unit and sources are presented in Table 1.

Intervention costs regarding time spent on team meetings, care planning, case management, and medication reviews were assessed by instructing practice and/or community nurses and social workers to fill in monthly time registration forms at participant level. To stimulate uniformity in and compliance with time registrations, structured timesheets with written instructions were sent each month as reminders. GPs and ECPs estimated their mean time spent on the intervention per GP practice, from which invested time per participant was calculated. Pharmacists

Table 1 Overview of the cost variables, sources, and cost prices per unit

Cost variable	Source of variable	Cost price per unit (in Euros)
Healthcare utilization costs:		
GP care[a] (per contact):		
Consultation	Structured interview	28
Consult > 20 min	Structured interview	56
Home visit	Structured interview	43
Home visit > 20 min	Structured interview	72
Consultation by phone	Structured interview	14
Prescription refill	Structured interview	14
GP care, out of office hours[b] (per contact)	Structured interview	101
Home care (per hour)	Structured interview	35
Domestic care (per hour)	Municipality registries	12,5
Hospital care, inpatient (per day)	Structured interview	457
Hospital care, outpatient (per contact)	Structured interview	72
Nursing home (per day)	Structured interview	238
Care home (per day)	Structured interview	90
Day care (per day)	Welfare organization registries	45
Physiotherapy (per contact)	Structured interview	36
Medication[c]	Electronic patient file	n/a
Intervention costs (per hour):	Time registrations	
General Practitioner[b]		103
Practice nurse[d]		30
Community nurse[d]		27
Social worker[d]		32
Elderly care physician[b]		103
Pharmacist[b]		85

Sources of cost prices per unit:
[a]Dutch guideline for costing research[30]
[b]Dutch Healthcare Authority
[c]Royal Dutch Society for Pharmacy[31]
[d]Collective Agreements

estimated a time investment of 30 min per participant per medication review.

Healthcare utilization variables, i.e. GP care, hospital care, institutionalization (i.e. nursing home admission, care home admission), home care, and physiotherapy were individually assessed at baseline and follow up through a structured interview by the nurse. Data on domestic care and day care were individually extracted from registries from the municipality of Nijmegen and welfare organizations. Last, data on medication costs (both reimbursed and non-reimbursed) were individually extracted from the electronic patient files (EPF).

Costs were calculated by multiplying volumes of care with their corresponding unit prices. In calculating costs of time invested by practice and/or community nurses and social workers we used their Collective Agreements. The thus generated hourly wages were raised with an estimated 45% for employers and overhead expenses and thus set on €30, €27, and €32 respectively [30]. We used hourly wages of €103, €103, and €85 in calculating costs of time invested by the GPs, ECPs, and pharmacists respectively, according to the fixed rates of the Dutch Healthcare Authority. Costs of healthcare utilization were valued according to the Dutch manual for costing research [30]. When no standardized unit cost prices were available, costs were derived from the Dutch Healthcare Authority. Medication costs were valued using prices of the Royal Dutch Society for Pharmacy [31], using minimum cost prices. All costs were presented in Euros, and indexed to the year 2011 using the consumer price index.

Statistical analysis

Katz-15 change scores and EQ-5D-3 L scores were analyzed using mixed model multilevel analyses, accounting for clustering of participants within GP practices and correcting for those variables that differed between groups at baseline and correlated to the primary outcome, as well as for baseline Katz-15 and EQ-5D-3 L scores to account for regression to the mean [18]. Quality adjusted life years (QALYs) were derived from the EQ-5D-3 L using the trapezium rule (i.e. an approximation of the area under the QALY curve). Mean healthcare utilization costs were analyzed with descriptive statistics and compared between groups using multilevel mixed model analyses, adjusting for clustering of participants within GP practices and for relevant covariates. The incremental Net Monetary Benefit (iNMB) statistic was used to evaluate cost-effectiveness [32] and consequently used as the dependent variable in the mixed model. The iNMB prevents several statistical drawbacks of an incremental cost-effectiveness ratio and enables the use of multilevel regression techniques including covariates in a convenient way [17]. It indicates the monetary gains or costs of an intervention at explicit Willingness to Pay (WTP) thresholds per gained unit of effect. In formula: iNMB = (WTP * Δ effects) − Δ costs. An iNMB (and 95% lower-level confidence interval) greater than zero indicates significant cost-effectiveness of the intervention. We used five WTP thresholds per point improvement on the Katz-15 change score, i.e. €0, €5000, €10,000, €15,000, and €20,000, where no reference values were readily available. Six commonly used WTP thresholds per QALY were used: €0, €20,000, €40,000, €60,000, €80,000, and €100,000 [33].

Results

Participants

In total, 536 participants (287 in the intervention group resp. 249 in the control group) were included in the effectiveness study [18]. At baseline, participants in the intervention group significantly more often lived alone, had more health-related limitations in social functioning, more cognitive deficits, and more social disadvantage, but showed less complex care [18]. No significant between-group differences in baseline Katz-15 scores and EQ-5D-3 L scores were found. We had a loss to follow up of 28. 9% participants in the intervention group and 33.7% in the control group, mainly due to death, institutionalization and declined consent for follow-up (Fig. 1). Additionally, we encountered a considerable number of missing cost variables, mainly medication cost data due to declined consent for use of EPF medication data and limited coverage of medication data in the EPFs. We adhered a complete case analysis with regard to missing values [34]. We analyzed costs and iNMB both with and without medication cost data, including 148 (51.6%) resp. 182 (63. 4%) participants in the intervention group and 103 (41. 3%) resp. 146 (58.6%) participants in the control group (Fig. 1), and considered the analyses including medication costs as the primary analysis. Participants included in the economic evaluation had a lower frailty index. This frailty index was calculated based on the accumulation of deficits in health (symptoms, morbidities, and/or functional abilities), and was used as an extra indicator of frailty next to the EasyCare-TOS [28]. It theoretically ranges from 0 (no indication of frailty) to 1 (extreme frailty), though frailty index scores in similar studies typically culminate at 0.7. Therefore, in addition to the covariates included in the effectiveness analysis, the frailty index was included as a covariate in this economic evaluation.

Outcome measures

At 12 months, we found no significant differences in functional dependence (adjusted mean difference of 0. 37, 95% CI -0.1 to 0.8) nor QALYs (adjusted mean difference of − 0.031, 95% CI -0.1 to 0.0) between the intervention and control group, but the control group did show less functional decline (Table 2) [18].

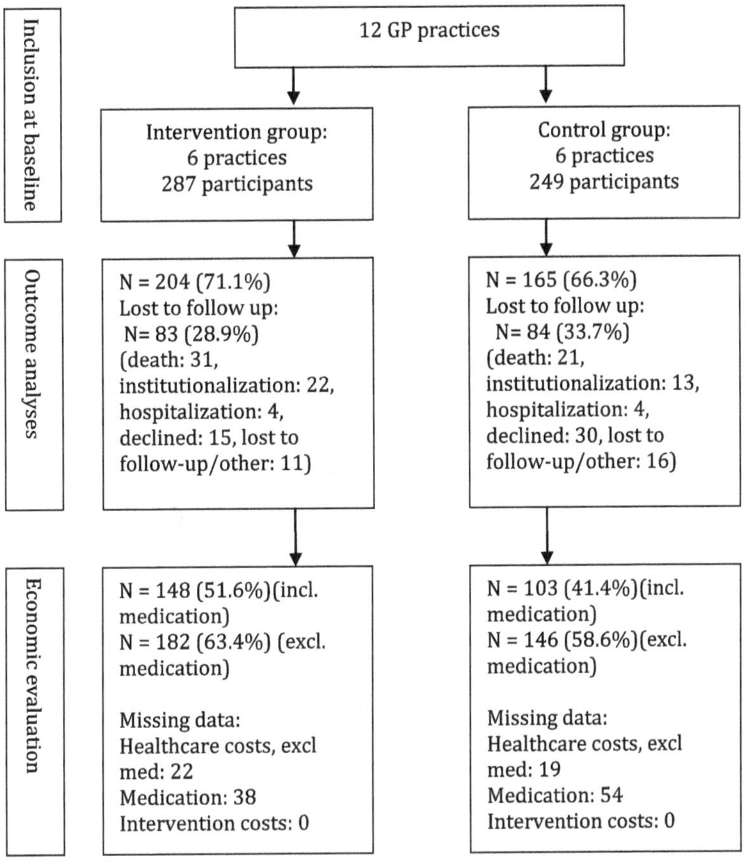

Fig. 1 Flow diagram of participants

Healthcare utilization costs and intervention costs

Mean intervention costs, adjusted for clustering and relevant covariates, were €456 (95% CI -512 to – 398). In the intervention group, mean total costs, i.e. intervention costs plus healthcare utilization costs, adjusted for clustering and relevant covariates, were €1583 (95% CI -4647 to 1481) higher than in the control group. Mean adjusted healthcare utilization costs, i.e. without the intervention costs, were €1143 (95% CI -4198 to 1912) higher in the intervention group. Of the healthcare utilization variables, only medication costs differed significantly, although mean costs of hospitalization, institutionalization, home care and physiotherapy in the intervention group exceeded those in the control group (Table 2).

Economic analysis

Figure 2 shows the iNMBs. It can be noticed that generally these iNMBs are negative, meaning that the intervention does not provide value for money compared to usual care, although the results are not significant. Sensitivity analysis, excluding medication costs, underlined these results.

Discussion

In this cluster controlled study with a follow up of 12 months, healthcare utilization costs and cost-effectiveness of the CareWell primary care program was compared to usual care. Earlier, effectiveness of the CareWell program on daily functioning and quality of life could not be demonstrated [18]. In this study, we found no statistically significant differences between groups in total costs and healthcare utilization costs, with the exception of higher medication costs in the intervention group. Moreover, cost-effectiveness analyses showed no significant differences between groups, but tended to favour usual care.

There are some possible explanations for the absence of cost-effectiveness. First, there is still a lively debate on the concept of frailty and the right timing of interventions [35, 36]. Possibly, the targeted population was too heterogeneous or, in part, too frail to respond to the intervention. Second, the Katz-15 index, measuring daily functioning, might be too restricted to capture the effects of our heterogeneous intervention. Possibly, more person- or goal centred outcomes, e.g. goal-attainment scaling, might suit better [37]. Moreover, the sensitivity

Table 2 Costs of care in intervention and control groups 0–12 months (in Euros)

	Intervention group		Control group		Adjusted mean difference[b] (95% CI)	*P* value
	Unadjusted mean[a]	SE[d]	Unadjusted mean[a]	SE[d]		
Outcome:						
Katz-15 change score[1]	0.80	0.13	0.50	0.16	0.37 (−0.10 to 0.80)	.10
QALY[2]	0.60	0.02	0.60	0.02	−0.03 (− 0.10 to 0.00)	.37
Intervention costs:	456	14	0	0	− 455 (− 512 to − 398)	<.001
Healthcare utilization costs, total:	10,125	983	8114	845	−1143 (− 4198 to 1912)	.46
GP care	163	13	169	18		
GP care, out of office hours	40	11	36	7		
Hospital care, inpatient	1557	510	1225	248		
Hospital care, outpatient	239	24	304	40		
Nursing home	943	399	198	118		
Care home	416	218	161	76		
Day care	422	102	342	101		
Home care	3712	423	2787	412		
Domestic care	1472	91	1417	113		
Physiotherapy	988	309	485	87		
Medication	1617	296	978	126		
Total costs[c]	10,576	983	8114	845	−1583 (− 4647 to 1481)	.31

[1]Katz-15 index (range 0 to 15); higher score indicates more functional dependence in (instrumental) activities of daily living
[2]Quality Adjusted Life Years (QALY), as derived from the EQ-5D-3 L.
[a]Unadjusted means, analyzed with descriptive techniques
[b]Multilevel mixed model analyses, accounting for clustering and covariates
[c]Total costs = intervention costs plus healthcare utilization costs
[d]*SE* standard error

to change of the EQ-5D-3 L in frail elders might have been (too) low [38]. The concept of 'capability wellbeing' has recently been suggested as an alternative, more sensitive measure [33]. However, further work on the validity and value of these capability indices in economic evaluations is needed [33, 39]. Third, it is likely that more profound effects of the intervention only become apparent after a longer follow up period that exceeds the time needed for implementation, individual and organizational learning effects, and efficient multidisciplinary collaboration [40, 41]. This lag-time in effectiveness is presumed to be even more important in complex interventions like our program [40]. Awareness to these short-run inefficiencies that might have resulted from the time limits set by the National Care for the Elderly Program is needed. Last, the selection of motivated professionals in the intervention group might have limited the room for improvement in the delivered care and possibly led to higher costs due to more proactive care, irrespective of the CareWell program. The overall increased awareness to the health care needs of frail elderly in Western countries in the last two decades together with the Dutch high-quality primary care might have further reduced the contrasts between the CareWell program and usual care. Possibly, our program would show clearer effectiveness in less well managed healthcare settings [12].

Our results are in line with comparable integrated care programs aimed at frail elderly, performed in other contexts [14, 42]. More recently, three cost-effectiveness studies of integrated care programs from the National Care for the Elderly Program demonstrated no effects on functioning nor quality of life, at unchanged or higher total costs mainly due to increased GP care and intervention costs without (expected) decreases in hospital and long-term care costs, after 12–24 months [43–45]. However, Van Leeuwen et al. did find increasing effects at lower costs compared to usual care in the last 18–24 months of follow up [45]. Previously, Counsell et al. demonstrated similar decreased costs in their third year of follow up, mainly through a shift away from emergency and hospital services towards more-desirable chronic and preventive care expenditures [14]. This supports our assumption of a lag-time in effectiveness. The results of the cost-utility analyses of the recent other Dutch studies, finding low probabilities of the intervention increasing QALYs at lower costs, correspond with our results [45, 46]. However, only Van Leeuwen et al. performed a formal cost-effectiveness analysis [45]. Like us, they found low probabilities of the intervention being cost-effective.

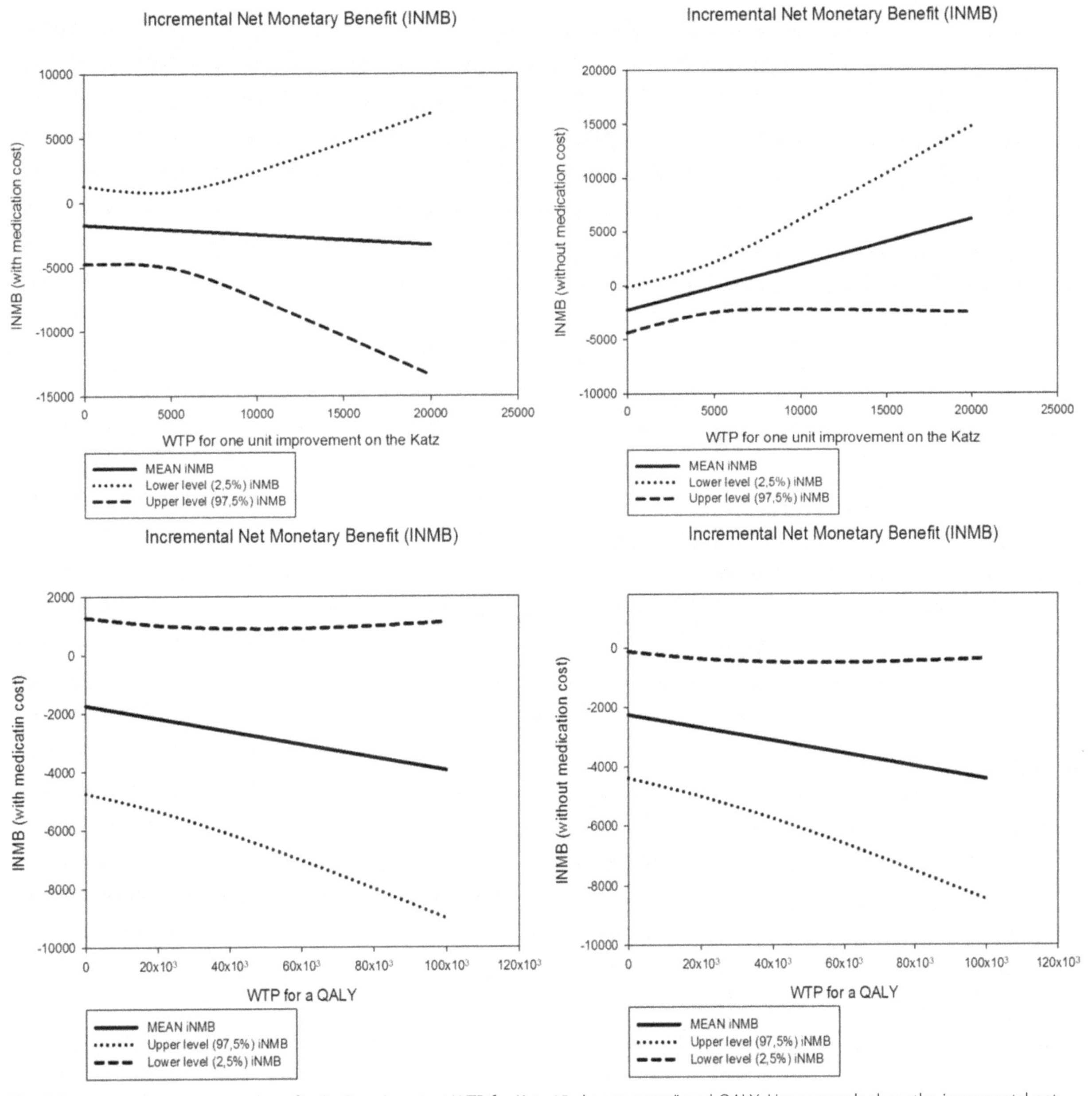

Fig. 2 Incremental net monetary benefits (in Euros) against WTP for Katz-15 change score* and QALY. Upper panels show the incremental net monetary benefits (in formula: iNMB = (WTP * Δ effects) – Δ costs) against WTP for Katz-15 change scores; lower panels show iNMBs against WTP for QALY. All iNMBs are negative, i.e. the intervention does not provide value for money compared to usual care (not significant). Sensitivity analyses, excluding medication costs, underline the results (right panels)WTP = Willingness to Pay. QALY = Quality Adjusted Life Year, derived from the EQ-5D-3 L, based on the Dutch tariff [29] using the trapezium rule.* Improvement on the Katz-15 change score is indicated by a lower score, meaning less functional decline regarding (Instrumental) activities of daily living

This study has several strengths. First, we used a comprehensive approach to costing, including a wide variety of cost variables that were assessed at participant level, thus enhancing internal validity. Next, robust multilevel techniques were used in analyzing both differences in costs and net monetary benefits. Last, since we used only a limited number of exclusion criteria and included participants from heterogeneous GP practices, our results should be generalizable to the population of frail elders in the Netherlands and comparable high-quality primary care settings.

We also should consider some limitations. First, we were unable to include informal care costs, since informal caregivers' willingness to participate was low and differed between groups. We were therefore not able to adhere to the societal perspective, as announced in our study protocol [20], but had to switch to a healthcare perspective. Since prior studies show contrasting results on the impact of informal care on total costs, the impact of this switch on our results is unclear [42, 45]. Next, since the extraction of data on healthcare use from external sources like healthcare insurance companies, as originally planned in the study design, was not possible, we had to collect these data through participants' retrospective self-report. This could have led to recall bias. Different studies showed self-report after 12 months to be an appropriate, reasonably accurate method for obtaining a wide range of healthcare utilization data in elderly people [47, 48]. More salient events in general suffer less from memory decay and thus recall bias [49]. Seidl et al. for example found the recall bias of hospital admissions of elderly people not to be influenced by applying various recall periods, although the probability of correctly self-reporting a single event was higher using a shorter recall period [48]. However, less salient events such as GP contacts could lead to both under- and over-reporting, and show less accuracy in self-report [49, 50]. Also, time registrations used to calculate intervention costs might be biased due to inaccuracies. However, we have no reason to assume unequal distributions of these potential biases between the groups. Last, we had to deal with a considerable number of missing medication cost data that had to be considered missing not at random. However, our additional sensitivity analysis without medication costs did not reveal other results.

Conclusions

After 12 months follow-up, no net monetary benefit of the CareWell program over usual care could be demonstrated.

This study adds to the currently scarce body of evidence regarding cost-effectiveness of integrated care programs targeting frail elderly. Future economic evaluations should account for pitfalls in their design with respect to the target population, outcome measures used, and adequate follow-up period. From a cost-effectiveness perspective, the CareWell primary program in its current form is not suited for widespread implementation.

Abbreviations

ECP: Elderly care physician; EPF: Electronic patient file; EQ-5D-3 L: EuroQol five-dimensional three-level instrument; GP: General practitioner; iNMB: Incremental net monetary benefit; MDT: Multidisciplinary team; QALY: Quality adjusted life years; WTP: Willingness to pay

Acknowledgements

We are most grateful to all participants and health care professionals that were involved in the study. Furthermore, we would like to thank all professionals, volunteers, and health care organizations that are involved in 'Netwerk 100' (https://www.netwerk100.nl/) for their contributions to the development of the CareWell-primary care program.

Funding

This study was funded by the Dutch National Care for the Elderly Program, as initiated by the Netherlands Organization for Health Research and Development (ZonMW: project no. 313050201). Health insurance companies (CZ and UVIT) and the municipality provided additional funding. Funding bodies were not involved in the design, methods, subject recruitment, data collection, analysis or preparation of the manuscript.

Authors' contributions

FR, HS, RK and SZ designed the study. FR acquired the data. FR, EA and SZ were responsible for the statistical analyses. FR, PA, HS, RK and SZ and contributed to the interpretation of data. FR wrote the first draft. PA, HS, RK and SZ critically revised this draft. FR wrote the final draft. All authors approved of the final version, and are accountable for all aspects of the manuscript.

Competing interests

The authors declare that they have no competing interests.

Author details

[1]Radboud Institute for Health Sciences, Department of Primary and Community Care, Radboud university medical centre, Nijmegen, the Netherlands. [2]Radboud Institute for Health Sciences, Department for Health Evidence, Radboud university medical centre, Nijmegen, the Netherlands. [3]Joachim and Anna, Centre for specialized geriatric care, Nijmegen, the Netherlands. [4]Department of General Practice and Elderly Care Medicine, University of Groningen, University Medical Centre Groningen, Groningen, Netherlands.

References

1. Ganguli I, Thompson RW, Ferris TG. What can five high cost patients teach us about healthcare spending? Healthcare (Amsterdam, Netherlands). 2016;
2. Joynt KE, Figueroa JF, Beaulieu N, Wild RC, Orav EJ, Jha AK. Segmenting high-cost Medicare patients into potentially actionable cohorts. Healthcare (Amsterdam, Netherlands) 2016.
3. De Lepeleire J, Iliffe S, Mann E, Frailty DJM. An emerging concept for general practice. Br J Gen Pract. 2009;59(562):e177–82.
4. Clegg A, Young J, Iliffe S, Rikkert MO, Rockwood K. Frailty in elderly people. Lancet. 2013;381(9868):752–62.
5. Collard RM, Boter H, Schoevers RA, Oude Voshaar RC. Prevalence of frailty in community-dwelling older persons: a systematic review. J Am Geriatr Soc. 2012;60(8):1487–92.
6. Clarkson P, Brand C, Hughes J, Challis D. Integrating assessments of older people: examining evidence and impact from a randomised controlled trial. Age Ageing. 2011;40(3):388–91.
7. Wagner EH, Austin BT, Davis C, Hindmarsh M, Schaefer J, Bonomi A. Improving chronic illness care: translating evidence into action. Health aff (Project Hope). 2001;20(6):64–78.
8. Markle-Reid M, Browne G, Weir R, Gafni A, Roberts J, Henderson SR. The effectiveness and efficiency of home-based nursing health promotion for older people: a review of the literature. Med Care Res Rev. 2006;63(5):531–69.
9. Eklund K, Wilhelmson K. Outcomes of coordinated and integrated interventions targeting frail elderly people: a systematic review of randomised controlled trials. Health Soc Care Community. 2009;17(5):447–58.
10. Beland F, Bergman H, Lebel P, Clarfield AM, Tousignant P, Contandriopoulos AP, Dallaire L. A system of integrated care for older persons with disabilities in Canada: results from a randomized controlled trial. J Gerontol A Biol Sci Med Sci. 2006;61(4):367–73.
11. Bernabei R, Landi F, Gambassi G, Sgadari A, Zuccala G, Mor V, Rubenstein LZ, Carbonin P. Randomised trial of impact of model of integrated care and case management for older people living in the community. *BMJ*. Clin Res. 1998;316(7141):1348–51.
12. Beswick AD, Rees K, Dieppe P, Ayis S, Gooberman-Hill R, Horwood J, Ebrahim S. Complex interventions to improve physical function and maintain independent living in elderly people: a systematic review and meta-analysis. Lancet (London, England). 2008;371(9614):725–35.
13. Counsell SR, Callahan CM, Clark DO, Tu W, Buttar AB, Stump TE, Ricketts GD. Geriatric care management for low-income seniors: a randomized controlled trial. JAMA. 2007;298(22):2623–33.
14. Counsell SR, Callahan CM, Tu W, Stump TE, Arling GW. Cost analysis of the geriatric resources for assessment and Care of Elders care management intervention. J Am Geriatr Soc. 2009;57(8):1420–6.

15. Stuck AE, Aronow HU, Steiner A, Alessi CA, Bula CJ, Gold MN, Yuhas KE, Nisenbaum R, Rubenstein LZ, Beck JC. A Trial of annual in-home comprehensive geriatric assessments for elderly people living in the community. N Engl J Med. 1995;333(18):1184–9.
16. Fairhall N, Sherrington C, Kurrle SE, Lord SR, Lockwood K, Howard K, Hayes A, Monaghan N, Langron C, Aggar C, et al. Economic evaluation of a multifactorial, interdisciplinary intervention versus usual care to reduce frailty in frail older people. J Am Med Dir Assoc. 2015;16(1):41–8.
17. Drummond MF, Sculpher MJ, Torrance GW, OB BJ, Stoddart GL. Methods for the economic evaluation of health care Programmes. New York: NY: Oxford university press; 2005.
18. Ruikes FG, Zuidema SU, Akkermans RP, Assendelft WJ, Schers HJ, Koopmans RT. Multicomponent program to reduce functional decline in frail elderly people: a cluster controlled trial. J Am Board Fam Med. 2016;29(2):209–17.
19. van Kempen JA, Schers HJ, Jacobs A, Zuidema SU, Ruikes F, Robben SH, Melis RJ, Olde Rikkert MG. Development of an instrument for the identification of frail older people as a target population for integrated care. Br J Gen Pract. 2013;63(608):e225–31.
20. Ruikes FG, Meys AR, van de Wetering G, Akkermans RP, van Gaal BG, Zuidema SU, Schers HJ, van Achterberg T, Koopmans RT. The CareWell-primary care program: design of a cluster controlled trial and process evaluation of a complex intervention targeting community-dwelling frail elderly. BMC Fam Pract. 2012;13:115.
21. Koopmans RT, Lavrijsen JC, Hoek JF, Went PB, Schols JM. Dutch elderly care physician: a new generation of nursing home physician specialists. J Am Geriatr Soc. 2010;58(9):1807–9.
22. Doran T, Roland M. Lessons from major initiatives to improve primary care in the United Kingdom. Health Aff. 2010;29(5):1023–9.
23. van Weel C, Schers H, Timmermans A. Health care in the Netherlands. J Am Board Fam Med. 2012;25(Suppl 1):S12–7.
24. Boeckxstaens P, De Graaf P. Primary care and care for older persons: position paper of the European forum for primary care. Qual Prim Care. 2011;19(6):369–89.
25. Weinberger M, Samsa GP, Schmader K, Greenberg SM, Carr DB, Wildman DS. Comparing proxy and patients' perceptions of patients' functional status: results from an outpatient geriatric clinic. J Am Geriatr Soc. 1992;40(6):585–8.
26. Krabbe PF, Stouthard ME, Essink-Bot ML, Bonsel GJ. The effect of adding a cognitive dimension to the EuroQol multiattribute health-status classification system. J Clin Epidemiol. 1999;52(4):293–301.
27. Karimi M, Brazier J. Health, health-related quality of life, and quality of life: what is the difference? PharmacoEconomics. 2016;34(7):645–9.
28. Lutomski JE, Baars MA, Schalk BW, Boter H, Buurman BM, den Elzen WP, Jansen AP, Kempen GI, Steunenberg B, Steyerberg EW, et al. The development of the older persons and informal caregivers survey minimum DataSet (TOPICS-MDS): a large-scale data sharing initiative. PLoS One. 2013;8(12):e81673.
29. Lamers LM, McDonnell J, Stalmeier PF, Krabbe PF, Busschbach JJ. The Dutch tariff: results and arguments for an effective design for national EQ-5D valuation studies. Health Econ. 2006;15(10):1121–32.
30. Hakkaart-van Roijen L, Tan S, Bouwmans C. Handleiding voor Kostenonderzoek, Methoden en Standaard Kostprijzen voor Economische Evaluaties in De Gezondheidszorg (Dutch manual for costing: methods and standard costs for economic evaluations in healthcare). College voor Zorgverzekeringen: Diemen, The Netherlands; 2011.
31. Z-index. In. *G-Standard.* The Hague, The Netherlands: Royal Dutch Society for Pharmacy; 2006. https://www.z-index.nl/g-standaard.
32. Hoch JS, Briggs AH, Willan AR. Something old, something new, something borrowed, something blue: a framework for the marriage of health econometrics and cost-effectiveness analysis. Health Econ. 2002;11(5):415–30.
33. Makai P, Looman W, Adang E, Melis R, Stolk E, Fabbricotti I. Cost-effectiveness of integrated care in frail elderly using the ICECAP-O and EQ-5D: does choice of instrument matter? Eur J Health Econ. 2015;16(4):437–50.
34. Sterne JA, White IR, Carlin JB, Spratt M, Royston P, Kenward MG, Wood AM, Carpenter JR. Multiple imputation for missing data in epidemiological and clinical research: potential and pitfalls. BMJ (Clinical research ed). 2009;b2393:338.
35. Marzetti E, Calvani R, Landi F, Hoogendijk EO, Fougere B, Vellas B, Pahor M, Bernabei R, Cesari M. Innovative Medicines Initiative: The SPRINTT Project. J Frailty Aging. 2015;4(4):207–8.
36. Lacas A, Rockwood K. Frailty in primary care: a review of its conceptualization and implications for practice. BMC Med. 2012;10:4.
37. Rockwood K, Howlett S, Stadnyk K, Carver D, Powell C, Stolee P. Responsiveness of goal attainment scaling in a randomized controlled trial of comprehensive geriatric assessment. J Clin Epidemiol. 2003;56(8):736–43.
38. Brazier JE, Walters SJ, Nicholl JP, Kohler B. Using the SF-36 and Euroqol on an elderly population. Qual Life Res. 1996;5(2):195–204.
39. Al-Janabi H, Flynn TN, Peters TJ, Bryan S, Coast J. Test-retest reliability of capability measurement in the UK general population. Health Econ. 2015; 24(5):625–30.
40. van de Wetering G, Olde Rikkert M, van der Wilt GJ, Adang E. Understanding and anticipating lag-time bias in cost-effectiveness studies: the role of time in cost-effectiveness analysis. Int J Technol Assess Health Care. 2014;30(6):608–11.
41. de Stampa M, Vedel I, Bergman H, Novella JL, Lechowski L, Ankri J, Lapointe L. Opening the black box of clinical collaboration in integrated care models for frail, elderly patients. The Gerontologist. 2013;53(2):313–25.
42. Sandberg M, Kristensson J, Midlov P, Jakobsson U. Effects on healthcare utilization of case management for frail older people: a randomized controlled trial (RCT). Arch Gerontol Geriatr. 2015;60(1):71–81.
43. Metzelthin SF, van Rossum E, Hendriks MR, De Witte LP, Hobma SO, Sipers W, Kempen GI. Reducing disability in community-dwelling frail older people: cost-effectiveness study alongside a cluster randomised controlled trial. Age Ageing. 2015;44(3):390–6.
44. Looman WM, Huijsman R, Bouwmans-Frijters CA, Stolk EA, Fabbricotti IN. Cost-effectiveness of the 'Walcheren integrated care Model' intervention for community-dwelling frail elderly. Fam Pract. 2016; 33(2):154–60.
45. van Leeuwen KM, Bosmans JE, Jansen AP, Hoogendijk EO, Muntinga ME, van Hout HP, Nijpels G, van der Horst HE, van Tulder MW. Cost-effectiveness of a chronic care model for frail older adults in primary care: economic evaluation alongside a stepped-wedge cluster-randomized trial. J Am Geriatr Soc. 2015;63(12):2494–504.
46. Looman WM, Huijsman R, Bouwmans-Frijters CA, Stolk EA, Fabbricotti IN. Cost-effectiveness of the 'Walcheren integrated care Model' intervention for community-dwelling frail elderly. Fam Pract. 2016;33(2):154–60.
47. Lubeck DP, Hubert HB. Self-report was a viable method for obtaining health care utilization data in community-dwelling seniors. J Clin Epidemiol. 2005; 58(3):286–90.
48. Seidl H, Meisinger C, Kirchberger I, Burkhardt K, Kuch B, Holle R. Validity of self-reported hospital admissions in clinical trials depends on recall period length and individual characteristics. J Eval Clin Pract. 2016;22(3):446–54.
49. Brusco NK, Watts JJ. Empirical evidence of recall bias for primary health care visits. BMC Health Serv Res. 2015;15:381.
50. Garcia PA, Dias JM, Silva SL, Dias RC. Prospective monitoring and self-report of previous falls among older women at high risk of falls and fractures: a study of comparison and agreement. Brazilian J Phys Ther. 2015;19(3):218–26.

8

Barriers and facilitators to HPV vaccination in primary care practices: a mixed methods study using the Consolidated Framework for Implementation Research

Jane M. Garbutt[1*], Sherry Dodd[2], Emily Walling[2,3], Amanda A. Lee[4], Katharine Kulka[2] and Rebecca Lobb[4]

Abstract

Background: In the United States, the effective, safe huma papilloma virus (HPV) vaccine is underused and opportunities to prevent cancer continue to be missed. National guidelines recommend completing the 2–3 dose HPV vaccine series by age 13, well before exposure to the sexually transmitted virus. Accurate characterization of the facilitators and barriers to full implementation of HPV vaccine recommendations in the primary care setting could inform effective implementation strategies.

Methods: We used the Consolidated Framework for Implementation Research (CFIR) to systematically investigate and characterize factors that influence HPV vaccine use in 10 primary care practices (16 providers) using a concurrent mixed methods design. The CFIR was used to guide collection and analysis of qualitative data collected through in-person semi-structured interviews with the primary care providers. We analyzed HPV vaccine use with data abstracted from medical charts. Constructs that most strongly influenced vaccine use were identified by integrating the qualitative and quantitative data.

Results: Of the 72 CFIR constructs assessed, seven strongly distinguished and seven weakly distinguished between providers with higher versus lower HPV vaccine coverage. The majority of strongly distinguishing constructs were facilitators and were related to characteristics of the providers (knowledge and beliefs; self-efficacy; readiness for change), their perception of the intervention (relative advantage of vaccinating younger vs. older adolescents), and their process to deliver the vaccine (executing). Additional weakly distinguishing constructs that were facilitators were from outer setting (peer pressure; financial incentives), inner setting (networks and communications and readiness for implementation) and process (planning; engaging, and reflecting and evaluating). Two strongly distinguishing constructs were barriers to use, one from the intervention (adaptability of the age of initiation) and the other from outer setting (patient needs and resources).

Conclusions: Using CFIR to systematically examine the use of this vaccine in independent primary care practices enabled us to identify facilitators and barriers at the provider, interpersonal and practice level that need to be addressed in future efforts to increase vaccine use in such settings. Our findings suggest that implementation strategies that target the provider and help them to address multi-level barriers to HPV vaccine use merit further investigation.

Keywords: HPV vaccine, Implementation strategies, CFIR

* Correspondence: jgarbutt@wustl.edu
[1]Departments of Medicine and Pediatrics, Washington University School of Medicine, St. Louis, MO, USA
Full list of author information is available at the end of the article

Background

A vaccine targeting oncogenic human papilloma viruses (HPV) is an important health innovation. The HPV vaccine is predicted to prevent ~ 70% of cervical cancers as well as other genitourinary and oral cancers and genital warts in men and women. [1, 2] The vaccine has been recommended for routine use in the United States for over ten years [1] and already has been shown to prevent up to 99% of HPV-related cervical dysplasia, a precursor of cervical cancer. [1–3] However, the full benefit of the HPV vaccine can only be realized if the vaccination series is completed prior to exposure to the sexually transmitted virus. National guidelines recommend giving the vaccine to all adolescents at their 11 to 12 year old check-up visit concurrently with the tetanus, diphtheria, pertussis booster (Tdap) and the meningococcal conjugate vaccine (MCV4), and completing the HPV vaccine series before their 13th birthday. [4] Until a few months ago, the recommended series comprised 3 doses given over 6 months. At the end of 2016, this changed to 2 doses of the 9-valent vaccine given over 6 to 12 months, if the series is initiated before the 15th birthday. [5]

Introduced in the United States (U.S.) for girls in 2006 and for boys in 2011, use of this effective vaccine is far below the Healthy People 2020 objective of 80% coverage by age 13 to 15 for both sexes. [6] In 2015, only 41. 9% of eligible females and 28.1% of eligible males aged 13–17 years had completed the 3-dose series, with marked variation among states. [7] Opportunities to prevent cancer continue to be missed. There is an obvious disparity in uptake of HPV vaccine when compared with coverage for Tdap (86.4%) and MCV4 (81.3%) in the same age-group. [7] Interventions to increase initiation of the HPV vaccine and series completion targeting both parents and providers that have been rigorously evaluated, have had at best a modest effect (~ 5% increase). [1, 8]' [9] Many studies showing larger effects have been criticized for being methodologically deficient. [1, 9, 10] Alternative approaches to increase use of HPV vaccine are urgently needed. Accurate characterization of the facilitators and barriers to full implementation of HPV vaccine recommendations in the primary care setting could inform effective implementation strategies.

Closing the gap between the national goal and current vaccine use requires improved uptake in primary care settings where the majority of children are vaccinated. We hypothesized that in these settings, factors that influence HPV vaccine use are multifactorial and complex. The objective of this study was to use a systematic approach based on the Consolidated Framework for Implementation Research (CFIR) [11] to identify and characterize factors that are facilitators of and barriers to implementation of the national recommendations for HPV vaccine use. We will use this information to inform development of a pragmatic and effective implementation strategy to increase timely use of this important oncogenic vaccine.

Methods

We assessed the implementation of HPV vaccine in ten community pediatric offices using a concurrent mixed methods design. Quantitative and qualitative data were analyzed separately and then were integrated to provide additional information. [12] Specifically, we conducted a retrospective analysis of HPV vaccine use data abstracted from medical charts and acquired during in-person semi-structured interviews with the pediatric primary care providers. The study was approved by the Washington University Human Research Protection Office.

The CFIR was used to guide development of the interview guide, data coding, and data analysis. Damschroder and colleagues developed the CFIR to consolidate and unify key constructs from 19 published implementation theories. [11] Seventy-two constructs are grouped under five major domains that influence successful implementation of evidence-based interventions. These include characteristics of the intervention (in this case, use of HPV vaccine in accordance with CDC guidelines), the inner setting (the pediatric practice), the outer setting (the context in which the pediatric practice resides), individual characteristics of the implementers (the healthcare providers), and the processes used for implementation of the intervention. [11] Definitions of the constructs within each domain can be found at 13012_2008_182_MOESM3_ESM.pdf [11].

Study participants

We invited all members of the Washington University Pediatric and Adolescent Ambulatory Research Consortium (WU PAARC) to participate. WU PAARC is a practice-based research network of 79 community pediatricians and 6 pediatric nurse practitioners associated with Washington University. A convenience sample of 16 providers from ten practices volunteered to participate. Each participant provided written consent and received $50 as a token of appreciation for their time.

Advisory board

The study was guided by an Advisory Board of three pediatricians, one pediatric nurse practitioner, and two parents. The three pediatricians volunteered to be study subjects. The group met five times over the 12-month study period to review materials, problem solve, and assist in interpretation of study findings.

Data collection

Quantitative data

For each provider, we abstracted data on vaccine coverage from medical charts for girls and boys who were 11 to 15 years old and had attended at least one office visit between January 1st, 2014 and December 31st, 2014. Data abstracted from the chart included: gender, date of birth, date of vaccine and type of vaccine (HPV, Tdap and MCV4).

Qualitative data

We developed an interview guide with a series of open-ended questions and probes to elicit examples that would clarify and illustrate the participant's responses. The guide included general and specific questions that addressed the main CFIR constructs to determine those that supported or created barriers to implementation. We explored how each of these constructs differed from that used for other adolescent vaccines to gather information to explain the higher coverage for the other childhood vaccines. The interviews were conducted between 1/27/2016 and 5/24/2016, by the principal investigator (JG) and co-investigator (EW). Interviews were designed to last about 30 min and were conducted at the practices. All were digitally recorded and transcribed verbatim by trained transcriptionists. After the qualitative interview, participants completed a short, structured survey describing their practice arrangements.

Data analysis

Quantitative data

For each practice and provider, we computed the overall coverage with HPV vaccine as the percentage of girls and boys who received three doses by their 13th birthday (a HEDIS measure for adolescent care). [13]

Qualitative data

We used a deductive approach to coding guided by the CFIR domains and constructs. We were also open to new themes that emerged inductively from the data. The transcripts were organized using NVivo software and each transcript was analyzed using consensual qualitative research methods with multiple analysts from diverse disciplines (e.g. pediatrician, implementation scientist, health services researcher) to foster multiple perspectives and validation. [14] We used an iterative process to develop a codebook that reflected each CFIR domain and its constructs, and key themes that emerged by refining the code definitions through consensus. The coding process began with two analysts who independently reviewed each transcript to identify the text units that were associated with each of the CFIR domains. Subsequently, they compared assessments, discussed differences and came to agreement on final text assignments. The text within each CFIR domain was further coded by three analysts to identify constructs within each CFIR domain. Thus, each transcript was subjected to a two-level consensus process.

Rating the CFIR constructs

Each transcript was subjected to a rating process. Five analysts used a deliberated consensus process to assign a rating to each construct within each transcript. The ratings reflected the valence (positive or negative influence) of the construct on implementation of HPV vaccine according to national guidelines (3 doses completed by the 13th birthday). Table 1 provides the criteria used to guide the rating process.

Integrating the rating of CFIR constructs and coverage rates

Next, for each provider, we integrated their construct ratings with their HPV vaccine coverage in a table (An example is provided in Table 2). We grouped physicians by coverage rates using tertiles: lower coverage < 5% (n = 5 providers), moderate coverage 6–19% (n = 6), and higher coverage > 20% (n = 5). This approach allowed us to observe patterns of ratings for CFIR domains and constructs among lower and higher coverage providers and generate hypotheses about constructs that distinguished between groups. We focused on extreme values of coverage to ascertain the most information. [14] Strongly and weakly distinguishing patterns were determined based on two dimensions within and across higher and lower coverage groups. We first assessed the pattern of positive and negative ratings for each construct within coverage groups (higher and lower) to determine if the factor was a facilitator or barrier to use of HPV vaccine. Next, we examined the difference in

Table 1 Criteria Used to assign Ratings to Constructs

Rating	Criteria
-1	A negative influence on providing HPV vaccine according to guideline recommendations i.e., complete the 3-dose series by the child's 13th birthday. The interviewee provides examples of how key aspects of the construct exert a negative impact on HPV vaccine use, reports an overall negative effect, or sufficient information is provided to make indirect inference about a negative effect.
O	Appears to have no effect on use of HPV vaccine according to guideline recommendations.
+ 1	A positive influence on providing HPV vaccine according to guideline recommendations i.e., complete the 3-dose series by the child's 13th birthday. The interviewee provides examples of how key aspects of the construct exert a positive impact on HPV vaccine use, reports an overall positive effect, or sufficient information is provided to make indirect inference about a positive effect.

Table 2 An example of the table of integrated data from qualitative and quantitative studies comparing ratings for CFIR constructs in the characteristics of individuals domain and HPV vaccine coverage data (completion of 3 doses by 13th birthday)

CHARACTERISTICS OF INDIVIDUALS	1013	1004	1007	1015	1005	1001	1009	1020	1019	1008	1014	1018	1010	1006	1011	1003
HPV vaccine coverage	25.5%	24.6%	24.0%	23.0%	20.5%	18.1%	16.5%	16.1%	8.7%	8.1%	6.1%	4.8%	4.6%	4.2%	3.7%	1.2%
Knowledge and Beliefs																
Value completing the vaccine by age 13	+	+	+	+	+	+	+	–	+	+	+	–	–	–	+	–
Believes benefit in bundling	+	+	+	+	+	+	+	–	+	+	–	+	+	–	+	–
Self-Efficacy																
Enthusiastic use of HPV vaccine	+	+	+	+	+	+	+	+	+	+	+	+	+	–	+	–
Familiarity with facts about HPV vaccine	+	+	+	+	+	+	+	+	+	+	+	+	+	–	+	+
Confident to recommend strongly at early age (11–12)	+	+	+	+	+	+	+	+	+	+	+	–	–	–	+	–
Confident in ability to convince hesitant parents	+	–	+	+	+	–	+	+	+	+	–	–	–	–	+	–
Readiness to change	+	–	+	+	+	–	+	–	–	–	+	–	–	–	+	–

positive or negative ratings in the higher and lower coverage groups to determine if the construct was an important distinguishing factor. If this difference was ≥ 60% (e.g.,5/5 or 100% positive in higher coverage and 1/5 or 20% positive in lower coverage), the construct was considered to be "strongly distinguishing." If this difference was between 40% to 59% (e.g., 5/5 or 100% positive in higher coverage and 3/5 or 60% positive in lower coverage), the construct was considered to be "weakly distinguishing." If the difference was < 40% (e.g. ,5/5 or 100% positive in higher coverage and 4/5 or 80% positive in lower coverage), the construct was determined to provide limited information about coverage rates. To support the validity of our conclusions, we checked with members of the Advisory Board. [14]

Results

Sixteen providers participated in both the quantitative and qualitative studies. They comprised 15 pediatricians and one pediatric nurse practitioner. Five were male, 11 were female, 13 were Caucasian, 2 were African American, and one was Asian. The 16 providers were drawn from ten practices, nine of which had multiple providers (2–6 providers per practice). Two practices were part of a healthcare group and had access to central support for information systems and quality improvement staff. Such resources were not available at other practices. Eight practices used an electronic medical record (EMR).

Quantitative data

Medical records from a total of 4592 teens were eligible for inclusion in the data analysis of coverage rates. Overall, 13.9% of eligible teens had received 3-doses of HPV vaccine before their 13th birthday (16.9% girls, 11.3% boys). This metric varied among practices from 2.3% to 25.5% and there was wide variability in HPV vaccine coverage among providers within the same practice (Table 3). Consequently, we chose to analyze the qualitative data at the level of the individual provider rather than at the level of the practice.

Qualitative data

CFIR constructs are not reported if we found limited text that could be coded within that domain construct. For intervention domain, this included the following constructs: intervention source, evidence strength and quality, trialability, design quality and packaging. For the inner setting domain, this included: structural characteristics, culture, compatibility, organizational incentives and rewards, and learning climate. For the characteristics of individuals domain, we found no text about individual identification with the organization. Within the process domain, we did not identify any opinion leaders, internal implementation leaders or champions.

Innovation characteristics domain

Relative advantage

The most commonly mentioned perceived advantages to providing HPV vaccine at age 11–12 years rather than to older teens were increased immunogenicity, successfully completing the series before exposure to HPV and accessing the child at their 11–12 year old check-up required by school. Although the vaccine can be given to children as young as 9, no providers did so routinely. Several providers offered it to younger children accompanying an older sibling to a check-up visit where they received HPV vaccine.

Table 3 Coverage Rates for HPV Vaccine by Practice and Provider

Practice	Number of children age 13	Electronic medical record (EMR) or paper records	Completed 3 doses HPV by 13th birthday	
			Practice coverage	Provider coverage
A	329	EMR	25.5%	25.5%
B	383	EMR	23.0%	23.0%
C[a]	299	EMR	18.1%	18.1%
D	726	EMR	18.6%	24.0%, 3.7%
E	441	Paper records	13.8%	24.6%, 16.1%, 4.2%
F[a]	940	EMR	10.6%	20.5%, 4.6%
G	636	EMR	9.6%	16.5%, 8.1%
H	416	EMR	8.7%	8.7%
I	293	EMR	6.1%	6.1%
J	129	Paper records	2.3%	4.8%, 1.2%
All	4592		13.9%	

[a]Practice was part of a healthcare group with access to information system assistance and quality improvement staff

Adaptability

All providers adapted the vaccine dosing schedule, most often to provide the 2nd and 3rd doses at subsequent annual checkup visits. Some providers also delayed the age of initiation beyond 11–12 years to prevent teens from having three vaccines concurrently or to avoid conflict with a family they thought might be uncomfortable discussing prevention of a sexually transmitted disease at this age.

Complexity

The majority of providers identified at least one difficulty with administering the 3-dose series. Many cited the resistance and hesitancy of parents, as exemplified by this quote:

> "Well, I think you have to go in more proactively with that one [HPV], because you expect a fight. You do, because nine times out of ten, you have a parent who has heard something about it who has a problem with it. You are trying to push the vaccine in a positive way before the negative parts come in from the parent."

Others mentioned that it took longer to discuss HPV vaccine than other adolescent vaccines and less frequent visits of older adolescents increased the difficulty of completing the series.

Cost

Few providers mentioned cost associated with providing HPV vaccine, although several noted that providing the 3-dose series was revenue generating.

Outer setting domain

Patient needs and resources

Most providers felt it was important to provide information about vaccine benefits as reported by this provider:

> "I think there are a lot of negative messages out there, so it's important for the families to hear the positive message from us."

To address this need, they routinely informed parents that HPV vaccine prevents cancer and sometimes they mentioned the prevention of warts. However, few routinely discussed vaccine safety, preferring to provide this information if parents expressed specific safety concerns. Few used parent educational materials apart from the required vaccine information sheets (VIS) from the CDC. Several providers noted that teenagers often were concerned about getting the HPV vaccine as they had heard it was more painful than other vaccines, and some teens were reluctant to get all three adolescent vaccines at the same visit.

Peer pressure

A few providers described pressure from a partner in their practice to change their approach to HPV vaccine implementation.

External policy and incentives

All providers were aware of the national guideline recommendations to complete the 3-dose series by age 13. Many parents chose to defer HPV vaccine as it is not required for school attendance. Few providers were aware of financial incentives including those offered by vaccine manufacturers to increase completion of the 3-dose series and by Medicaid to promote meaningful use of clinical information.

Cosmopolitan

All providers reported that they learned about the recommendations for HPV vaccine from external sources, most commonly through membership with the American Academy of Pediatrics (AAP) list serve. They also received information from "throw away" medical journals, drug representatives, and the internet, and were unlikely to seek or receive information about the vaccine from local infectious disease experts.

Inner setting domain

Networks and communication

Except for the solo-practitioner, all providers reported formal or informal opportunities for communication with other providers in their practice, typically through formal meetings or shared office space. However, the majority of providers were unaware of how their colleagues approached delivery of HPV vaccine.

Readiness for implementation

Few providers reported leadership engagement in system-level improvement activities or use of available resources (such as their EMR and reminder calls) to increase use of HPV vaccine. Only one provider reported training for office staff involved with vaccine delivery.

Implementation climate

In some practices that delivered both the other adolescent vaccines at the 11–12 year old check-up visit, delivery of HPV vaccine fit well with existing workflows. In others, delivery required additional work at a subsequent check-up visit. More than half of providers reported that increasing use of HPV vaccine was a relatively high priority for improvement within their practice, but there were no statements that demonstrated a tension for change. Although all aspired to 100% vaccine coverage, none had any formal goals for themselves or their practice, or monitored vaccine coverage.

Characteristics of individuals domain

Knowledge and beliefs

All providers believed that HPV vaccine was an important vaccine and had a personal investment in providing the vaccine. Several routinely provided vaccine-related facts about HPV vaccine to parents such as usage data to address safety concerns. The majority of providers were aware that earlier vaccination resulted in an increased immune response. They varied in their belief that the vaccine should be initiated at age 11–12 years, and that there was benefit to initiating the HPV series by bundling with Tdap and MCV4. While some were very supportive of this "bundling," others thought it was "a harder sell." Several providers were reluctant to immunize pre-pubertal teens and tailored their recommendation to their perception of the child's risk of sexual activity. One provider mentioned concern that the duration of protection may not be adequate if provided at age 11–12.

Self-efficacy

Providers varied in their confidence to strongly recommend HPV vaccine at the 11–12 year visit and to convince hesitant parents to accept it. Many expressed frustration with hesitant parents as demonstrated by this quote:

> "You can talk until you're blue in the face and give every ounce of evidence and research behind what you do and why you do it. They don't listen. It just—it's frustrating as a provider. Extremely frustrating."

Readiness to change

Several providers had engaged in informal efforts to change their approach to increase vaccine use. An example is described by this provider.

> "I used to say, "I have an optional vaccine." And, I found that when I said that, I had a very, very low, um, percentage of patients who agreed to take it. So, I don't use the word 'optional' anymore."

Process domain

Planning

No-one used a formal planning process initially to implement HPV vaccine or subsequently to change their approach to vaccine use.

Engaging

Few providers had actively engaged staff members in problem solving to increase vaccine use or expected their Medical Assistants (MAs) to endorse vaccination.

> "[The MA's] don't really influence the parents' decisions about vaccines...They administer the vaccines, but they're not counseling."

Executing

Providers universally assumed responsibility for vaccine delivery and reported the same approach for girls and boys. Typically, they recommended the HPV vaccine at the 11–12 year old visit, although the strength of this recommendation varied. Some providers routinely shared personal information about vaccinating their children or grandchildren, while others only provided this information if asked. One provider had the MA present all three vaccines as "the vaccines recommended today," and only discussed benefits and concerns if requested by the parent. He suggested that this MA-driven process of presenting this vaccine as "no different from any other vaccine" was very effective. He thought that the more traditional approach of "We're gonna do this vaccine today, this vaccine today, and your doctor will discuss this vaccine with you today. ..." both "justified the concern that families have if they came in with it and it created concern in families that didn't."

Teamwork to deliver the vaccine series was uncommon. Many providers were unaware of the approach their MA took with parents regarding follow-up doses after they had immunized them with the first dose.

All providers reported that they had vaccine-only visits and offered follow-up doses at acute care visits. Few used practice-level strategies to support subsequent doses such as routinely booking follow-up appointments or making reminder calls to parents. Most often the responsibility to schedule the 2nd and 3rd doses was left to the parent.

Reflecting and evaluating

No providers reviewed HPV vaccine coverage data. One provider commented that, "it's not as easy as you think to get the data out of here [the EMR]."

Integrated data results

Of the 72 CFIR constructs assessed in the table with the coverage rates, seven strongly distinguished and seven weakly distinguished between providers with higher versus lower HPV vaccine coverage. These constructs are briefly described here and are summarized in Table 4 as facilitators and barriers to vaccine use.

Intervention characteristics domain

Within the intervention characteristics domain, relative advantage and adaptability of the age of initiation were strongly distinguishing constructs, one acting as a facilitator and one as a barrier to vaccine use. All providers in the higher coverage group had positive ratings for perceiving a relative advantage to providing the vaccine at age 11–12 years as suggested by the guidelines compared to delaying until the teen is older, as characterized in this quote.

> "We would recommend the Tdap, the Menactra, as well as the HPV. ...We recommend starting the HPV at that age, simply because the earlier you start it, the more effective it becomes. You want to start it because you want to get the kids before there's any concern for any exposure. You wanna make sure that they complete their series. We always routinely recommend that at 11."

Table 4 Facilitators and Barriers for completing the HPV vaccine series by 13th birthday

CFIR Domain	Facilitators	Barriers
Characteristics of HPV vaccine recommendations	*Perceived advantage to vaccinate at age 11/12 compared to older: • Increased immunogenicity • Efficient; Can bundle • Complete series before exposure • Easier patient access	*Adapt recommendation to initiate at older age
External environment and context	Financial incentives for series completion: • Increased billing • Meaningful use for Medicaid	*Not mandated by school therefore offer as optional at age 11/12
Internal context of practice	• Communication across staff and providers to coordinate series completion • Leadership engaged in system level improvements e.g., EMR • Use of multiple available resources e.g., EMR alert, outreach calls	
Characteristics and attitudes of providers	• *Perceive value in completing series by age 13 • Perceive value in bundling 3 adolescent vaccines • *Confident to strongly recommend HPV vaccine and to convince hesitant parents • Enthusiastic about HPV vaccine • *Already made efforts to increase HPV vaccine use	
Process for implementation of HPV vaccine recommendations	• *Routinely provide strong recommendation for HPV vaccine at age 11/12 and bundle 3 vaccines • Involve staff in meaningful problem-solving • Reflect on HPV vaccine use with a view to making changes	

*Strongly distinguishing factor

None of the providers with higher coverage routinely adapted the recommended age of vaccine initiation. Providers with lower coverage routinely initiated the vaccine series at a later age when they described the parents as "more accepting."

Outer setting domain

Within the outer setting domain, patient needs and resources was a strongly distinguishing construct. Providers who anticipated that parents wanted to know which vaccines offered at the 11–12 year old checkup were mandatory for school attendance routinely suggested HPV vaccine as optional at that visit. These providers also had lower vaccine coverage suggesting this construct is a barrier to HPV vaccine use. One provider described her typical approach:

> "Because the Menactra is, and the Tdap are required by school, I guess I introduce them by saying these are the vaccines they get at 11, in order to go to school. The other one I say we highly encourage that your child gets the HPV."

None of the providers with higher coverage adjusted the adolescent vaccine recommendation in this way and they were more likely to routinely discuss vaccine safety than those with lower coverage. Other factors in this domain weakly distinguished between higher and lower vaccine coverage. Providers with higher coverage were less likely to feel peer pressure to change their implementation approach and were more likely to have positive ratings for responding to financial incentives as demonstrated by this quote:

> "...... we're imagining that a lot of the parameters they're using for meaningful-use will also be for pay for performance... and so we wanna make sure our percentages are up there so, we're, we're always very cognizant of those red flags (*... to indicate a vaccine is due)* and, and that they need to be checked off." ... "That, that's the main incentive. Um, you know. Meaningful use."

These findings suggest that a statement of vaccine safety and awareness of financial incentives can facilitate vaccine use.

Inner setting domain

Within the inner setting domain, patterns of ratings in the dimensions of networks and communications and readiness for implementation weakly distinguished provider-level vaccine coverage, acting to facilitate use. Providers who communicated with staff to coordinate vaccine use; reported a consistent approach across providers in their practice; described leadership engagement in system-level improvement activities and use of available resources to provide HPV vaccine had higher vaccine coverage than those who did not report these features.

Characteristics of individuals domain

Within the characteristics of the individual domain, many factors distinguished between higher and lower vaccine coverage, all facilitating vaccine use. The knowledge and beliefs of the providers about HPV vaccine was a strongly distinguishing construct. Providers with higher coverage were more likely to believe there was value in completing the vaccine series by age 13 and in bundling the three recommended adolescent vaccines at the 11–12 year checkup visit. Provider self-efficacy was a strongly distinguishing construct as was readiness to change of individual providers. Providers with higher coverage were more likely to be enthusiastic and confident in strongly recommending the vaccine at age 11–12 and in their ability to convince hesitant parents to accept the vaccine as demonstrated by this quote:

> "...I feel like I'm able to work through their concerns, rebut any inaccuracies that they come in with, and give them the right information they need to make a decision to proceed."

In contrast, those with lower coverage did not share this confidence as demonstrated by this quote:

> "...typically, if they're not going to give it, nothing you're going to tell them is going to change their mind."

Those with higher coverage were more likely to already have engaged in personal efforts to increase HPV vaccine use such as adding provider reminders to the EMR.

Process domain

Within the process domain, executing was a strongly distinguishing construct. All providers with higher coverage routinely strongly recommended and routinely provided the vaccine at the 11–12 year old check-up visit, and bundled the three adolescent vaccines. Also, they were more likely to provide personal information about HPV vaccine use as described by one provider:

> "I give a quick spiel about how I think it's really important, how it helps protect against cancer, how it's safe, we've given lots of doses, nationwide lots of doses have been given, it's effective, it prevents cancer, I give it to my kids and lots of kids every day, I think it's really important..."

Several constructs weakly distinguished between providers with higher and lower coverage. Evidence of planning, engaging, and reflecting and evaluating was most often associated with higher coverage, suggesting these constructs facilitate use.

Discussion

Study findings both confirm that effective strategies to increase HPV vaccine use are urgently needed and inform their development. By systematically examining the complex web of factors that influence use of this vaccine in the primary care setting, we identified important facilitators and barriers to following National guidelines. We learned that a multi-level approach is needed to markedly increase use of this important vaccine. At the provider-level, buy-in to vaccination by age 13 is critical as is the provider's confidence to address parental hesitancy. At the interpersonal-level, our findings suggest several strategies the provider could use with the patient, parents and staff to increase vaccine use. These include recommending the three adolescent vaccines as a bundle and addressing parental hesitation with a strong and persistent recommendation for timely HPV vaccine use. Better co-ordination between the provider and staff who administer the vaccine could standardize communication messages for patients and parents and ensure opportunities for vaccination are not missed. At the practice-level, collaboration among providers could improve efficiency by standardizing use of reminder systems and maximize benefit from financial incentives.

Our findings confirm that the provider's approach to HPV vaccine personally, interpersonally and at the practice level, strongly influences uptake. [15, 16] Providers in these independent community practices universally assumed responsibility for vaccine delivery, and reported they routinely recommended HPV vaccine, Tdap and MCV4 to their patients at their 11–12 year-old checkup visit. Our analysis demonstrated that the quality of their recommendation varied widely as did HPV vaccine coverage by age 13. These findings are consistent with national studies with larger samples [17, 18] and likely reflect the complexity of communication about this vaccine. [18] Failure to require HPV vaccine for school attendance influenced some providers to suggest that the vaccine could be delayed [19] and anticipation of parental resistance caused them to feel compelled to have a conversation about the vaccine. This likely contributed to reduced vaccine uptake as parents are more likely to resist vaccination recommendations if the provider uses a participatory, conversational approach rather than a more directive approach (a presumptive or announcement approach). [20, 21] It is likely that providers' lack of buy-in to vaccination by age 13 and their low self-efficacy to address parental hesitancy further compromised their ability to provide a strong recommendation. At the practice-level, reminder and recall systems that can increase vaccine series initiation and completion, [9, 10, 22, 23] were infrequently used. Many providers in our sample lacked resources such as information technology (IT) support to augment their EMR with these systems. [24]

Effective implementation strategies must help providers to change their approach to HPV vaccine. However, changing provider behavior is difficult. Educational interventions targeting providers have not been successful, [9] and reminders and audit and feedback have had mixed results. [9] Although lack of a strong provider recommendation is reputed to be the most common barrier to use of HPV vaccine, [15–17, 25] few studies have tried to improve the quality of provider communication. One randomized trial conducted in the primary care setting showed that training providers to use an announcement approach increased vaccine coverage by 5%, [8] but the broader literature of message framing has yielded mixed results. [18] In addition to changing provider behavior regarding the timing and quality of their recommendation for HPV vaccine, our findings suggest the need for providers to develop an adolescent vaccine delivery system. While a systematic approach was effective in a large healthcare system with access to staff and technical support for implementation, [19] most interventions to systematize vaccination in primary care practices have been disappointing and expensive. [9] [26] A recent randomized controlled trial showed an intervention comprised of provider education, audit and feedback and EMR reminders increased vaccine initiation by 8% and the intervention was relatively inexpensive, but may not be scalable without IT support. [27] Effective, scalable interventions to encourage and support providers in independent practices to deliver HPV vaccine to all eligible teens in a timely fashion are needed. [10]

Our findings inform an implementation strategy to change provider behavior regarding this complex vaccine. An acceptable approach will be simple to use, save time, and alleviate the stress associated with dealing with vaccine hesitant parents. [28] Key ingredients might include the following: 1) Education to motivate behavior change and increase self-efficacy. Providers must be convinced of the benefits of early initiation of the vaccine series and able to succinctly and comfortably address parental concerns. 2) To facilitate change, additional pragmatic resources such as a communication strategy to increase the quality of vaccine recommendation are needed. 3) Targeting increased coverage for any age before the 15th birthday may engage more providers in the change process and capitalize on the latest recommendation for a 2-shot series. [5] It would also significantly impact the Healthy People 2020 goal of 80% coverage for 13–15 year olds. 4) Finally, engaging staff in developing and implementing a new vaccine delivery system to increase vaccine use would be beneficial. Failure to simultaneously address all these factors may explain why prior interventions to improve use of HPV vaccine have had at best a modest effect and changes have not been sustained.

Our study is limited by several considerations. Although we believe the study sample is representative of providers working in independent, community-based pediatric practices in our community with considerable variation in the context of where and how the providers practiced, our convenience sample of 16 providers is small and from one geographic area and may not be representative of other populations. Completion of the 3-dose series before the 13th birthday was low among participants, consistent with national data. [7] As no providers had high vaccine uptake, our findings regarding barriers and facilitators for HPV vaccine uptake should be considered as exploratory. The time span for collecting the quantitative and qualitative data were different (2014 and 2016 respectively. National data show the increase in HPV vaccine coverage from 2014 to 2015 was minimal, and suggest that a dramatic change between 2014 and 2016 is unlikely. [7, 29] However, if changes in coverage were large and not equal across providers, then our assessment of barriers and facilitators may be inaccurate. Finally, our qualitative data was retrospective and we did not interview parents or patients.

Conclusions

In conclusion, study and national data suggest that many teens are not protected against HPV-related cancers prior to exposure to the virus and that widespread efforts to increase HPV vaccine use are urgently needed. Using CFIR to systematically examine the use of this vaccine in independent primary care practices enabled us to identify facilitators and barriers at the provider, interpersonal and practice level that need to be addressed in future efforts to increase vaccine use in such settings. Our findings suggest that implementation strategies that target the provider and help them to address multi-level barriers to HPV vaccine use merit further investigation.

Abbreviations

AAP: American Academy of Pediatrics; ACIP: Advisory Committee on Immunization Practices; CDC: Centers for Disease Control and Prevention; EMR: Electronic Medical Record; HEDIS: Healthcare Effectiveness Data and Information Set; HPV: Human Papillomavirus; IQR: Inter-quartile range; MCV4: Quadrivalent meningococcal vaccine; NCATS: National Center for Advancing Translational Sciences; NIH: National Institutes of Health; Tdap: Tetanus, diphtheria and pertussis vaccine; U.S.: United States; VIS: Vaccine information sheet; WU PAARC: Washington University Pediatric and Ambulatory Research Consortium

Funding

This study was supported by the Washington University Institute of Clinical and Translational Sciences grant UL1 TR000448 from the National Center for Advancing Translational Sciences (NCATS) of the National Institutes of Health (NIH), with co-funding from St. Louis Children's Hospital. This study's contents are solely the responsibility of the author and do not necessarily represent the official view of NCATS or NIH. The sponsors had no involvement in the design and conduct of the study; collection, management, analysis, and interpretation of the data; preparation, review, or approval of the manuscript; and decision to submit the manuscript for publication.

Author's contributions

JMG designed the study, conducted interviews, analyzed and interpreted the qualitative and quantitative data, and drafted the manuscript. SD analyzed and interpreted the qualitative data and critically reviewed and edited the manuscript. EW conducted interviews, analyzed and interpreted the qualitative data, and critically reviewed and edited the manuscript. AAL analyzed and interpreted the qualitative data, and critically reviewed and edited the manuscript. KK analyzed and interpreted the qualitative data, and critically reviewed and edited the manuscript. RL designed the study, analyzed and interpreted the qualitative data, and critically reviewed and edited the manuscript. All authors read and approved the final manuscript.

Consent for publication

We confirm that the consent form signed by all participants provides consent to publish anonymous quotes within the manuscript.

Competing interests

The authors declare that they have no competing interests.

Author details

[1]Departments of Medicine and Pediatrics, Washington University School of Medicine, St. Louis, MO, USA. [2]Department of Pediatrics, Washington University School of Medicine, Campus Box 8116, 660 S. Euclid Ave, St. Louis, MO 63110, USA. [3]Department of Pediatrics, Michigan Medicine, C.S. Mott Children's Hospital, Ann Arbor, USA. [4]Department of Surgery, Washington University School of Medicine, St. Louis, MO, USA.

References

1. Fu LY, Bonhomme LA, Cooper SC, Joseph JG, Zimet GD. Educational interventions to increase HPV vaccination acceptance: a systematic review. Vaccine. 2014;32(17):1901–20.
2. President's Cancer Panel Annual Report 2012-2013 [http://deainfo.nci.nih.gov/advisory/pcp/annualReports/HPV/PDF/PCP_Annual_Report_2012-2013.pdf]. Accessed 30 Apr 2018.
3. Gertig DM, Brotherton JM, Budd AC, Drennan K, Chappell G, Saville AM. Impact of a population-based HPV vaccination program on cervical abnormalities: a data linkage study. BMC Med. 2013;11:227.
4. Markowitz LE, Dunne EF, Saraiya M, Chesson HW, Curtis CR, Gee J, Bocchini JA Jr, Unger ER, Centers for Disease C, Prevention. Human papillomavirus vaccination: recommendations of the Advisory Committee on Immunization Practices (ACIP). MMWR Recomm Rep. 2014;63(RR-05):1–30.
5. Meites E, Kempe A, Markowitz LE. Use of a 2-dose schedule for human papillomavirus vaccination - updated recommendations of the advisory

committee on immunization practices. MMWR Morb Mortal Wkly Rep. 2016;65(49):1405–8.
6. Healthy People 2020 [http://healthypeople.gov/]. Accessed 30 Apr 2018.
7. Reagan-Steiner S, Yankey D, Jeyarajah J, Elam-Evans LD, Curtis CR, MacNeil J, Markowitz LE, Singleton JA. National, regional, state, and selected local area vaccination coverage among adolescents aged 13–17 years - United States, 2015. MMWR Morb Mortal Wkly Rep. 2016;65(33):850–8.
8. Brewer NT, Hall ME, Malo TL, Gilkey MB, Quinn B, Lathren C. Announcements Versus Conversations to Improve HPV Vaccination Coverage: A Randomized Trial. Pediatrics. 2017;139(1):e20161764.
9. Smulian EA, Mitchell KR, Stokley S. Interventions to increase HPV vaccination coverage: a systematic review. Human vaccines & immunotherapeutics. 2016;12(6):1566–88.
10. Niccolai LM, Hansen CE. Practice- and community-based interventions to increase human papillomavirus vaccine coverage: a systematic review. JAMA Pediatr. 2015;169(7):686–92.
11. Damschroder LJ, Aron DC, Keith RE, Kirsh SR, Alexander JA, Lowery JC. Fostering implementation of health services research findings into practice: a consolidated framework for advancing implementation science. Implementation science : IS. 2009;4:50.
12. Fetters MD, Curry LA, Creswell JW. Achieving Integration in Mixed Methods Designs - Principles and Practices. Health Serv Res. 2013;48:1–23.
13. Immunization and Infectious Diseases [https://www.healthypeople.gov/2020/topics-objectives/topic/immunization-and-infectious-diseases/objectives]. Accessed 30 Apr 2018.
14. Palinkas LA. Qualitative and mixed methods in mental health services and implementation research. J Clin Child Adolesc Psychol. 2014;43(6):851–61.
15. Holman DM, Benard V, Roland KB, Watson M, Liddon N, Stokley S. Barriers to human papillomavirus vaccination among US adolescents: a systematic review of the literature. JAMA Pediatr. 2014;168(1):76–82.
16. Perkins RB, Clark JA, Apte G, Vercruysse JL, Sumner JJ, Wall-Haas CL, Rosenquist AW, Pierre-Joseph N. Missed opportunities for HPV vaccination in adolescent girls: a qualitative study. Pediatrics. 2014;134(3):e666–74.
17. Gilkey MB, Calo WA, Moss JL, Shah PD, Marciniak MW, Brewer NT. Provider communication and HPV vaccination: the impact of recommendation quality. Vaccine. 2016;34(9):1187–92.
18. Gilkey MB, McRee AL. Provider communication about HPV vaccination: a systematic review. Human vaccines & immunotherapeutics. 2016; 12(6):1454–68.
19. Farmar AM, Love-Osborne K, Chichester K, Breslin K, Bronkan K, Hambidge SJ. Achieving High Adolescent HPV Vaccination Coverage. Pediatrics. 2016;138(5):e20152653.
20. Opel DJ, Mangione-Smith R, Robinson JD, Heritage J, DeVere V, Salas HS, Zhou C, Taylor JA. The influence of provider communication behaviors on parental vaccine acceptance and visit experience. Am J Public Health. 2015; 105(10):1998–2004.
21. Opel DJ, Heritage J, Taylor JA, Mangione-Smith R, Salas HS, Devere V, Zhou C, Robinson JD. The architecture of provider-parent vaccine discussions at health supervision visits. Pediatrics. 2013;132(6):1037–46.
22. Szilagyi PG, Albertin C, Humiston SG, Rand CM, Schaffer S, Brill H, Stankaitis J, Yoo BK, Blumkin A, Stokley S. A randomized trial of the effect of centralized reminder/recall on immunizations and preventive care visits for adolescents. Acad Pediatr. 2013;13(3):204–13.
23. Tierney CD, Yusuf H, McMahon SR, Rusinak D, OB MA, Massoudi MS, Lieu TA. Adoption of reminder and recall messages for immunizations by pediatricians and public health clinics. Pediatrics. 2003;112(5):1076–82.
24. Wolfson D, Bernabeo E, Leas B, Sofaer S, Pawlson G, Pillittere D. Quality improvement in small office settings: an examination of successful practices. BMC Fam Pract. 2009;10:14.
25. Darden PM, Thompson DM, Roberts JR, Hale JJ, Pope C, Naifeh M, Jacobson RM. Reasons for not vaccinating adolescents: National Immunization Survey of teens, 2008-2010. Pediatrics. 2013;131(4):645–51.
26. Perkins RB, Zisblatt L, Legler A, Trucks E, Hanchate A, Gorin SS. Effectiveness of a provider-focused intervention to improve HPV vaccination rates in boys and girls. Vaccine. 2015;33(9):1223–9.
27. Fiks AG, Grundmeier RW, Mayne S, Song L, Feemster K, Karavite D, Hughes CC, Massey J, Keren R, Bell LM, et al. Effectiveness of decision support for families, clinicians, or both on HPV vaccine receipt. Pediatrics. 2013;131(6):1114–24.
28. Kempe A, O'Leary ST, Kennedy A, Crane LA, Allison MA, Beaty BL, Hurley LP, Brtnikova M, Jimenez-Zambrano A, Stokley S. Physician response to parental requests to spread out the recommended vaccine schedule. Pediatrics. 2015;135(4):666–77.
29. Laurie D, Elam-Evans DY, Jeyarajah J, Singleton JA, Robinette Curtis C, MacNeil J, Hariri S. National, Regional, State, and Selected Local Area Vaccination Coverage Among Adolescents Aged 13–17 Years — United States, 2013. In: Morbidity and Mortality Weekly Report (MMWR), vol. 63. Atlanta: Centers for Disease Control and Prevention; 2014. p. 625–33.

9

A focus group study to understand biases and confounders in a cluster randomized controlled trial on low back pain in primary care in Norway

Erik L. Werner[1*], Ida Løchting[2], Kjersti Storheim[2] and Margreth Grotle[3]

Abstract

Background: Cluster randomized controlled trials are often used in research in primary care but creates challenges regarding biases and confounders. We recently presented a study on low back pain from primary care in Norway with equal effects in the intervention and the control group. In order to understand the specific mechanisms that may produce biases in a cluster randomized trial we conducted a focus group study among the participating health care providers. The aim of this study was to understand how the participating providers themselves influenced on the study and thereby possibly on the results of the cluster randomized controlled trial.

Methods: The providers were invited to share their experiences from their participation in the COPE study, from recruitment of patients to accomplishment of either the intervention or control consultations. Six clinicians from the intervention group and four from the control group took part in the focus group interviews. The group discussions focused on feasibility of the study in primary care and particularly on identifying potential biases and confounders in the study. The audio-recorded interviews were transcribed verbatim and analyzed according to a systematic text condensation. The themes for the analysis emerged from the group discussions.

Results: A personal interest for back pain, logistic factors at the clinics and an assessment of the patients' capacity to accomplish the study prior to their recruitment was reported. The providers were allowed to provide additional therapy to the intervention and it turned out that some of these could be regarded as opposed to the messages of the intervention. The providers seemed to select different items from the educational package according to personal beliefs and their perception of the patients' acceptance.

Conclusion: The study disclosed several potential biases to the COPE study which may have impacted on the study results. Awareness of these is highly important when planning and conducting a cluster randomized controlled trial. Procedures in the recruitment of both providers and patients seem to be key factors and the providers should be aware of their role in a scientific study in order to standardize the provision of the intervention.

Background

The nature of primary health care creates challenges for clinical trials that are different from the specialized health care. A limited number of eligible patients at each site in primary care require a greater number of clinicians at different locations involved in the trial than in a hospital department with referred patients.

* Correspondence: e.l.werner@medisin.uio.no
[1]Department of General Practice, Institute of Health and Society, Faculty of Medicine, University of Oslo, Oslo, Norway
Full list of author information is available at the end of the article

Therefore cluster randomized controlled trials (cRCT) are often used in primary care settings because the randomization procedure is then performed on the health care providers and not on the subjects producing the data [1]. However, both ethics and validity of the data have been questioned in the cRCT study design [2, 3].

We have recently conducted and published a study on a treatment of low back pain (LBP) among general practitioners (GPs) and physiotherapists (PTs) in Norway, using cRCT as the study method [4]. The COPE study aimed to produce a simple tool for GPs and PTs in primary care for treatment of patients with LBP. The providers in the intervention group were thoroughly trained for performing the intervention appropriately, while the providers in the control group were instructed to follow their best practices as usual care. Also in the intervention group, additional care according to the provider's or the patient's wish was allowed (i.e. physiotherapy, medication etc.) [5].

Although we observed great improvements in both disability and sickness absence in both the intervention group and the control group, we were unable to report significant differences between the groups [4]. We therefore wanted to investigate whether there were factors related to the study design that were accountable for this result. In scientific literature such process evaluation are more often asked for [6].

As opposed to a randomized controlled trial (RCT) where the subjects in question are facing a randomization procedure, the cRCT involves an extra level [1]. The randomization procedure is normally conducted on a number of providers who in turn will provide the intervention on the subjects who produce the data. While an intervention in studies on drugs may be easily accomplished regarding blinding and administration and dosage of the actual drug in study, this is more complicated when people constitutes the intervention. This may be even more complicated when the health care providers involved are not working at the same department and have different backgrounds, experiences and attitudes. How may we ensure that the subjects actually receive an identical intervention provided by different providers at different locations?

The challenges with differences between providers providing a specific procedure in clinical practice may also be valid in ordinary RCTs conducted at different locations or by different providers as in multicenter studies. However, we assumed that the extra level of the recruitment procedure (providers and patients) in a cRCT poses more possible biases to the study. Therefore, we invited all participating clinicians in the COPE study [4] to a focus group discussion on this theme. The aim of this study was to understand how the participating health care providers themselves influenced on the study and thereby possibly on the results.

Methods

The COPE study

In 2008 20 general practitioners (GPs) and 20 physiotherapists (PTs) were recruited through an information meeting at Oslo University Hospital Ullevål, to participate in a clinical trial in primary health care on LBP patients. Through a randomization procedure, half of the GPs and PTs were randomized to perform the intervention while the other half constituted the control group. All providers should include consecutively LBP patients with more than 4 weeks duration of pain, but less than 1 year. All patients in both intervention and control group would meet with their provider for 30 min every week for 4 weeks, but only those in the intervention group would be provided with the specific content of the trial.

A manual based on the "Explain Pain" concept of Butler & Moseley [7] was developed adjusted to the setting and aims of the study. The "Explain Pain" concept is a simple education of patients in pain physiology, and the idea is that if the LBP patient understands these mechanisms he or she will be better capable to draw right conclusions on health behavior and consequently cope with the pain until it eventually fades away [7]. The providers in the intervention group were thoroughly trained in the manual while the concept was not communicated to the control group. The protocol for the study is previously described in detail [5] and the results are presented elsewhere [4].

According to the protocol, the recruitment of 300 patients was planned to take place during 2009 and 2010. For several reasons, the recruitment period lasted for 4 years and was not closed until January 2013 with 220 included patients [4].

The focus group study

We conducted a generic qualitative study as the aim of our study was to understand the processes of the COPE study [8, 9]. All 36 participating clinicians in the COPE study were in spring 2013 invited by e-mail or a phone call to take part in a focus group study on their experiences with the study. Six clinicians from the intervention group and four from the control group participated in two separate focus group interviews. Four of the participants from the intervention groups were PTs while two were GPs. In the control group, three of the participants were PTs while one was a GP. Each of the two group sessions lasted for 90 min (the participants were gathered only once) and took place at the location of the Research and communication unit for musculoskeletal health (FORMI) at Oslo University Hospital.

The participants were invited to share their experiences from their participation in the COPE study, from recruitment of patients to accomplishment of either the intervention or control consultations. In the group discussions we focused on feasibility of the study in primary care and particularly on identifying potential biases and confounders in the study. An interview guide was produced prior to the interviews and the groups were moderated by ELW with MG and IL as observers (see Additional file 1). ELW is experienced by three former qualitative studies (of which two focus group studies) while MG and IL had limited experience with this methodology. The themes of the interview guide followed each step of the study from recruitment and randomization of health care providers, to recruitment of patients at each site. We also discussed the content of the four sessions in both the intervention and the control groups. Also the providers' adherence to the manual in the intervention group was discussed and for all participants, their personal views on the study were asked for.

The audio-recorded interviews were transcribed verbatim and all authors collaborated on analysis conducted as systematic text condensation [10]. The four steps comprised: (i) reading all the material to obtain an overall impression, (ii) identifying units of meaning, representing different aspects of participants' experiences with the study according to the aims of the study, and coding for these, (iii) condensing the contents of each of the coded groups, and (iv) summarizing the contents of each group to generalize the findings.

The systematic text condensation starts with all researchers reading all the audio-recorded interviews separately. Following a discussion of these, we started to group statements and experiences into units of meaning. Then we looked at our units and found several that could be combined. The coding procedure had the four steps of the COPE study as starting point and units of meaning were placed according to these steps. We thoroughly checked that all important statements found their place in one of the categories.

Ethics

All GPs and PTs participating in the COPE study were invited to take part in the focus group study. We included all those who volunteered and due to the limited number of participants we were unable to balance the groups according to age, gender, years of practice. The participants were informed about the study and gave their consent orally. We found the study not to be subject to approval by the Ethical Committee due to the participants' professional status. The tape recordings and the transcriptions are all anonymized and stored at FORMI, Oslo University Hospital.

Results

The results were categorized into four important aspects of the accomplishment of the COPE study: (i) recruitment of participating clinicians, (ii) recruitment of participating patients, (iii) conducting the intervention (or control), and (iv) the health care providers' own benefits from having participated in the study. Within all these aspects, the responses were analyzed in respect of any impact on the study results.

Specific interest in back pain among the participating professionals

All participants agreed that a genuine interest for back pain was an absolute requirement for their participation. To be a part of research and being in an environment that shared the same interest was described as exciting and interesting. Several also found it developing and felt that participation increased their knowledge about back pain. Several also highlighted that the intervention gave them a practical tool for their management of LBP patients.

> *"It was exciting with a new way to address back pain. That was my motivation." (GP in intervention group).*

Selections based on good chemistry?

Recruitment of patients was reported to be facilitated by the fact that participation provided four sessions with the provider free of charge. In addition, it was necessary that the provider felt a good chemistry with the patients and that the provider himself or herself had confidence in the content of the intervention.

Due to slow recruitment process of the patients, a small number of patients were recruited through advertising in newspapers during the study period. This was also appreciated by several of the participants, and it seemed that patients recruited through this advertising were more prepared for an intervention containing education rather than physical treatment.

> *"It was fantastic to have these that were recruited actively, versus those we picked ourselves. Some of these, they had....they took all the points, they were so ready for it." (GP in intervention group)*

Some providers disclosed that lack of good chemistry with a patient could exclude patients from the study because the clinician was uncomfortable with the idea of spending so much time with the patient, or was unsure of the patient's acceptance of the messages. In addition, the providers seemed to conduct an active selection of patients according to their own perceptions of the patient's language skills and intellectual capacity. It was assumed that the intervention required a certain level of understanding of the messages.

Also general logistics at the clinic seemed to influence the recruitment. Sometimes the secretary or colleagues forgot to refer eligible patients, but also if it was late on the working day the provider felt it too bothersome to inform and in some way persuade the patient to take part in the study.

For some reason all participating providers experienced a general lack of eligible patients which made recruitment slow and difficult. They also experienced the intervention as more demanding and time consuming than ordinary treatment, which may have declined the interest for recruiting patients.

Difficult to adhere to the manual accurately

Most of the clinicians experienced that providing the intervention was easier across time, indicating improved skills with exercise. They were also encouraged if they experienced that the patient really benefited from the education and improved in health. Some started to use elements of the treatment also for patients with other unspecific pain conditions. However, despite several meetings and a DVD providing accurate accomplishment of each of the four sessions, some of the participants called for more training in the intervention.

According to the participants, patients' expectancies to the treatment could be both a facilitator and an obstacle. If the patient expected a physical treatment, they could sometimes have a hard time to accept a treatment based on education. Several professionals presented this as specifically challenging. On the other hand, some patients seemed to receive a new understanding of their pain and were grateful for the new coping strategy, which in some way could give more energy to the sessions.

> *"The patients expected a treatment – a new treatment. And so they came and received conversations..... about matters they may be already knew. They expected more. And all we said, they did it already...." (GP in intervention group)*

Some of the PTs provided manual therapy as an additional care to the intervention, and the clinicians were asked if this could represent a conflicting communication. On the one hand to explain the pain within the frames of expectations and sensitization and on the other hand provide manipulation on a perceived physical cause for the pain. The clinicians argued with referral to the patients' expectations and wishes and regarded the manipulation as more complementary treatment than conflicting messages.

One GP illustrated the difficulties with the provision of the messages in the space between psychological and physical aetiology:

> *"I think that across time one moved within a very narrow space between somatic and psychological and cognitive..... As "no, it is nothing mental", "no, you're not depressed", "no, there is no injury in the back". You should, in a way, wedge the message between all these things." (GP in intervention group)*

Some providers were unsure of their personal qualifications and authority to provide the intervention properly. The discussions even revealed some uncertainty among the providers themselves whether they believed in the messages. Across time, it seemed that many providers selected some of the messages to be included and others, that were perceived too difficult, were excluded.

> *"The messages (of the study) seem to be in an outer edge, it is very popular to believe that the cause of the pain is not local but sensitization of the central nerve system.... But there might be cases of combinations..... patients may have a local problem with their recruitment of muscles that may provoke a local pain...." (PT in intervention group).*

While some PTs seemed to experience the 30 min intervention to be insufficient for conducting the study because many patients also wanted additional physical treatment, many of the GPs felt the intervention were too much time consuming. Particularly in the control group the GPs had difficulties with talking about the back pain for 30 min every week.

> *"...so when they met at the meetings, you start with the back and "how are you doing" etc. etc.. But I had to be aware not to put any cognitive approach into it because this should be a control group. (.....) So we did a little chatting, yes." (GP in control group)*

Making a strategy for the management of a complex group of patients

All intervention providers participating in the focus group interviews underscored the value of transferring elements of the intervention to other patients with unspecific pain conditions. They also appreciated the new knowledge they had received, which gave them tools for management of a variety of patients. They felt they had increased their consciousness on wordings in general in their communication with patients, and the long term contact with the patients had particularly for the GPs provided a broader insight in the patient's life.

> *"I have learned a lot about pain. When you explain, you learn for yourself...you have to think about what you say. (....) .... Which I probably use when I talk with patients." (PT in intervention group)*

> *"Previously, pain was something that I did not have any tool for talking about or address or explain, but now... I believe I can defuse the pain to a great extent." (PT in intervention group).*

On the other hand, the providers of the control groups hardly found any benefit from their participation a part from the award of having free training in the intervention after the closure of the study.

Discussion

This focus group study has disclosed a number of challenging factors that may impact on the results of a cRCT in primary care. The most important one is probably the great possibility of a selection bias. The findings might indicate that some of the clinicians did not include patients from the trial if they did not believe that he or she would be able to accept the content of the messages. Also simple logistic factors at the clinics could result in a selection bias in recruitment of the patients.

The risk of selection bias in cRCT is well known from previous research [11]. Farrin et al. argue that individuals should be recruited to the study before randomizing the professionals as this procedure will more likely ensure equality between the groups [12]. If that is not possible, the cluster allocation could be performed by someone independent by the study [13]. Neither of these procedures could have been possible in the COPE study as the recruitment was based on the providers' patient population and the patients were recruited consecutively as they visited their provider for back pain. This procedure was chosen in order to have the trial setting as close to normal practice as possible, as development of a tool for the management of back pain in primary care was the aim of the COPE study [4]. However, information according to a risk of bias tool in reporting from a cRCT is helpful to the reader to assess the validity of the study [14].

The participating health care providers also highlighted the importance of their personal interest for LBP and the felt need of a tool for best management of this patient group as necessary for their own enthusiasm and interest for learning this treatment strategy. This possible selection bias both on recruitment of patients and also on the recruitment of health care providers to the study questions the external validity of the study.

On the one hand, the possible selection bias on the recruitment of health care provider to the study may reflect real life: best practice is most likely provided by those with interest and knowledge in the field. However, this may complicate the delivery of the messages of a trial as these may be colored by the providers' personal attitudes and knowledge to a greater extent than by providers not particularly familiar with the field. This is somewhat exemplified by the PTs offering manual therapy as additional therapy, which was accepted in the study protocol, but still is based on a different view on back pain, being a physical injury in need for specific therapy. Furthermore, several of the PTs in the control group were familiar with the concept of Explain Pain and may unwillingly have provided messages in line with this.

Also adherence and compliance with the trial manual in the COPE study was questioned in the present study. Strategies for improving compliance among the providers have been presented [15]. Such strategies comprise thorough education of the participants not only on the intervention but also about their role as research participants, having continuous contact with the providers, and the provision of incentives for participation. Regarding the COPE study the providers' understanding of their role as research participants may have been insufficient according to the findings of the present study. The incentives provided (refund of the actual patient cost) may have been too small.

Process evaluation is highly recommended in the literature on cRCTs [15]. Obviously it would be helpful in the management of the study. For the COPE study the continuing meetings with the providers and the provision of a DVD recording the actual delivery of the messages may be regarded as a process evaluation. Following the trial, two separate master thesis have demonstrated a difference in ability to recall the messages of the sessions among the patients, in favor of those in the intervention group, and that the patients found the messages in the two groups equally favorable.

How much training is needed for the providers to be able to conduct a trial in accordance with the study manual? There is no accurate answer to that. In a study comparing three different training conditions, statistically significant differences favoring a seminar plus supervision over review of a manual or manual plus a training web site, were found [16]. The providers in the COPE study underwent an initial seminar and several meetings throughout the study period in addition to a DVD presenting the sessions. They did not have a specific individual supervision [4, 5].

Difficulties with patient recruitment in primary care studies have been reported previously. Therefore a subtype of cRCT named professional-cluster trial has been suggested [17, 18]. Also in this design, the providers are the target of the intervention but they do not provide any specific intervention towards their patients. It is the impact of the intervention on the providers that may alter their treatment and management of their patients across time that possibly will produce a better outcome on the patients.

Applied on our study, a professional-cluster trial could be that a number of health care providers received a thorough training in the guidelines for the management of LBP. They would not have to recruit patients specifically to a trial but outcomes on patients with LBP could be measured retrospectively at a later stage. The advantage of this design is that the providers do not have to actively recruit patients and by this the selection bias in recruitment is avoided. Possibly it would also have been more in accordance with the ethics suggested by the Ottawa Statement on the Ethical Design and Conduct of Cluster Randomized Trials [19]. A recent study on improved antibiotic prescription among Norwegian GPs has demonstrated success with this method [20]. In this study, the GPs were trained in groups to reduce inappropriate prescribing for older patients. Data was collected through extraction from the GPs electronic patient record system and no patients were actively recruited to the study [21].

There are limitations with this study. One is a lack of data saturation due to a limited number of participants in the focus groups. Although we invited all providers who had participated in the COPE study, only a few were willing to spend time on this. Also only three GPs were attending the groups. Nevertheless we believe that most items were disclosed during the group talks. Furthermore, aiming to explore possible biases in the COPE study by a qualitative study, the systematic text condensation does not necessarily demand "a complete description of all aspects of the phenomenon we study" [10].

For the analysis of this focus group study we chose to follow Malterud's systematic text condensation [10]. The procedure is presented in the Method section. The aim of the study was to explore the participants' views on the conduct of the COPE study, in order to understand the results of that trial. A methodology based on phenomenology seemed to be appropriate to that purpose.

Conclusion

Although the research design cRCT seems somewhat ideal for the structure of primary health care, our experiences disclose several potential serious biases which may be valid for all RCTs but possibly even more for cRCTs. Particularly it seems to be selection biases and uncertainty about the messages delivered. In our opinion the ways to overcome these biases suggested at present in the literature do not easily comply with the infrastructure of primary care. Researchers planning cRCT should pay attention to tools like the Cochrane risk of bias tool, the PRECIS-2 tool and The Ottawa statement on the ethics of cRCTs.

Abbreviations

COPE: The COgnitive patient education trial; cRCT: Cluster randomized controlled trial; FORMI: Research and communication unit for musculoskeletal health; GP: General practitioner; LBP: Low back pain; PT: Physiotherapist; RCT: Randomized controlled trial

Acknowledgements

Thanks to the participants of the focus groups for their valuable reflections and comments in the group sessions.

Authors' contributions

ELW was the leading manager of the study and took part in all parts of the study. IL was involved in planning the study, the accomplishment of the focus groups, analyzing the material and as co-author of the manuscript. KS was involved in planning the study, analyzing the material and as co-author of the manuscript. MG was involved in planning the study, the accomplishment of the focus groups, analyzing the material and as co-author of the manuscript. All authors had co-authored the papers of the COPE study. All authors read and approved the final manuscript.

Competing interests

The authors declares that they have no competing interests.

Author details

[1]Department of General Practice, Institute of Health and Society, Faculty of Medicine, University of Oslo, Oslo, Norway. [2]Research and Communication Unit for Musculoskeletal Health (FORMI) Clinic for Surgery and Neurology, Oslo University Hospital, Oslo, Norway. [3]Department of Physiotherapy, Oslo Metropolitan University/FORMI, Clinic for Surgery and Neurology, Oslo University Hospital, Oslo, Norway.

References

1. Murphy AW, Esterman A, Pilotto LS. Cluster randomized controlled trials in primary care: an introduction. Eur J Gen Pract. 2006;12:70–3.
2. Taljaard M, McRae AD, Wejer C, et al. Inadequate reporting of research ethics review and informed consent in cluster randomized trials: review of random sample of published trials. BMJ. 2011;342:d2496. https://doi.org/10.1136/bmj.d2496.
3. Eldridge SM, Ashby D, Feder GS, et al. Lessons for cluster randomized trials in the twenty-first century: a systematic review of trials in primary care. Clin Trials. 2004;1:80–90.
4. Werner EL, Storheim K, Løchting I, et al. Cognitive patient education for low back pain in primary care: a cluster randomized controlled trial and cost-effectiveness analysis. Spine. 2016;41(6):455–62.
5. Werner EL, Storheim K, Løchting I, et al. The COPE LBP trial: cognitive patient education for low back pain – a cluster randomized trial in primary care. BMC Musculoskeletal Dis. 2010;11:33.
6. Moore GF, Audrey S, Barker M, et al. Process evaluation of complex interventions: Medical Research Council guidance. BMJ. 2015;350:h1258. https://doi.org/10.1136/bmj.h1258.
7. Moseley L, Nicholas M, Hodges P. A randomized controlled trial of intensive neurophysiology education in chronic low back pain. Clin J Pain. 2004;20:324–30.
8. Caelli K, Ray L, Mill J. 'Clear as mud': towards greater clarity in generic qualitative research. Int J Qual Methods. 2003;2:2.
9. Merriam SB. Qualitative research and case study applications in education. San Fransisco: Jossey-Bass. ISBN-13: 978–0787910099.
10. Malterud K. Systematic text condensation: a strategy for qualitative analysis. Scand J Public Health. 2012;40:795–805.
11. Diaz-Ordaz K, Froud R, Sheenan B, Eldridge S. A systematic review of cluster randomized trials in residential facilities for older people suggests how to improve quality. BMC Med Res Methodol. 2013;13:127.
12. Farrin A, Russell I, Torgerson D, et al. Differential recruitment in a cluster randomized trial in primary care: the experience of the UK back pain, exercise, active management and Manipulatikon (UK BEAM) feasibility study. Clin Trials. 2005;2:119–24.
13. Eldridge S, Kerry S, Torgerson D. Bias in identifying and recruiting participants in cluster randomized trials: what can be done? BMJ. 2009;339:b4006.
14. Higgins JPT, Sterne JAC, Savović J, et al. A revised tool for assessing risk of bias in randomized trials. In: Chandler J, McKenzie J, Boutron I, Welch V, editors. Cochrane methods. Cochrane Database of Systematic Reviews; 2016, Issue 10 (Suppl 1). dx.doi.org. https://doi.org/10.1002/14651858.CD201601. Accessed 14 May 2018.
15. Grant A, Treweek S, Dreischulte T, et al. Process evaluation for cluster-randomised trials of complex interventions: a proposed framework for design and reporting. Trials. 2013;14:15.
16. Sholomskas DE, Syracuse-Siewert G, Rounsaville BJ, et al. We Don't train in vain: a dissemination trial of three strategies of training clinicians in cognitive-behavioral therapy. J Consult Clin Psychol. 2005;73(1):106–15.

17. Moberg J, Kramer M. A brief history of the cluster randomized trial design. JLL Bull: Comment History Treat Eval. 2015; http://www.jameslindlibrary.org/articles/a-brief-history-of-the-cluster-randomized-trial-design/. Accessed 14 May 2018.
18. Page MJ, French SD, McKenzie JE, et al. Recruitment difficulties in a primary care cluster randomised trial : investigating factors contributing to general practitioners' recruitment of patients. BMC Med Res Methodol. 2011;11:35. http://www.biomedcentral.com/1471-2288/11/35. Accessed 14 May 2018.
19. Weijer C, Grimshaw JM, Eccles MP, McRae AD, White A, Brehaut JC, et al. The Ottawa statement on the ethical design and conduct of cluster randomized trials. PLoS Med. 2012;9(11):e1001346. https://doi.org/10.1371/journal.pmed.1001346. Accessed 14 May 2018.
20. Rognstad S, Brekke M, Fetveit A, et al. Prescription peer academic detailing to reduce inappropriate prescribing for older patients: a cluster randomised controlled trial. Br J Gen Pract. 2013;63(613):e554–62.
21. Gjelstad S, Fetveit A, Straand J, et al. Can antibiotic prescriptions in respiratory tract infections be improved? A cluster-randomized educational intervention in general practice – the prescription peer academic detailing (Rx-PAD) study. BMC Health Serv Res. 2006;6:75. https://doi.org/10.1186/1472-6963-6-75. Accessed 14 May 2018.

10

The needs of informal caregivers and barriers of primary care workers toward dementia management in primary care

Meirong Wang[1†], Shuang Shao[1†], Jing Li[2], Yingjie Liu[1], Xiaojingyuan Xu[1] and Juan Du[1*]

Abstract

Background: Informal caregivers of people with dementia in Beijing are increasingly called upon to provide home-based care for their patients due to the increasing number of dementia patients and the shortage of standardized institutional solutions of care for patients in China. This study aimed to clarify the needs of informal caregivers and barriers of primary care workers toward dementia management in primary care in Beijing to provide references that may help to improve the care and services provided to individuals with dementia and their family caregivers residing in urban China.

Methods: A mixed-methods approach was used in this study. We performed individual in-depth interviews with 10 informal caregivers. Moreover, we carried out focus group interviews with 29 primary care workers. Content analysis was used to separately identify themes and codes. Discrepancies were discussed until final agreement was achieved.

Results: Three themes representing the core attitudes of informal caregivers and primary care workers were identified: care knowledge and skills, psychological counseling, and collaborative management. Most primary care workers believed that the management of dementia patients in primary care was necessary. However, due to the heavy work load and different medical specialties involved, these workers were unable to manage it.

Conclusions: Professional training focused on dementia for primary care workers should be strengthened. At the same time, the establishment of a community-based dementia team management model that includes specialists, community health service centers (CHSCs), and community committees should be explored.

Keywords: Dementia, Primary care, Qualitative approach, Beijing

Background

Estimates show that the number of people with dementia will increase from approximately 46.8 million in 2015 to 131 million by 2050 worldwide. In 2016, the global societal economic cost of dementia was estimated to be US$818 billion [1]. This situation challenges governments and health care providers to develop and improve services to people with dementia, with an emphasis on earlier diagnosis, the provision of support in the community, and the role of primary care services [2, 3]. Case management is described as a collaborative process of assessment, planning, facilitation and advocacy for options to meet an individual's health needs through communication and available resources to promote quality, cost-effective outcomes [4]. Dementia case management interventions are becoming a major way to manage dementia patients in primary care in North America and Europe [5, 6]. A systematic review had demonstrated that some needs (e.g., education about the disease) of patients and caregivers were well targeted by dementia case management, while some very common needs (e.g.,

* Correspondence: cuckoo@ccmu.edu.cn
†Meirong Wang and Shuang Shao contributed equally to this work.
[1]School of General Practice and Continuing Education, Capital Medical University, No.10 Xitoutiao, You An Men, Beijing 100069, China
Full list of author information is available at the end of the article

early diagnosis) were still overlooked [7]. Furthermore, general practitioners (GPs) often lack knowledge about dementia, and confidence in recognizing the symptoms, they are unsure about how - or if - cognitive screening should be conducted, and often harbor beliefs that little can be done therapeutically in any case [8].

Compared with other countries worldwide, China is experiencing the greatest overall increase in its population of elderly residents. There were approximately 240 million people, or 17.3% of the population, who were aged 60 years or above in 2017 [9]. The number of people in China with dementia is also expected to increase from approximately 9.5 million in 2015 to 16 million by 2030 [1]. There is high-quality evidence suggesting that the total annual cost of dementia will increase from US$900 million in 1990 to US$114.2 billion in 2030 in China [10].

The current medical treatment and management of dementia in China is not promising. Only 10% of people with dementia have been diagnosed, while only 21% diagnosed dementia patients have received medical treatment in urban China [11]. Most people with dementia in China live at home, supported by informal caregivers [12]. The heavy care burden easily leads caregivers to have depression, anxiety and other negative emotions [13], which can cause them to vent their difficult emotions on their patients [14]. But there were also surveys [15, 16] shown that a strong sense of family responsibility might reduce the perception of care burden. Alternative care (respite service, institutional care, etc.) and professional support (professional knowledge and skills guidance, rehabilitation services for dementia patients, psychological support for caregivers, etc.) are important aspects of caregivers' care needs. However, these needs have not been met effectively [17].

The World Health Organization states that it would be challenging to intervene without the effective involvement of primary care, and dementia should be the priority of public health [18]. However, the national basic package of public health services which was promulgated by National Health and Family Planning Commission of China in 2017 only covered the management of hypertension, diabetes, psychosis and tuberculosis in community health services setting [19]. In 2015, the State Council of the People's Republic of China promulgated the National Five-year plan for Mental Health (2015–2020), which focused on four brain diseases (autism, schizophrenia, depression and dementia) occurring in different stages of life; the plan includes the development of integrated services, training of mental health specialists, improvement of rehabilitation services and community- and family-based support, as well as the promotion of social awareness [20]. Studies showed that community-care interventions (dietary adjustments, regular home visits, etc.) provided by primary care workers for dementia patients and their caregivers could improve the quality of life for patients and reduce the mental stress of caregivers and the burden of families [21–23]. However, qualified primary care workforces are not sufficient in China. Take GPs for example, there were only 1.82 licensed GPs per 10,000 people in 2017 [24]. Furthermore, a study in Shanghai showed that most GPs still lack training and related knowledge about dementia, and their attitudes toward the care of dementia are pessimistic [25].

As an aging city, there were approximately 150 thousand to 200 thousand dementia patients in Beijing in 2015 [26]. The population of people with dementia is still growing [27]. This qualitative study aimed to clarify the needs of informal caregivers and barriers of primary care workers toward dementia management in primary care in Beijing to provide references that may help to improve the care and services provided to individuals with dementia and their family caregivers residing in urban China.

Methods

A descriptive approach was chosen because the goal of the study was to elicit the needs of informal caregivers and barriers of primary care workers toward dementia management that would directly and pragmatically show their reality [28].

The topics for the caregivers and primary care workers were designed and modified based on the *expert consensus on long-term healthcare of patients with cognitive disorders in China* by academy of cognitive disorder of China - effective support by caregivers and physicians at lifestyle changes, cognitive maintenance and training [29]. At first the questions were roughly listed based on our literature review and status quo of primary care in China. Then they were categorized by the specific topics that represent the key components of the needs of informal caregivers and barriers of primary care workers' toward dementia management. We created the topics to ascertain a diversity of perceptions about the needs and barriers mentioned above to make consistent and reliable integration of perspectives from caregivers and primary care workers.

Participants and recruitment

The study was conducted in four CHSCs in Chaoyang district, Beijing. Twenty-five individuals who were diagnosed with dementia by neurologists in secondary or tertiary hospital were approached by the general practitioner of our research group via electronic health records.

Twenty-five main informal caregivers were approached by the inclusion criteria as follows: (1) minimum 2 h of daily care and the longest duration of care per day for patients at home over 6 months; (2) willingness to be interviewed as part of the study; and (3) could answer the interviewer's questions clearly and logically.

We purposively sampled primary care workers from the inner city and suburbs with a mix of primary care workers, sexes, ages and years of experience. Inclusion criteria were general practitioner or nurse qualifications, a current primary care practice and at least one patient with dementia.

Data collection

Individual in-depth interviews

In-depth interviews with caregivers were conducted from September to December 2017 by interviewers who received training and supervision in conducting qualitative interviews. The interviews were structured and included predetermined topics and associated probes. These predetermined topics were chosen by the research team to elicit, in an open-ended fashion, an exploration of caregivers' attitudes. The topics included who else provided support and assistance for you in the community during the care period, what else do you need while providing care, and who would you tend to ask for help if you run into trouble in the process of care. Field notes included difficulties encountered during the interviews and the interviewer's impressions of participants' reactions to the study. Participants were advised that the whole interview could be completed in 30 min but were not discouraged from extending the interview duration if willing. The interviews ranged from 30 to 90 min in length, which mostly lasted for approximately one hour.

Focus groups

To explore issues identified in the interviews, we conducted focus group with GPs and community nurses from January to February 2018. The objectives were to answer the following questions about primary care workers with respect to dementia: (a) the understanding of knowledge and skills of dementia care; (b) the attitudes, ability and difficulty in dementia management; (c) their advice on dementia care in the community.

After informing participants of the purpose of the study and obtaining written consent, four experienced moderators led the four groups simultaneously. An experienced researcher in qualitative study observed the groups' discussions and took notes. Each group was given the same task, namely, to identify the barriers to managing dementia in primary care and to suggest effective approaches that could overcome these barriers. Each session was approximately 90 min in length and was held in a private meeting room located in the health clinics.

Data analysis

All interviews and focus group discussions were audio recorded with consent from participants. Digital recordings were stored in a password-protected, secure system. Audio-taped data were transcribed verbatim. Transcripts were reviewed and analyzed by six members of the research team. To bring a wide variety of knowledge and preconceptions to the analysis process, the team comprised professionals with different research backgrounds, including an associate professor and a lecturer of general practice, three graduate students and a general practitioner. The team members read all the material through several times to obtain the whole sense and then independently coded transcripts to identify themes by condensing and summarizing the contents. When no new topics were identified, data saturation was considered [30].

We conducted a content analysis by analyzing the verbatim transcripts and identifying specific meanings and potential implications, in accordance with the topics. A second researcher conducted a second transcription after a researcher independently transcribed each audiotape. A third researcher then compared the first and second transcriptions for disparities. A final transcription was developed after the researchers collectively discussed the most accurate interpretation of the disparities. No new categories emerged in the analysis after the 8th interview, as interview no. 9 and 10 only added minimal information. Saturation of themes was reached after the fourth focus group and data-collection was stopped. We then reviewed the coded data for different approaches, which led to the combination of some codes, the identification of new subcodes and the production of a narrative summarizing the key themes of the discussions. A back-translation approach was also used, which involved translation to English and then double-checking for errors by a second independent researcher to ensure equivalence in both languages.

Results

Sample

According to the severity of the patient's condition, 12 informal caregivers of people with dementia were selected in Chaoyang district, Beijing. Only 10 caregivers were interviewed; 2 declined because they did not want to talk about their work. Most caregivers were either spouses (6/10, $n = 6$) or adult children (3/10, $n = 3$) (see Table 1 for additional characteristics). The primary care workers were recruited from 8 districts in Beijing, 75% of which were metropolitan. The 29 primary care workers (overall age range, 30–62 years; mean, 38.9 ± 8.3 years) represented a wide range of practice sizes and length of experience (range, 4–29 years; mean, 12.7 ± 6.7 years), and included 20 GPs and 9 community nurses. The ratio of male to female GPs in the groups was 3:17. Twenty GPs were divided into three groups of 7, 8 and 5 GPs; nine community nurses were in a group.

Table 1 Characteristics of interviewed caregivers and care recipients

Items	Caregivers ($n = 10$)	Care recipient ($n = 10$)
Mean age	66.9 ± 16.6	79.0 ± 4.1
Sex		
Female	9	2
Male	1	8
Self-reported general health		
Excellent/very good	0	N/A
Good	0	N/A
Fair	3	N/A
Poor	7	N/A
Relationship		
Spouse	6	N/A
Child	3	N/A
Other family relative	1	N/A
Marital status		
Married	9	8
Widowed	1	2
Education		
Elementary school	0	2
Secondary school	6	3
Higher education	4	5
Severity of dementia		
Mild	N/A	5
Moderate	N/A	3
Severe	N/A	2

Qualitative findings

Analysis of the interviews with the caregivers and the focus groups with primary care workers led to the identification of three themes related to the needs of informal caregivers and barriers of primary care workers: care knowledge and skills, psychological counseling, and collaborative management.

Quotes are shown in italics. "C" stands for caregiver who participated in the interview, "GPA" stands for the first group of general practitioners, "GPB" stands for the second group of general practitioners, "GPC" stands for the third group of general practitioners, and "ND" stands for community nurse.

Care knowledge and skills

Urgent needs for care knowledge

To provide more appropriate care, almost all informal caregivers mentioned that they needed GPs or community nurses to provide professional care guidance. People caring for patients with mild dementia wanted to obtain care guidance about how to prolong the early process of the condition, how to address patients with abnormal behavior problems, how to enhance the patient's memory and how to improve the patient's ability to live. People caring for patients with severe dementia wanted to obtain skills to address dietary and toileting difficulties of their patients and wanted to know how to prevent the occurrence of complications or how to address them, etc. They also hoped that the primary care workers could offer home care services, such as injections.

My father-in-law's condition is not very severe, but we are not good at taking care of him. I hope to grasp some knowledge to prolong the process of the disease.(C8)

We need some professional care knowledge because we are not professional. (C7)

I learned stomach intubation care from nursing workers when my father was hospitalized. (C6)

I take care of my husband. He is bedridden now. I do not know whether it is good to take care of him like before. I am afraid to touch him. (C2)

He always gets inflamed. It's not easy for us to bring him to the CHSC because of his mobility problems. If the medical workers could do some follow-up regularly and offer injection services, it would be more convenient. (C6)

Willing to help but lack professional training

As for the primary care workers, they could provide only a small amount of help because of their heavy workloads and their lack of expertise related to dementia. The help provided to caregivers was mainly focused on the advice regarding usual care for the patients, such as dietary care, the prevention of accidents, and the prevention of complications for bedridden patients. Only three GPs said they had received training related to dementia, but they had already forgotten the specific details. Almost all the interviewees said they only had a preliminary understanding of the knowledge and skills of dementia. For them, the experience mostly came from clinical practice, books, and the web. All interviewees agreed that they lacked confidence regarding the management of dementia patients in primary care.

I like to help them. I educate the care providers by providing some care knowledge, such as pressure sores care, lung infection care. (N3)

I see almost 100 patients every day. It is difficult for me to guide the caregivers particularly. The specialists have a deeper understanding of dementia than us. I think they could provide more targeted advice. (GPB1)

As a general practitioner, I pay more attention to the patients' physical diseases, such as high blood pressure and diabetes, not dementia. (GPC3)

The main thing we can do is to provide care for complications during dementia, such as lung infection and high blood pressure. (GPA1)

I did not accept any systematic training about dementia during residency. (GPB1)

I had managed patients with dementia during residency training of GPs, but my knowledge about dementia is not comprehensive. (GPA1)

Psychological counseling

Needs for psychological support

The heavy care burden and pressure could easily lead caregivers to irritability, anxiety and other negative emotions. This might lead to a reduction in their ability to provide care and to the quality of the care services provided to the dementia patients. Caregivers need psychological consultations to ease the pressures they felt and to maintain their good emotional state.

I feel better now. I adjusted myself slowly... I felt helpless and anxious at the beginning. (C10)

Sometimes I get angry at my husband. He says he wants to separate from me. He always says something weird like that. (C4)

My mum fell in the bathroom a few days ago. Her head wedged in the crack of close stool and pillar. I called her, but she did not respond to me. If I discovered her later, she would never be saved. I am so scared. (C10)

His illness really bothers me. My condition was good before, but I feel uncomfortable with my heart recently. He depends on me for everything. I take care of him all day. I am really irritated. (C4)

He is stronger than me. He wanted to hit me that day. I was so grieved. (C3)

I would be extremely delighted to chat with someone. Nobody talks to me because they are busy. (C1)

Limited help provided by primary care workers

Primary care workers could give informal caregivers only limited psychological guidance and support because of the different medical specialties. Actually, there were already some patients with dementia and their caregivers who had established telephone contact, WeChat (a mobile text and voice messaging communication service) and other contacts with their GPs to accept personalized guidance about psychological problems.

I think it is still necessary for the specialists to see patients in CHSCs. Sometimes when we say something to the caregivers or patients to express our empathy, they refute us. They think that we cannot understand their feelings. Psychologists have specialized knowledge and they know how to deal with it. (GPB1)

Some caregivers are in my WeChat list. If there is any special situation, he can consult me directly on WeChat. I will give him a reply when I have time. I think this is a more personalized guide, but the help I provide is very basic and limited. (GPB2)

As a community health worker, we should increase the public awareness of dementia, help the patients and caregivers as much as possible in various ways. (GPC2)

Collaborative management

Expectations of respite services

Lack of social contact was a common situation among caregivers. They rarely arranged leisure or social activities, especially those caring for patients who could not take care of themselves. To improve the quality of care, collaboration was necessary. Most informal caregivers were spouses; they were older, and their body functions degenerated gradually. They felt physically overextended and exhausted, and their health condition was becoming gradually worse in the process of taking care of their patients.

The main thing is that I do not have any time to socialize. I have no energy and I'm tired all the time. (C7).

I have to take care of my dad. I really do not have time to take care of my own family. I feel sorry for them. (C6)

He likes to go out for a walk, but my body is in a bad situation. I am unable to follow him, and I hope there is someone to follow him. (C1)

Team-based management model

Almost all the primary care workers in the interview indicated that a team-based management model should be established. GPs should be mainly responsible for the early identification and the monitoring of dementia, maintaining the overall physical condition of patients and the overall coordination of the team. Community nurses would undertake care guidance, including life guidance and regular follow-up. In addition, the team also needed to have specialists, such as neurologists or psychiatrists. They could offer professional guidance to the GPs and provide support to the caregivers by seeing patients in CHSCs regularly.

I think it should be a team. Apart from GPs and community nurses, specialists should be involved according to the patients' situation and caregivers' needs. GPs are mainly responsible for the overall physical condition of patients and specialists solve the specific problems. In addition to providing care guidance, community nurses can also do some follow-up. (GPB4)

As the most accessible social resource for patients, community committees should cooperate with the CHSCs to play an active role in organizing patient exchange activities and other events and in coordinating available social resources to help the patients and their caregivers, such as helping to contact care institutions.

Community nurses provide some care guidance of patients' daily life for caregivers, such as prevention of accidental injury. GPs and specialists maintain the patients are in a stable physical condition and provide some psychological support for caregivers. I think this is the best way. It is also good for community committees and care institutions to provide some help because taking care of such patients is not unilateral. More participants, better quality of care work. (N1)

Discussion

In this study, two caregivers of people with dementia declined. The possible reasons tended to be either lack of knowledge on the part of the families/patients or the stigma sometimes attached to dementia. There is an overall low level of understanding of the condition of dementia among the public and the nonspecialist domain, which, alongside the stigma that might be attached, makes it difficult for people to discuss. One strategy to enhance attendance and eliminate stigma is by educating society [31]. The public health system in China has been working hard on promoting the social awareness through mental health propaganda and education in hospitals, communities and schools to reduce or eliminate stigma [12]. Since 2012, the appellation of "lao nian xing chi dai" with derogatory meaning in Mandarin has been gradually replaced by "cognitive disorder" in Chinese health care system [32].

People with dementia need help with challenging changes in behavior, memory, physical disability, and mood [33]. Informal caregivers need to know the characteristics of dementia and have knowledge of disease-related therapies and care. The needs for related knowledge persist from the early stages of the patients' disease; as the disease progresses, the focus of caregivers' needs change as well. An intervention that examined care skills was carried out in the caregivers of elderly patients with dementia; the research looked at skills that included coping styles, cognitive rehabilitation training and daily life care principles. The results showed that anxiety and depression of the caregivers were relieved and that the life quality score improved after the intervention [34]. Technology such as face-to-face interactions via various secure video connection platforms, and devices that monitor the health status or function of an older adult can be helpful for individuals who are caring for someone at home, especially to those who have heavily care duties and have difficulty leaving the home. In addition, the guidance and application of predictive care can also help to minimize further harm, risk and cost for the patient and the psychological burden on caregivers [35]. In China, GPs are often inadequately trained and may be reluctant or unable to detect, diagnose or manage dementia [36]. The results of the interviews also showed GPs were more focused on the physical diseases of their dementia patients and paid insufficient attention to their dementia, similar to a previous survey conducted in Shanghai, China [25]. Guidelines for the management of dementia in primary care have been established in Australia and Canada [37, 38]. These guidelines are intended to be used by health professionals and policy makers who plan, organize and deliver care for people who have dementia and their caregivers. Therefore, the domestic management of dementia in primary care should focus on strengthening the professional training regarding dementia for medical workers and establishing guidelines that suit the national culture.

Psychological counseling for caregivers is an important part of care. The caregivers' positive mental attitudes are the basis for the implementation of care. In America, GPs periodically assess caregivers for the level of perceived burden, presence of depression and anxiety, and coping strategies, and they help the patient and caregiver with care planning in advance. Community nurses, social workers, rehabilitation specialists, and psychologists provide support services such as health education, psychological counseling, and emotional support for caregivers [39]. Therefore, given the needs of caregivers in China, it is recommended that this model be used as a reference. Meanwhile, hospitals and CHSCs provide psychological counseling and care guidance for the caregivers collectively and organize gatherings for caregivers on a regular basis to promote the sharing of feelings and care skills. In addition, respite service is necessary according to the caregiver's work and physical condition to deliver an individualized, simple, flexible, and adaptable response to caregivers' needs [40].

Community management of dementia involves a wide range of areas, requiring multidisciplinary collaboration. Various social resources in addition to primary care support should also be noted. Community committees, neurologists and psychologists in secondary and tertiary hospitals should be available to collaborate. A clear and robust multidisciplinary expert group will enable diagnosis and management [41] and enhance patient and caregiver satisfaction [42]. This integration of medical and social services, emphasizing multidisciplinary and multi-domain team communication and collaboration of the personalized management model, fully embodies the principle of being "patient centered".

In North America and Europe, case management has become an important way for primary care providers to manage dementia in communities. Case managers are mostly nurses who care for the dementia patients; they work with GPs, assisting physicians in conducting examinations around the diagnosis, coordinating treatment plans, providing health education on diseases, suggesting available resources and reporting the health status and needs of patients and caregivers regularly. The GPs are responsible for providing medical treatment, developing a care plan, and adjusting the plan according to the feedback of the case managers [7]. Domestic case management was first introduced in Taiwan and Hong Kong and has a short development history in the mainland. The current application in community schizophrenia is relatively mature and has achieved a significant effect [43]. Prior work showed that patients' cognitive ability, self-care ability and quality of life were all improved through the application of dementia case management [44]. Case management not only had a positive impact on dementia patients and caregivers themselves but also improved the utilization of community health resources and reduced the cost of health care [45]. To some extent, services provided will be dependent on local provisions, demography, and geography, but even if the services are available, if the understanding or relationship of expectations between the GPs and specialists is dysfunctional, then patients will not receive the high quality of care that they deserve [46]. At present, the case management of dementia in China is still at an exploratory stage. There is no clear definition of team formation rules, implementation processes of case management and evaluation of management effectiveness. Based on these concerns, the establishment of a community-based dementia team management model that suits the national culture should be explored.

It became clear that there were many similar aspects about the needs of informal caregivers and barriers of primary care workers toward dementia management in primary care between China and some Western countries. More-general expectations were described by informal caregivers (e.g., sharing the responsibility of caring for dementia patients and making joint decisions regarding the care) [47] and primary care workers (e.g., time constraints and lack knowledge about dementia) [48]. Different aspects were also existed. General practitioners in Western countries perceived lack of knowledge of early diagnostic, and some of them seemed to attach stigma to the condition of dementia by assuming that the caregiver/patient did not want a diagnosis until the symptoms were so severe that it was inevitable [48]. However, these contents were not reflected in our study. We think there are two potential reasons. First, the GPs working in CHSCs are generally less educated in China. Only 44.8% GPs had a bachelor degree or above compared with 69.9% physicians in the secondary and tertiary hospitals [49]. The perceived low quality of primary care is a major reason why people prefer to use hospital care. Second, the management of specific chronic diseases required by the government is an important job for CHSCs. Therefore, primary care workers rarely show more initiative on diseases not required by the government.

After the researchers collectively discussed the most accurate interpretation of the disparities, a final transcription was developed to make consistent and reliable integration of perspectives from caregivers and primary care workers, which increases the confidence in our findings. But this study has its limitations. It is an exploratory study, only the informal caregivers in Chaoyang district were recruited. The representativeness of informal caregivers in this study was relatively limited. We plan to do further studies in other districts of Beijing.

Abbreviations

C: Caregiver who participated in the interview; CHSCs: Community Health Service Centers; GPA: The first group of general practitioners; GPB: The second group of general practitioners; GPC: The third group of general practitioners; GPs: General practitioners; N: Community nurse

Acknowledgments

The authors thank Guanghui Jin for his editorial help. To all the caregivers and primary care workers who participated in this research, the authors convey their sincere thanks and respect for their contribution and sharing of experiences.

Funding

This work was supported by the Capital General Practice Research Project (17QK05). The funding organization had no role in the design, conduct, analysis and interpretation or preparation of the report of this study.

Authors' contributions
MRW, SS, JL, YJL, XJYX and JD contributed to the conception and design of this study. MRW SS, JL, YJL and XJYX were involved in data collection. MRW, SS, JL, YJL, XJYX and JD analyzed and interpreted the data. The manuscript was drafted by MRW and SS and edited by JD. The final version was reviewed and approved by all authors.

Consent for publication
Not applicable.

Competing interests
The authors declare that they have no competing interests.

Author details
[1]School of General Practice and Continuing Education, Capital Medical University, No.10 Xitoutiao, You An Men, Beijing 100069, China. [2]Dongfeng Community Health Service Center, Chaoyang District, Beijing, China.

References

1. Prince M, Comas-Herrera A, Knapp M, Guerchet M, Karagiannidou M. World Alzheimer report 2016. In: The global voice on dementia. Alzheimer's disease international. 2016. https://www.alz.co.uk/research/WorldAlzheimerReport2016. Accessed 22 Aug 2018.
2. Global Alzheimer's Disease Charter. In: The global voice on dementia. Alzheimer's disease international. 2008. https://www.alz.co.uk/global-charter. Accessed 22 Aug 2018.
3. Alzheimer Europe. Policy in practice: Paris declaration. 2015. http://www.alzheimer-europe.org/EN/Policy-in-Practice2/Paris-Declaration. Accessed 22 Aug 2018.
4. Case Management Society of America. What is a case manager? 2016. http://www.cmsa.org/who-we-are/what-is-a-case-manager/. Accessed 22 Aug 2018.
5. Bamford C, Poole M, Brittain K, Chew-Grahamet C, Fox C, Iliffe S, et al. Understanding the challenges to implementing case management for people with dementia in primary care in England: a qualitative study using normalization process theory. BMC Health Serv Res. 2014;14(1):549.
6. Iliffe S, Robinson L, Bamford C, Waugh A, Fox C, Livingston G, et al. Introducing case management for people with dementia in primary care: a mixed-methods study. Br J Gen Pract. 2014;64(628):735–41.
7. Khanassov V, Vedel I. Family physician-case manager collaboration and needs of patients with dementia and their caregivers: a systematic mixed studies review. Ann Fam Med. 2016;14(2):166–77.
8. Spenceley SM, Sedgwick N, Keenan J. Dementia care in the context of primary care reform: an integrative review. Aging Ment Health. 2015;19(2):107–20.
9. National Bureau of Statistics of the People's Republic of China. Beijing: The National Bureau of Statistics. The national economic and social development statistical bulletin 2017. 2017. [in Chinese], http://www.stats.gov.cn/tjsj/zxfb/201802/t20180228_1585631.html. Accessed 22 Aug 2018.
10. Xu J, Wang J, Wimo A, Fratiglioni L, Qiu C. The economic burden of dementia in China, 1990–2030: implications for health policy. Bull World Health Organ. 2017;95(1):18–26.
11. Yu X, Chen S, Chen X, Jia J, Li C, Liu C, et al. Clinical management and associated costs for moderate and severe Alzheimer's disease in urban China: a Delphi panel study. Transl Neurodegener. 2015;4(1):15.
12. Chen Z, Yang X, Song YT, Song BB, Zhang Y, Liu JW, et al. Challenges of dementia care in China. Geriatrics. 2017;2(1):7.
13. Arango Lasprilla JC, Moreno A, Rogers H, Francis K. The effect of dementia patient's physical, cognitive, and emotional/behavioral problems on caregiver well-being: findings from a Spanish-speaking sample from Colombia, South America. Am J Alzheimers Dis Other Demen. 2009;24(5):384.
14. Yang PP, Shen J. Abuse tendency among dementia caregivers: a qualitative research. Chin J Prac Nurs. 2013;29(1):27–30 (in Chinese).
15. Tang Y. The establishment of mental health and long-term care system for the main caregivers of the disabled elderly. Academic Forum. 2012;35(9):168–73 (in Chinese).
16. Abdollahpour I, Nedjat S, Salimi Y. Positive aspects of caregiving and caregiver burden: a study of caregivers of patients with dementia. J Geriatr Psychiatry Neurol. 2017;31(1):34–8.
17. Hao W, Wu J, Zhang H, Zou BH, Wang ZW. Supportive care demands of family caregivers of community-dwelling patients with dementia. Chin Nurs Manag. 2015;15(11):1294–7 (in Chinese).
18. World Health Organization. Dementia: a public health priority. 2012. http://apps.who.int/iris/bitstream/handle/10665/75262/WHO_NMH_MSD_2012.3_eng.pdf?sequence=1&isAllowed=y. Accessed 22 Aug 2018.
19. National Health Commission of the People's Republic of China. National Basic Public Health Service Regulations (the Third Edition). 2017. [in Chinese], http://www.nhfpc.gov.cn/ewebeditor/uploadfile/2017/04/20170417104506514.pdf. Accessed 28 Oct 2018.
20. The State Council of the People's Republic of China. The National Five-year plan for mental health (2015-2020). 2015. [in Chinese], http://www.gov.cn/zhengce/content/2015-06/18/content_9860.htm. Accessed 22 Aug 2018.
21. Lu FH, Zeng H, Ji SY, Zhu HR, Lv XF. A review of community nursing interventions for Alzheimer's disease. J Nurs Sci. 2016;31(13):110–3 (in Chinese).
22. Xiao WY, Zheng SH, He XZ. The effect of community nursing intervention on quality of life of Alzheimer patients and caregivers. Chin J Gen Pract. 2016;14(1):150–2 (in Chinese).
23. Zhang WL, Zhao LJ. Effect of community nursing intervention on dementia patients and their caregivers. J Clin Med. 2014;1(12):2254 (in Chinese).
24. Planning Development and Information Technology Division. The national development of health care statistical bulletin in 2017. 2017. [in Chinese], http://www.nhfpc.gov.cn/guihuaxxs/s10743/201806/44e3cdfe11fa4c7f928c879d435b6a18.shtml. Accessed 28 Oct 2018.
25. Yu L, Xu Q, Wang ZY, Chen G, Cao WY, Mi JH, et al. A survey on the attitudes and confidence of GPs in handling dementia and its related problems. Natl Med J China. 2013;93(35):2794–8 (in Chinese).
26. National Health Commission of the People's Republic of China. Beijing: 150 thousand to 200 thousand dementia patients, many hospitals have a memory loss clinic. 2015. [in Chinese], http://health.china.com.cn/2015-04/17/content_7835452.htm. Accessed 22 Aug 2018.
27. Central People's Government of the People's Republic of China. There are 3. 29 million elderly people registered in Beijing, and the aging population has exceeded 24%. 2017. [in Chinese], http://www.gov.cn/xinwen/2017-10/31/content_5235685.htm. Accessed 22 Aug 2018.
28. Jiggins CK, Evans B. Qualitative descriptive methods in health science research. Herd. 2016;9(4):16–25.
29. Academy of Cognitive Disorder of China. Expert consensus on long-term healthcare of patients with cognitive disorders in China. Chin J Geriatr. 2016;35(10):1051–60 (in Chinese).
30. Caelli K, Ray L, Mill J. 'Clear as mud': toward greater clarity in generic qualitative research. Int J Qual Method. 2003;2(2). https://doi.org/10.1177/160940690300200201.
31. Department of Health. Living well with dementia: a national dementia strategy. 2009.https://www.gov.uk/government/publications/living-well-with-dementia-a-national-dementia-strategy. Accessed 22 Aug 2018.
32. China Central Television. Caring for the elderly, dementia changed its name to cognitive disorder. 2012. [in Chinese], http://tv.cntv.cn/video/C10616/d3fa304b2ae94e399c6061ec19812d00. Accessed 1 Nov 2018.
33. Hg VDR, Meiland FJ, Maroccini R, Comijs HC, Jonker C, Dröes RM. Subjective needs of people with dementia: a review of the literature. Int Psychogeriatr. 2007;19(3):559–92.
34. Dong CF. Nursing intervention for the main caregivers of dementia patients. Chin J Trauma and Disability Med. 2012;20(5):107–9 (in Chinese).
35. Hu P, Liu Q. Effects of predictive nursing on elderly patients with Alzheimer's disease. Nurs J Chin PLA. 2013;30(10):32–4 (in Chinese).
36. Patel V, Xiao S, Chen H, Hanna F, Jotheeswaran AT, Dan L, et al. The magnitude of and health system responses to the mental health treatment gap in adults in India and China. Lancet. 2016;388(10063):3074–84.
37. Palk E, Carlson L, Parker D, Abbey JA. Clinical practice guidelines and care pathways for people with dementia living in the community. In: Cognition/dementia care system. 2008. https://www.researchgate.net/publication/27476359. Accessed 22 Aug 2018.
38. Diagnosis and Management in Primary Care. Cognitive Impairment-Recognition. British Columbia. 2016. https://www2.gov.bc.ca/gov/content/

health/practitioner-professional-resources/bc-guidelines/cognitive-impairment. Diagnosis and Management in Primary Care. Accessed 22 Aug 2018.
39. Dang S, Badiye A, Kelkar G. The dementia caregiver--a primary care approach. South Med J. 2008;101(12):1246–51.
40. Yang XL, Chen M, Zhang H, Tian AJ, Li L. Application of Plato analysis in negative influencing evaluation of Alzheimer caregivers. J Nurs Train. 2014; 22:2046–7 (in Chinese).
41. De LJ, Wind AW, Iliffe S, Moniz-Cook ED, Wilcock J, González VM. The primary care diagnosis of dementia in Europe: an analysis using multidisciplinary, multinational expert groups. Aging Ment Health. 2008; 12(5):568–76.
42. Hinton L, Franz CE, Reddy G, Flores Y, Kravitz RL, Barker JC. Practice constraints, behavioral problems, and dementia care: primary care physicians' perspectives. J Gen Int Med. 2007;22(11):1487–92.
43. Liu JH, Hao, Chen H, Xiang YQ, Qiu D, Li YJ Community social function of schizophrenia application case management interventions to improve performance evaluation J Int Psychia 2016; (1):72–6. (in Chinese).
44. Li W, Zhang XY, Zhao ZR. Study on the effect of case management on improving the quality of life of patients with dementia. Chin J Clin Rat Drug Use. 2014;27:163–4 (in Chinese).
45. Pimouguet C, Lavaud T, Dartigues JF, Helmer C. Dementia case management effectiveness on health care costs and resource utilization: a systematic review of randomized controlled trials. J Nutr Health Aging. 2010;14(8):669–76.
46. Iliffe S, De LJ, Van HH, Kenny G, Lewis A, Vernooijdassen M. Understanding obstacles to the recognition of and response to dementia in different European countries: a modified focus group approach using multinational, multi-disciplinary expert groups. Aging Ment Health. 2005;9(1):1–6.
47. Stephan A, Bieber A, Hopper L, Joyce R, Irving K, Zanetti O, et al. Barriers and facilitators to the access to and use of formal dementia care: findings of a focus group study with people with dementia, informal carers and health and social care professionals in eight European countries. BMC Geriatr. 2018;18(1):131.
48. Iliffe S. Rapid appraisal of barriers to the diagnosis and management of patients with dementia in primary care: a systematic review. BMC Fam Pract. 2010;11:52.
49. China Ministry of Health. Yearbook of Chinese health statistics 2018. 1st ed. Beijing: Peking Union Medical College; 2018.

Piloting electronic screening forms in primary care: findings from a mixed methods study to identify patients eligible for low dose CT lung cancer screening

Mary Ann O'Brien[1*], Frank Sullivan[1,2,3,5], Andrea Carson[1], Rabiya Siddiqui[1], Saddaf Syed[1] and Lawrence Paszat[4,5]

Abstract

Background: Recent evidence suggests that screening with low dose computed tomography (LDCT) scans significantly reduces mortality from lung cancer. However, optimal methods to identify potentially eligible patients in primary care are not known. Using brief electronic screening forms administered prior to a primary care visit is a strategy to identify high risk, asymptomatic patients eligible for LDCT screening. The objective of this study was to compare the acceptability and feasibility of using brief electronic versus paper screening forms to identify eligible patients at high risk of developing lung cancer in primary care.

Methods: A mixed method pilot comparative study was conducted in primary care. Practices were allocated to an electronic form (e-form) group or a paper-based form (p-form) group. Allocation was randomly assigned for the first practice then by alternation. Patients in the e-form practices completed forms at home via the web or in the waiting room on a tablet. Patients in p-form practices completed forms in waiting rooms. Interviews were conducted with patients, administrators, and primary care physicians (PCPs) about their experiences.

Results: Six of 30 (20%) eligible practices agreed to participate. Over the 16-week study period, a total of 831 of an expected 1442 patients (58%) aged 55–74 years were enrolled; 573/690 (83%) patients in the e-form group and 258/752 (34%) in the p-form group. Of the 573 participants in the e-form group, 335 (58%) completed forms via the web; 238 (29%) did so via tablet. Twenty-four interviews were conducted with 15 patients, 5 administrative staff and 4 PCPs. Patients were willing to discuss lung cancer screening eligibility with their PCP. Staff members expressed low administrative burden except for an extra step to link appointment information to patient demographics to identify eligible patients. PCPs indicated that forms were reminders to discuss smoking cessation. PCPs in the e-form group reported that patients asked questions about screening.

Conclusion: There was fairly low uptake by primary care practices. For e-forms to be feasible in practice workflow, electronic medical record software needs to link appointment information with patient eligibility requirements. The use of brief pre-consultation electronic screening forms for LDCT eligibility encouraged PCPs to discuss smoking cessation with patients.

Keywords: Lung cancer screening, Primary care, Health services research, Low dose computed tomography (LDCT)

* Correspondence: maryann.obrien@utoronto.ca
[1]Department of Family and Community Medicine, University of Toronto, 500 University Avenue, Fifth Floor, Toronto, ON M5G 1V7, Canada
Full list of author information is available at the end of the article

Background

The National Lung Screening Trial in the United States and the Lung Cancer Screening Trial in the United Kingdom have demonstrated that screening with low dose computed tomography (LDCT) scans significantly reduces mortality from lung cancer [1, 2]. Optimal methods to identify potentially eligible asymptomatic patients in primary care are not known, although web-based technologies may be useful. For example, software is now available which allows patients attending primary care appointments to receive and respond to electronic questionnaires before their consultation. Responses to electronic questionnaires can then be used for different purposes such as determining eligibility for clinical studies, populating the electronic medical record (EMR) and providing an opportunity for 'just-in-time' counseling by primary care providers (PCPs). For example, in New Zealand, researchers developed an electronic tool for primary care called eCHAT (electronic case-finding and help assessment tool) [3]. The tool was used by patients in the waiting room prior to a visit or via the Internet in the community. The goal of the tool was to encourage active participation by patients in decision-making and self-management practices.

In the context of LDCT lung cancer screening, pre-consultation software could be used to facilitate identification of potentially eligible patients. This software may also help to remedy physician inconsistencies in recommending high-risk patients to LDCT that was identified as problematic in a previous study [4], by contributing to a more formalized screening process. Information from pre-consultation screening forms may help PCPs to counsel their patients about their risk for lung cancer and the potential benefits and risks of LDCT lung cancer screening, and refer appropriate patients to a screening program.

Identifying and describing the potential impact of electronic technologies on health care is necessary to better prepare for the potential myriad of challenges that come with implementing such technologies in primary care [5]. The goal of the current study was to assess two pre-screening strategies to identify eligible patients for LDCT should a lung cancer screening program become available in Ontario. At the time of this study, an organized LDCT screening program for lung cancer was not available in Ontario although pilot work for a potential program is underway (https://www.cancercareontario.ca/en/guidelines-advice/cancer-continuum/screening/lung-cancer-screening-pilot-people-at-high-risk).

The design and implementation of this study were based on our views of how the primary care clinical process would unfold. The pre-screening form used in this study was not intended to determine eligibility for LDCT screening; instead, it was intended to identify patients who were at high risk for lung cancer, who could then potentially be referred to a more detailed screening assessment and possible LDCT screening. This paper reports the acceptability and feasibility of electronic and paper-based strategies to make a preliminary assessment of lung cancer risk in asymptomatic patients in primary care.

Methods

Pilot comparative study (quantitative component)

Participants

Family physicians affiliated with a single community hospital in Ontario were identified using the College of Physicians and Surgeons of Ontario database (http://www.cpso.on.ca/Public-Information-Services/Find-a-Doctor/). The research team identified and contacted 30 physicians from this list; 6 physicians representing 6 practices agreed to participate. Patients were eligible to participate if they were between 55 and 74 years (y) and had a scheduled appointment with a clinician in one of the six practices that enrolled in the study. Based on the number of patients aged 55–74 y seen in 2015 in each practice and given a study period of 16 weeks, we estimated that about 1442 patients would be eligible during the study period.

Design

Six practices were assigned to either an electronic form (e-form) group (completion of screening forms via pre-consultation software) or a paper form (p-form) group (completion of paper forms in the waiting room). To avoid unconscious selection bias, the first consenting practice was assigned by coin toss; thereafter, practices were assigned to groups by alternation. All six practices completed the study (Fig. 1).

Data collection

All patients completed a questionnaire that included three questions pertaining to lung cancer screening (Table 1), demographics, and Internet preferences; administrative staff and physicians completed a demographic form. Information regarding primary practice setting, type of practice, and practice fee structure was obtained from physicians at four out of six practices. For the remaining two practices, information was obtained using the websites of the College of Physicians and Surgeons in Ontario and the North York Family Health Team. To estimate the number of potentially eligible patients in each practice over the 16-week study period, we used the Canadian Primary Care Sentinel Surveillance Network (CPCSSN) database for five of six practices. We obtained the actual number of eligible patients aged 55–74 y seen in 2015 and prorated this value to 16 weeks. For the sixth practice, we imputed the number of eligible patients seen in one year based upon the average of the actual number of eligible patients divided by

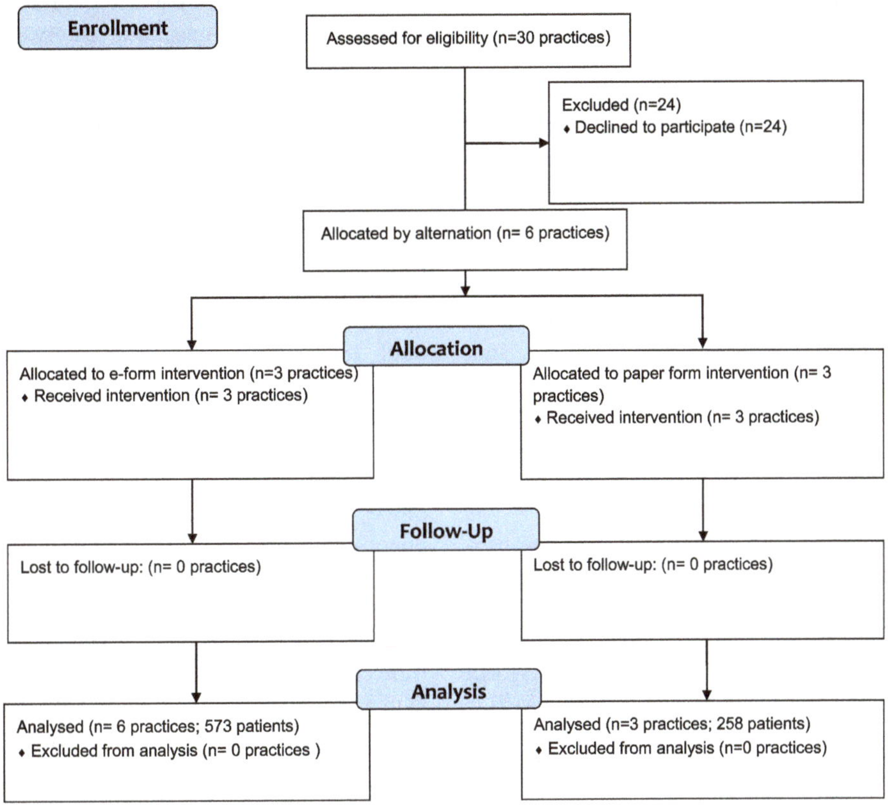

Fig. 1 Study Flow

the practice size for the other practices and multiplied by the practice size of 2000 patients.

Interventions

Two pre-consultation strategies were compared. The intent of a pre-consultation strategy was that physicians would receive just-in-time information about the patient's responses on the pre-screening form and would discuss lung cancer screening or smoking cessation in the visit. In the e-form group, pre-screening forms were sent electronically to eligible patients to complete at home via the Internet. This strategy was intended to place minimal demands on administrative staff. If the EMR indicated that the form was not completed, patients were asked to complete the form on a tablet in the waiting room prior to their visit. The e-form strategy was pilot-tested with 12 patients in one practice. In the p-form group, eligible patients were asked to complete a paper version in the waiting room. Brief descriptions of the implementation of each strategy are provided below.

Table 1 Pre- Screening Questions

The three questions below were included on the lung cancer screening form. The response options were "yes" or "no".

1. Are you between the ages of 55 and 74?
2. Have you smoked cigarettes for at least 20 years in your lifetime?
3. Have you usually smoked 10 or more cigarettes per day?

E-form practices

The implementation of the e-form varied depended on each practice's EMR capability and compatibility with Oceanwave software (CognisantMD http://www.cognisantmd.com/). In two of three practices, the following procedure was used: At the beginning of the week, all eligible patients with a scheduled appointment and with a cell phone number or email address on file were sent a study invitation by email or text. Patients were then sent a url link via the Oceanwave software to a web version of the lung cancer screening form, as well as a demographic and Internet preferences questionnaire. When patients checked in for their appointment, the EMR would indicate if the screening form was complete. Patients who had not yet completed the form were invited to participate by clinic staff and given a tablet on which to complete the form in the waiting room prior to their appointment. Data from the tablet were uploaded to the EMR. The third practice lacked EMR and Oceanwave software compatibility, and had few patient emails and cell phone numbers on file. Eligible patients at this clinic were approached by a practice research facilitator to complete the screening form via tablet in the waiting room.

P-form practices

The implementation process at p-form practices varied and depended on administrative staff preference and daily office functioning. Each practice displayed study information on posters in the waiting room. In one practice, the receptionist provided forms to eligible patients. If they agreed to participate, patients were asked to return completed forms to the receptionist or to a collection box in the waiting area. In the remaining two practices, staff waited for interested patients to approach them. However, staff at one of these two clinics reported low participation and thereafter actively invited patients to the study.

Outcomes

The primary study outcome (acceptability) was the proportion of practices who agreed to participate of those approached. The secondary outcomes (feasibility) were: 1) the proportion of patients with completed forms in each group; 2) the proportion of patients in the e-form group who completed the forms via the Internet versus a tablet. Acceptability of completing pre-consultation forms was also explored during interviews with patients, administrative staff, and physicians.

Analysis

Data were analyzed descriptively using counts and proportions.

Qualitative study component

Patients

After completing the screening form, patients in both e-form and p-form groups were invited to participate in a brief semi-structured telephone interview about their experience with the form. A purposeful sampling strategy was used to select the patients for interviews [6]. Two or three patients from each clinic who had completed the forms were contacted. A mix of patients at high risk, low risk (as determined by their responses to the smoking questions), and who indicated both low and high comfort using technology were contacted for an interview. Patients who completed a telephone interview were mailed a $25.00 gift card.

In the interviews, patients were asked about their overall experience completing the lung cancer pre-screening form, whether or not they had difficulties, if they would be willing to answer follow-up questions based on the form, and their general views on having lung cancer screening forms in primary care.

Administrative staff and physicians

Staff members were asked about their experiences implementing the screening forms, the impact on clinical functioning, and their interactions with patients. Physicians were asked about their overall impressions of the clinical process of having screening forms in their offices, and whether this had an impact on the subsequent clinic visit.

Analysis

Two research team members analyzed the interview transcripts using an editing style of coding [7] using data management and analysis software (NVivo 9, QSR International). Three interviews were coded and results were compared until team members reached an agreement on the preliminary codes. The interview guide was revised throughout the analytic process as new codes were identified. Qualitative analytic techniques were used to inductively identify the main themes [8–10]. An audit trail including interview summaries and memos were used to document all major decisions taken during the study [11].

Results

Quantitative study results

Demographics

Estimates for the number of patients in each practice and the number of eligible patients are provided in Table 2. The estimated practice size varied from approximately 2000 to 7400 patients in the e-form group and 5000 to13500 patients in the p-form group. The estimated number of eligible patients in the practices

Table 2 Description of primary care practices by pre-screening strategy to identify potentially eligible patients for lung cancer screening

	Electronic Form			Paper Form		
	Practice 1	Practice 3	Practice 4	Practice 2	Practice 5	Practice 6
Estimated practice size	7400	2000	5700	13,500	8100	5000
Estimated number of eligible patients	1600	Not known[a]	1400	2000	1700	1100
Actual number of eligible patients seen per year (2015)	1052	242[b]	948	1044	811	589
Number of physicians per practice	5	1	3	6	5	4

[a]Estimated number of eligible patients was not available from this practice

[b]Actual number of eligible patients seen in 2015 was not available from this practice. The number was imputed from the average of the actual number of eligible patients divided by the practice size for the other practices and multiplied by the practice size of 2000 patients

ranged from 1400 to 1600 in the e-form group and 1100 to 2000 in the p-form group. All six practices were in a community-based setting. Five of six practices were part of a family health team. All six practices were structured based on an alternative payment plan.

Across all practices in the 16-week study period, 831 of an expected 1442 patients (58%) aged 55–74 y were enrolled with 573/690 (83%) patients in the e-form group and 258/752 (34%) in the p-form group.

Table 3 describes patient participation by practice and by intervention group. The number of patients who would be potentially eligible for LDCT screening based on their smoking history as assessed by patient responses was 116/831 (14%) overall with 74/573 (13%) in the e-form group and 42/258 (16%) in the p-form group (Table 3).

Internet preferences

Results from the Internet preferences form (data not shown) indicated that 75% of participants were comfortable or very comfortable using computers and 80% used the Internet 1–7 h per day. Almost 80% of participants were comfortable using email and 56% were comfortable using smartphones. Almost 90% of participants indicated that they had a computer at home as well as Internet access.

Outcomes

Primary outcome (acceptability): Six of 30 (20%) practices agreed to participate.

Secondary outcomes (feasibility):

1. Proportion of patients with completed forms in each group: In the e-form group, 68% of patients completed all questions as did 78% in the p-form group. Of the three questions related to lung cancer risk, 99% and 93% of patients in the e-form and p-form practices respectively, completed all three questions.
2. Proportion of patients in the e-form group who completed the forms via the Internet versus a tablet: Of the 573 patients in the e-form group, 335 (58%) completed the forms at home via the web and 238 (42%) completed the forms in the waiting room via tablet.

Implementation of pre consultation screening strategies

During implementation of the electronic screening strategy, we found that the Oceanwave was not as compatible with EMR systems as we had anticipated despite pre-testing. In addition, the EMR capability for searching and identifying eligible patients was not as expected. For all e-form practices, we assumed that we would be able to identify patients within the specified age range who had an upcoming appointment. We assumed that all eligible patients would be sent the information and web link to the forms in a batch. However, this was not possible. The appointment search and email invitation had to be done manually each week by the front desk staff by searching the practice's appointment schedule for patients who fit the age range and sending them email invitations for the study a few days before their scheduled visit.

Qualitative results

Twenty-four interviews were conducted with 15 patients, 5 administrative staff and 4 PCPs. Of the 15 patients, three completed the form via the web, three completed the tablet version, and 8 completed the paper version. One patient could not recall the version that they had completed. Although we pre-specified that patients be able to read and understand English, one

Table 3 Patient recruitment by practice and pre-screening strategy ($n = 831$ patients)

	Electronic Form (573 patients)				Paper Form (258 patients)				
	Practice 1	Practice 3	Practice 4	Total	Practice 2	Practice 5	Practice 6	Total	Overall Total
Number of patients	361	14	198	573	54	193	11	258	831
Email link (at home)	235	0	100	335	N/A	N/A	N/A	N/A	N/A
Tablet (in waiting room)	126	14	98	238	N/A	N/A	N/A	N/A	N/A
Sex									
Male	146	10	52	208	20	69	3	92	300
Female	166	4	104	274	33	112	7	152	426
Lung Cancer Risk Category									
High Risk[a]	47	4	23	74	13	27	2	42	116
Low - Moderate Risk[b]	61	2	34	97	7	21	0	28	125
Low Risk[c]	250	8	141	399	32	133	6	171	570

[a]Represents patients who answered Yes (Y) to all three screening questions
[b]Represents patients who answered Y to age range and Y to one of the other two screening questions
[c]Represents patients who are within the eligible age range and answered No (N) to the second and third screening questions

patient preferred to complete the telephone interview with the assistance of a translator. Of the 15 patients interviewed, 10 were women and 5 were men. All patients were between the ages 55 and 74 y. Of the 15 patients, 7 indicated that they smoked for a period of more than 20 y, and 5 indicated that during that time they had smoked more than 10 cigarettes per day.

Of the 5 administrative staff members, four were from p-form practices and one staff member was from an e-form practice and had experience with both web and tablet versions. All 5 administrative staff members were female; mean age was 35 y. Of the four physicians, two were from e-form practices and the other two were from p-form practices. All four physicians were male; mean age was 50 y.

Theme 1: Patients found screening forms easy to complete

Patients expressed little to no difficulty completing the lung cancer pre-consultation screening form. For example, patients described their experience with the form as "fast", "easy", "efficient", and "nothing to it". All patients said that they would be willing to complete these types of screening forms prior to their primary care visit if they were implemented into practice. All patients were willing to answer follow-up questions and to discuss lung cancer screening eligibility with their PCPs.

Theme 2: Screening forms caused minimal administrative burden for staff members

Administrative staff members expressed little administrative burden as a result of having these forms at their offices. The extra time that was required to participate in the study was primarily related to identification of eligible patients who had an appointment and either (i) making a list of patients to approach at the practice (p-form) or (ii) sending the survey via email (e-form). For example, in a p-form practice, an administrator noted:

> "*Our office manager would go through the schedule like maybe at the beginning of the week, and any patients that fell within that age category ... she would put a 'Q' [questionnaire] in the schedule. So anytime I saw the 'Q'...I was prompted to hand out a questionnaire...As long as the office manager was there to do it, then it wasn't an issue. [But] she wasn't always able to add the questionnaires, so sometimes we would miss it if we weren't paying attention while we were checking them in.*" (Admin 5)

In a practice that used both web and tablet versions, an administrator explained:

> "*We kind of developed on our own...system of ... going through all our appointments a few days in advance and seeing who was eligible, emailing them, and then the day of, every morning looking through all the ones that we had e-mailed to see if they had responded yet, so then we knew exactly who we had to ask so that ended up working out very well.*" (Admin 3)

One practice described more success implementing the web versus tablet version of the form because of the nature of their office work flow.

> "*We had a lot more success reaching [patients] by email I believe than tablet. Because of the nature of our office, we tend to get patients into rooms very quickly, and so, a lot of time, we didn't have time to get them the tablet before the nurse was calling them in... The whole process, I think, was very positive. We did get a lot of responses. Just the tablet part didn't work very well for us*" (Admin 3).

Theme 3: Screening forms served as a reminder for physicians to discuss smoking cessation with patients

While the screening forms did not necessarily provide new information to physicians, they agreed that forms acted as a reminder to discuss smoking cessation and served as a reaffirmation to patients that smoking is harmful. For example: "*We've been working on smoking cessation for so long...so we've been incorporating it for a long time. So it's hard to know about the degree to which this has an incremental impact on top of that. It's certainly yet another reminder*" (Physician 1). Additionally: "*[The survey] would allow me to say that screening is not yet widely available but they would be an appropriate candidate if they met the criteria. So I think it got the discussion started*" (Physician 2).

Discussion

The aim of this study was to assess the acceptability and feasibility of pre-consultation electronic screening forms to identify high-risk patients eligible for LDCT lung cancer screening. We targeted patients with a scheduled appointment only so that information would be 'just-in-time' and would be fresh in the minds of both patients and physicians [12]. We hypothesized that providing information just prior to the consultation could potentially facilitate a discussion about lung cancer screening and/or smoking cessation between physician and patient. However, several of the interviewed PCPs expressed that they would have preferred to target all eligible patients at their practices and not just those with a scheduled appointment.

The current study had a fairly low acceptance rate by practices of 20%. We do not know if low acceptance was related to lack of enthusiasm toward the pre consultation screening forms specifically on behalf of patients or practice administrative staff or lack of interest in participating in a research study. However, both patients and physicians who agreed to be interviewed expressed positive views about the electronic screening forms. With respect to feasibility, we found a high rate of completion of the three questions related to lung cancer risk. We were also interested whether the web version would be feasible as we had hypothesized that there would be less administrative burden as the EMR system could query the upcoming appointments list and automatically send invitations to eligible patients. Of the 573 patients in the e-form group, 63% completed the forms via the web link and 42% completed the forms via a tablet in the waiting room. We believe that this result can be attributed to technical difficulties with the EMR and/or the availability of cell phone numbers and email addresses in the practices. These problems could be resolved in the future with advances in EMR technology and improvements in capturing cell phone numbers and email addresses. In the current study, approximately, 88% of patients reported having Internet access at home and patients may be willing to provide email addresses to their primary care physicians.

Other studies have assessed the feasibility of introducing various computer-based software programs into primary care. For instance, Voncken-Brewster et al. assessed the feasibility of introducing a web-based self-management application into primary care in the Netherlands for patients living with chronic obstructive pulmonary disease. The authors argued that integrating this particular application in primary care could benefit patients and the organization of care. However, the authors found that patient interest in the application was not sustained through multiple revisits to the application [13]. Fleisher et al. assessed a web-based intervention to improve colorectal cancer screening in the United States (average risk and noncompliant to current screening recommendations). Using a randomized controlled trial design, they compared Internet versus print format of the intervention, and implicitly assumed that participants would embrace the web format. However, the authors found that the web intervention was underused in a "real world" setting [14]. It is possible that the lack of engagement in this web-based intervention was due to the unique password given to each participant that was required to log in to the program each time, and dwindling interest in the intervention. In the current study, patient completion of the three screening questions was high. This could be due to the brief nature of the form, as well the one-time only form completion. The frequency of administration of such screening forms in day-to-day practice is uncertain. Once a patient is referred to a lung cancer screening program, it is anticipated that the program itself would be responsible for follow up of patients.

The current study also reveals important insights regarding the 'real world' application of web-based software in primary care. Using normalization process theory, Mair et al. (2012) argue that the e-health literature has largely focused on organizational issues related to implementation, and neglected consideration of the wider social framework when introducing such technologies into practice [15]. The Normalization Process Model is a theoretical model that can be used to help conceptualize and understand the implementation of complex interventions in primary care. It raises such questions as: How effectively are practices able to organize and carry out a complex intervention in conjunction with their day-to-day activities? How does a complex intervention integrate into the organization in which it is set? [16]. Mair et al. (2012) suggest more empirical investigation is needed to examine how these e-services will affect the clinical interaction, performance, and work allocation, as well as different ways of engaging with professionals prior to and during their implementation [15]. In relation to the current study, by piloting an electronic pre-screening form (or "e-health intervention") prior to the availability of LDCT screening, we gained important insights into the ways that this particular electronic strategy was implemented in practices, its perceived effect on practice functioning, and the willingness of patients to complete screening forms.

Limitations

There are five limitations of this pilot study. First, we were unable to determine the actual number of eligible patients in each practice during the study period. Estimates of eligibility were based on the actual number of eligible patients seen in each practice in one year prorated to the 16-week study period. We do not know if the estimate we calculated was an over or under estimate of the actual number of patients seen in each practice.

The inability to obtain actual numbers of eligible patients during the study period was related to difficulties in linking the patients' demographic information to the list of upcoming appointments. Improvements in EMR software capabilities will be needed to reduce barriers to the implementation of this type of pre-consultation screening strategy in primary care.

Second, this pilot study was conducted in six primary care practices affiliated with one community hospital. We do not know if our findings would be similar in other types of practice settings. Third, in the quantitative component of study, the first practice was assigned by coin toss and subsequent practices were assigned by alternation. The results of our study need to be interpreted with these design limitations in mind. In the future, a stronger design is warranted by including practices affiliated with more than one hospital and with random allocation to groups.

Fourth, patient recall during the qualitative interviews was limited. Although we attempted to avoid recall issues by selecting patients who had completed the survey within the previous three weeks, this was not always possible. The median number of days between form completion and interview was 70 days. Delays in contacting patients occurred because of non-responses to phone calls, incorrect numbers, and waiting for written consent forms to be returned by post rather than accepting verbal consent by phone. In the future, a shorter time span between form completion and interviews would be preferable.

Fifth, in this study, all forms were written and completed in English. Although one interview was conducted with the assistance of a translator, it is possible that we missed patients who may not have been able to read the pre-screening form, and who may have felt uncomfortable participating in an interview. Pre-screening forms that are distributed only in English are not able to capture data from diverse linguistic populations. Translated versions of the pre-screening form should be made available if a screening program were to be implemented in primary care in Ontario.

Conclusions

Brief pre-consultation electronic forms for LDCT screening eligibility completed at home via the web, or on tablets in the waiting room were acceptable and feasible when software and clinical process were contextually tailored to each practice environment. If brief lung cancer pre-screening forms are to be implemented, practice contextual factors such as technological capabilities/ available software and day-to-day practice functioning would need to be considered.

The current study provides insight into the potential future implementation of electronic lung cancer pre-screening forms in primary care. It is important that research continue to be conducted on potential screening processes in primary care to anticipate and remedy potential issues before a LDCT screening program is widely available.

Abbreviations

eCHAT: Electronic case-finding and help assessment tool; e-form: Electronic form; EMR: Electronic medical record; LDCT: Low-dose computed tomography; PCPs: Primary care physicians; p-form: Paper form; y: years old

Acknowledgements

We wish to thank the physicians and staff who participated in the study. We thank Michelle Greiver, MD, Ivanka Pribramska, and Rahim Moineddin, PhD for their advice and support.

Funding

This study was funded by The Ontario Cancer Screening Research Network.

Authors' contributions

MAO conceived the study with FS and LP, led the qualitative study component, interpreted the data, and was a major contributor to writing and revising the manuscript. FS conceived the study with MAO and LP, led the quantitative study component, interpreted the data, and critically reviewed the manuscript. AC was responsible for qualitative data collection and analysis, including all participant interviews, coding and analysis of transcripts. AC was a major contributor to writing the manuscript. RS was responsible for assisting with data collection in primary care practices, data analysis, and critically reviewed the manuscript. SS was responsible for assisting with data collection in primary care practices, and critically reviewed the manuscript. LP conceived the study with MAO and FS and critically reviewed the manuscript. All authors read and approved the final manuscript.

Consent for publication

Not applicable

Competing interests

The authors declare that they have no competing interests.

Author details

[1]Department of Family and Community Medicine, University of Toronto, 500 University Avenue, Fifth Floor, Toronto, ON M5G 1V7, Canada. [2]North York General Hospital, Toronto, ON, Canada. [3]Medical School, University of St Andrews, Scotland, UK. [4]Sunnybrook Research Institute, Toronto, ON, Canada. [5]Institute for Clinical Evaluative Sciences, Toronto, ON, Canada.

References

1. Aberle DR, Adams AM, Berg CD, Black WC, Clapp JD, Fagerstrom RM, Gareen IF, Gatsonis C, Marcus PM, Sicks JD. For the National Lung Screening Trial Research Team. Reduced lung-cancer mortality with low-dose computed tomographic screening. N Engl J Med. 2011;365(5):395–409. https://doi.org/10.1056/NEJMoa1102873.
2. Field JK, Duffy SW, Baldwin DR, Whynes DK, Deveraj A, Brain KE, Eisen T, Gosney J, Green BA, Holemans JA, Kavanagh T, Kerr KM, Ledson M, Lifford KJ, McRonald FE, Nair A, Page RD, Parmar MKB, Rassl DM, Rintoul RC, Screaton NJ, Wald NJ, Weller D, Williamson PR, Yadegarfar G, Hansell DM. UK lung cancer RCT pilot screening trial: baseline findings from the screening arm provide evidence for the potential implementation of lung cancer screening. Thorax. 2016;71:161–70.
3. Goodyear-Smith F, Warren J, Elley CR. The eCHAT program to facilitate healthy changes in New Zealand primary care. Family Medicine World Perspective. 2013;26:177–82.
4. Henderson S, DeGroff A, Richards TB, Kish-Doto J, Soloe C, Heminger C, Rohan EA. Qualitative analysis of lung cancer screening practices by primary care physicians. J Community Health. 2011;36:949–56.
5. Sittig DF. Potential impact of advanced clinical information technology on cancer care in 2015. Cancer Causes Control. 2006;17:813–20.
6. Devers KJ, Frankel RM. Study design in qualitative research- 2: sampling and data collection strategies. Education for Health. 2000;13:263–71.
7. Crabtree B, Miller W. Doing qualitative research. 2nd ed. London: Sage Publications; 1999.
8. Glaser BG, Strauss AL. The discovery of grounded theory: strategies for qualitative research. Chicago. Aldine. 1967;
9. Charmaz K: Constructing grounded theory. London; Thousand Oaks, Calif.: Sage Publications, 2006.
10. Boeije HA. Purposeful approach to the constant comparative method in the analysis of qualitative data. Quality & Quantity. 2002;36:391–409.
11. Guba EG, Lincoln YS. Fourth generation evaluation. Newbury Park: Sage Publications; 1989.

12. Naughton F. Delivering "Just-In-Time" Smoking cessation support via mobile phones: current knowledge and future directions. Nicotine Tob Res. 2016 May 28.
13. Voncken-Brewster V, Tange H, Moser A, Nagykaldi Z, de Vries H, van der Weijden T. Integrating a tailored e-health self-management application for chronic obstructive pulmonary disease patients into primary care: a pilot study. BMC Fam Pract. 2014;15:1–10.
14. Fleisher L, Kandadai V, Keenan E, Miller SM, Devarajan K, Ruth KJ, Rodoletz M, Bieber EJ, Weinberg DS. Build it, and will they come? Unexpected findings from a study on a web-based intervention to improve colorectal cancer screening. J Health Commun. 2012;17:41–53.
15. Mair FS, May C, O'Donnell C, Finch T, Sullivan F, Murray E. Factors that promote or inhibit the implementation of e-heath systems: an explanatory systematic review. Bulletin world health. Organization. 2012;90:357–64.
16. May C, Finch T, Mair F, Ballini L, Dowrick C, Eccles M, Gask L, MacFarlane A, Murray E, Rapley T, Rogers A, Treweek S, Wallace P, Anderson G, Burns J, Heaven B. Understanding the implementation of complex interventions in health care: the normalization process model. BMC Health Serv Res. 2007;7:148–54.

12

Family-centered depression treatment for older men in primary care

Ladson Hinton[1*], Andrés F. Sciolla[2], Jürgen Unützer[3], Edward Elizarraras[4], Richard L. Kravitz[5] and Ester Carolina Apesoa-Varano[6]

Abstract

Background: Family members often play important roles in the lives of depressed older men and frequently attend primary care visits with their loved ones, yet surprisingly little is known about how to most effectively engage and include family members in depression treatment. However, including family in depression treatment may be difficult due to several factors, such as depression stigma and family conflicts. The objective of this study was to describe challenges in engaging family members in older men's depression treatment and potential strategies to overcome those challenges.

Methods: A cross-sectional, qualitative descriptive interview study was conducted in a safety-net, Federally Qualified Health Center in California's Central Valley. A total of 37 stakeholders were recruited, including 15 depressed older (i.e. age ≥ 60) men, 12 family members, and 10 clinic staff. Depressed men were identified through mail outreach, waiting room screening, and referral. Depressed men identified family members who were later approached to participate. We also recruited a purposeful sample of clinic staff. Interviews explored stakeholder perspectives on family involvement in men's depression treatment as part of a primary care intervention. Interviews were conducted using a semi-structured interview guide, tape-recorded, transcribed verbatim, and translated if the interview was conducted in Spanish.

Results: Four themes were identified representing core challenges: engaging men at the right time; preserving men's sense of autonomy; managing privacy concerns; and navigating family tensions. Stakeholders also provided practical suggestions and advice about how each of these challenges might be addressed.

Conclusions: While engaging family is a promising approach to strengthen depression care for older men in primary care settings, several potential challenges exist. Family- centered depression intervention development and clinical practice need to anticipate these challenges and to develop approaches and guidelines to address them.

Keywords: Depression, Older men, Family, Qualitative

Background

Advancing depression care for depressed older men is a public health priority because older men are less likely than older women to receive depression treatment and are also more likely to commit suicide [1]. While prior research has demonstrated the challenges in getting depressed men to seek help for depression [2], relatively little is known about how to tailor treatments to more effectively engage and treat depressed men [3]. Mobilizing family members, who are often already assisting older adults in their healthcare, to support depression treatment has been suggested as one possible strategy that may help to improve outcomes and more effectively engage under-served groups such as older men and minorities [4–6]. Despite the possible value of including family members as a strategy to close gaps in care for depressed older men, little is known about the most effective ways to do this in primary care settings.

* Correspondence: lwhinton@ucdavis.edu
[1]Department of Psychiatry and Behavioral Sciences, University of California Davis, 2230 Stockton Blvd., Sacramento, CA 95618, USA
Full list of author information is available at the end of the article

The potential value of family involvement in supporting older men's depression treatment is supported by both observational studies and intervention studies. Men often rely on family members, particularly their wives and daughters, for assistance with managing their health and health care, including medication management, health-care decision-making, transportation to doctor's appointments, and participating in healthcare visits [7–11]. More than one third of older adults who present for care in primary care settings are accompanied by family members, usually a spouse or adult child [12, 13]. Families often play a very influential role in getting depressed or suicidal men into formal treatment [1, 14–16]. Primary care providers view family members as potential allies in depression treatment [5] and a majority of older men prefer to have family involved in their care [6]. While we are not aware of any depression intervention studies that have systematically incorporated family members into treatment, one review of the literature found that family involvement in psychosocial interventions for chronic illness can improve outcomes [17].

Family members may also hinder depression care [4]. Family communication patterns that are critical, controlling or overprotective are associated with negative health and mental health outcomes [18, 19]. When family members view depression as a highly-stigmatized condition, a normal response to loss or aging, or as a part of co-occurring medical conditions, they may discourage help-seeking or be critical of the older man with depression [20–22]. Families may also view depression as "unmanly" and encourage men to "tough it out" rather than seek help [23]. Family attitudes towards antidepressants and endorsement of depression-related stigma can negatively influence patient adherence [24, 25].

While the literature highlights the potential value and challenges of engaging family to support older men's depression care, little is known about how to address these challenges. In this manuscript, we describe the results of formative work (i.e. qualitative interviews with key stakeholders) as part of a larger effort to develop and test a family-centered intervention for ethnically diverse older men with depression in primary care settings. Specifically, we describe stakeholder perspectives on both the challenges in engaging family members in men's depression treatment and the potential strategies to address those challenges. The larger goal of the project was to develop and test a primary-care based intervention to strengthen evidence-based depression treatments (e.g. behavioral activation, anti-depressant medications) for older men through the involvement of family members.

Methods

Setting

Participants were recruited from two primary care clinics at San Joaquin General Hospital (SJGH), a large county hospital in California's Central Valley that provides care for underserved populations including a high proportion of Mexican Americans.

Participant selection and recruitment

Three different stakeholder groups were recruited: depressed older men, their family members, and clinic staff, including those with administrative responsibilities.

Recruitment of depressed older men

Fifteen men were recruited from the San Joaquin General Hospital primary care clinics. The study inclusion criteria were as follows: (1) age 60 or older; (2) English or Spanish speaking; (3) non-demented; (4) non-psychotic; and (5) have a PHQ-9 score ≥ 10 [26]; and (6) expressed a willingness to have a family member be interviewed as part of the study. Three different recruitment approaches were used. Letters were mailed to 115 men with a chart diagnosis of depression or a PHQ-9 score ≥ 10 in the past year, 15 of whom returned the postcard expressing interest in participating and 10 were successfully interviewed. We also screened 123 men age 60 and above at the time of their primary care appointments and 23 had a score of ≥10. Of those 23, 4 were interviewed (13 did not have a family member, 5 declined, and one was lost to follow-up). Finally, 7 patients were referred directly from primary care physicians (PCPs) and 1 was successfully interviewed (2 declined, 2 were ineligible, and 2 were lost to follow-up).

Recruitment of family members

Of the 15 depressed men who were interviewed, 12 identified family members who were then successfully recruited and interviewed. For the remaining 3 men, their family members either could not be reached or declined to be interviewed.

Recruitment of clinic staff

We conducted a purposive sampling to identify 10 staff including administrators, primary care physicians, social workers and physician assistants. Because insights regarding the topic of engaging family in men's depression care might vary depending on staff role and training, we chose to interview a variety of different types of staff to generate a wider range of perspectives.

In-depth interviews

A qualitative approach was chosen to allow us to elicit and better understand stakeholder attitudes and concerns related to engaging family in older men's depression care, a topic about which very little is known. In-depth interviews with stakeholders were conducted by interviewers who were bilingual/bicultural and who received training and supervision in conducting qualitative interviews. The interviews were semi-structured and included pre-determined topics and associated probes. These pre-determined topics were chosen by the research team to elicit in an open-ended fashion stakeholder perspectives on involving family in men's depression treatment and to explore stakeholders' perspectives on specific aspects of the research team's anticipated intervention approach. For older men and family members, the topics included family relationships and living situation, depression explanatory model and views of treatment, attitudes and experiences related to family involvement in depression care, and best approaches to involve family in older men's depression care. For clinic staff, the topics included background and role in clinic, attitudes and experiences in having family involved in depression treatment, and best approaches to involve family in older men's depression treatment. The interviewer had latitude to explore topics and emerging themes as they arose during the interview.

Interviews were conducted separately with depressed older men and their identified family members. Interviews were conducted in the interviewee's home and in their language of choice, either English or Spanish, and lasted 0.5 to 2.0 h. We interviewed clinic staff in their offices or by phone. Clinic staff interviews lasted 0.5–1.5 h. All interviews were digitally audio-recorded, transcribed verbatim into text by bilingual research staff and de-identified. Interviews conducted in Spanish were transcribed into English by bilingual research staff.

Data analysis

Computer-assisted data analysis (i.e. data management and coding) was conducted using NVIVO® 10.0 (QSR International) and involved multiple steps that included open-coding and constant comparison, following an accepted approach for qualitative descriptive studies [27–29]. A descriptive approach was chosen because the goal of the study was to generate knowledge that would directly and pragmatically inform intervention development and implementation [30, 31]. First, three members of the research team, including two who were bilingual in Spanish and English, independently read and coded the interviews to identify emergent themes (i.e. meaning units of text) that related to family involvement in men's depression care. The entire research team, which included a sociologist and two clinicians, then met to discuss their coding and through a consensus process grouped conceptually related themes. This process led to the identification of four themes representing core challenges related to family involvement in men's depression treatment. A code book was developed and used by two members of the research team to systematically code the data for each of these core challenges. In this second round of coding we also identified mentions of possible strategies relevant to address each challenge in intervention development and clinical practice. Data saturation was reached for each of the four core challenges described in this study [32].

Results

Participant characteristics

Older men had a mean age of 63.5 years, were ethnically diverse (47% Latino) and 8 (53%) were married. Most family caregivers were either spouses (50%, n = 6) or adult children (25%, n = 3) and 42% (n = 5) were Latino (see Table 1 for additional characteristics). Clinic staff included physicians, social workers, nurses, physician assistants and clinic administrators (see Table 2 for additional characteristics).

Qualitative findings

Analysis of the interviews with key stakeholders (i.e., depressed men, family members of depressed older men, and clinic staff) led to the identification of four themes related to core challenges in the implementation of a family-centered intervention for depressed older men in primary care: engaging men at the right time, preserving men's sense of autonomy, managing privacy concerns, and navigating family tensions. In their discussions of these themes, stakeholders also made practical suggestions about how these challenges might be overcome.

"They got to be ready": engaging men at the right time

Stakeholders emphasized that the right time to engage men in a family-centered treatment is after they recognize that they are depressed and accepted the need for treatment. The wife of a depressed man told us that it would be difficult to engage her husband because *"I guess he thinks he doesn't have a problem."* Minimizing depressive symptoms or attributing them to other causes were cited as reasons men might not self-identify as depressed. Stakeholders emphasized that depression might need to be severe (e.g., *"they have to be willing, they have to hit rock bottom"*) before men are willing to accept any treatment: *"I think the person has to have a desire to do something. You know, it's like that saying I heard before, too. It's I'm sick and tired of being sick and tired" (depressed older man).* Stigma may also play an important role in men's reluctance to recognize their depression and seek help: *"Well you have to get past the stigma of depression first..." (social worker).* Once they have accepted the diagnosis of depression, it may also take men time to warm up to the idea of family involvement. As one older man told us: *"But I wouldn't force that [family involvement] because I do kind of believe is when you are ready and the reason why is for example like I would've rebelled if I didn't, if you tried to force me with people."*

Table 1 Characteristics of interviewed depressed older men and their family members

	Men (*N* = 15)	Family (*N* = 12)
Mean age	63.5	53.7
Ethnicity		
Latino	7 (46.66%)	5 (41.67%)
White non-Hispanic	4 (26.67%)	5 (41.67%
Other	4 (26.67%)	2 (16.66%)
Language		
English	12 (80%)	11 (91.67%)
Spanish	3 (20%)	1 (8.33%)
Country of birth		
United States	11 (73.34%)	11 (91.67%)
Mexico	2 (13.33%)	1 (8.33%)
Other	2 (13.33%)	0
Self-reported general health		
Excellent/very good	0	4 (33.34%)
Good	5 (33.33%)	5 (41.67%)
Fair	6 (40%)	2 (16.66%)
Poor	4 (26.67%)	1 (8.33%)
Relationship		
Spouse/partner	N/A	6 (50%)
Child	N/A	3 (25%)
Other family relative	N/A	2 (16.67%)
Family friend	N/A	1 (8.33%)
Marital status		
Married	8 (53.33%)	6 (50%)
Living in a marriage-like relationship	0	1 (8.33%)
Separated/divorced/widowed	4 (26.67%)	3 (25%)
Never married	3 (20%)	2 (16.67%)
Education		
< 12 years	4 (26.67%)	4 (33.33%)
12 years	5 (33.33%)	4 (33.33%)
> 12 years	6 (40%)	4 (33.33%)
Employment		
No, retired	9 (60%)	5 (41.67%)
No, unemployed but seeking work	5 (33.33%)	2 (16.67%)
Yes, part-time	0	1 (8.33%)
Yes, full-time	1 (6.67%)	4 (33.33%)
Income		
Less than $10,000	7 (46.67%)	3 (25%)
$10,000–$25,000	7 (46.67%)	5 (41.67%)
$25,000–$50,000	1 (6.66%)	4 (33.33%)

Table 2 Interviewed clinic staff characteristics

Characteristics	N (%)
Age	
20–29 years	2 (20%)
30–39 years	1 (10%)
40–49 years	4 (40%)
50–59 years	3 (30%)
60+ years	0
Gender	
Female	5 (50%)
Male	5 (50%)
Ethnicity	
Latino	5 (50%)
White non-Hispanic	5 (50%)
Role in clinic	
Non-MD clinical staff	5 (50%)
Physicians	4 (40%)
Administrators	1 (10%)
Years in practice	
1–10 Years	5 (50%)
11–20 Years	3 (30%)
> 20 Years	2 (20%)

Stakeholders suggested that for the reasons cited above, some men are unlikely to accept family involvement at the beginning of their depression treatment. As one primary care physician told us: *"I have to kind of work with them and initially gain their trust to even introduce the possibility of depression."* Another clinic staff emphasized the need for a more gradual approach that begins by helping men gain insight before engaging family members: *"I think we need to work with a patient first to help them gain a better insight to their situation, to move them from, say pre-contemplative to contemplative stage, so that they're more willing to hear their family and accept their support that they would have from their family."* This was echoed by a depressed older man who said: *"First the person gets to know what's going on with me and then they you know", "would you mind if I ask your wife or somebody from your family to participate in the next visit?"* Thus, for a subgroup of men, it might make sense to broach the topic of family involvement after several sessions or even in the middle stages of treatment.

"They have to know they're in charge": preserving men's sense of autonomy

Stakeholders also stressed that involving family members might be off-putting or threatening to some men who may perceive it as undermining their sense of autonomy and control. The value placed on autonomy by men was viewed as closely connected to men's masculine self-identity, as illustrated in the following quote from a clinician: "*You're telling the patient, 'I don't think you can handle this on your own, I want to bring someone else to help you handle it'. And this is a gentleman who's been living for sixty years plus, some or most of it on his own, you know." Even if he's had a family, he's been at the head of the family, he's been at the top of his game, now you're telling him, "you're going to need some help"*. Some participants viewed older men as particularly vulnerable to real or perceived threats to their autonomy because they often experienced other losses that undermined their independence and sense of usefulness, such as physical disabilities or job loss. A wife graphically described the importance of independence for her depressed husband: "*Sometimes a man is hard to help cause they, they want to do it or, you know, they don't want to have you do it for them. And so that's one thing I kind of have to keep holding myself back a lot of times when he's eating. [...] I want to help him out, but uh, I realized that him being a man he wants to try, he wants to do it himself.*" Another potential obstacle is that men might perceive family members as too controlling: "*... and the bottom line is this man feels as though his family member attempts to control what he does and that it's under the guise of I'm trying to help you.*"

While emphasizing men's need for control as a challenge, stakeholders also suggested that a family-centered intervention could be effective if it valued and addressed men's need for control while negotiating a role for family involvement. As a clinic provider told us: "*I think that [family involvement] can be helpful as long as that doesn't take the control and autonomy away from the patient.*" Along the same lines, a family member stressed that for the model to work, "*...the person who has depression has to know that they have that they're in charge.*" One depressed older man emphasized that allowing men to feel that they are "in charge" might begin by respecting their preferences in who to involve in their care and for the clinician not to make assumptions about which family member to involve. Clinic staff suggested other possible strategies for helping men feel in charge of their treatment, such as managing their own medications: "*try to work out a system that the older man is in charge of their own medication, so that you empower them to be in charge.*" Asked if family might assist men in identifying side effects and remembering to take their medication, another clinician said, "*Yeah I think that that can be helpful as long as that doesn't take the control and autonomy away from the patient to, you don't want to feel like they're belittled.*"

"Some stuff is personal": managing privacy concerns

A variety of concerns were expressed about how the presence of a family member might interfere with the older men to discuss sensitive or "personal" issues with their healthcare provider. As one man said: "*I don't know if, um, I have such mixed emotions, but I don't know if we should have the family member involved in their meeting. I just don't think that's productive myself, and I'm going to explain to you why: because then the person might not open up to things, that is very private.*" This man went on to give an example of something he wouldn't want to share with his family: "*I had kept secret that I was almost killed working for the FBI in (the) US Marshalls office, and never told them to what degree, that I could've been killed, and I never shared to them that I had suffered emotionally from that.*" Additional reasons for not wanting to share things with family members included not wanting to "burden" them or feeling uncomfortable about showing emotions. As one man said "*Well, because no one wants to hear about your little problems when they got problems of their own.*" Stakeholders provided other topics that men might not feel comfortable discussing with family in the room, such as drug or alcohol use or sexual dysfunction. One provider echoed these concerns about the need for privacy around mental health issues: "*Yes, so the one thing is that there's somebody else that they trust to that level that they are going to allow [them] to be in that circle of privacy, of knowing their mental or health issues. That's number one: is there's somebody there they can trust? Sometimes even their very close partners spouse may not be the right person for them to trust, because there might be some issues.*" Finally, some providers expressed concerns about sharing information with a family member from a medical-legal perspective (e.g., signing a HIPPA form or verbal consent). While some insisted patients would be required to sign a "release of information form", others indicated that it was sufficient for the patient to give verbal consent when a family member was present.

To address the concerns about privacy in the context of a family-centered intervention, stakeholders said it would be important to give men the opportunity to spend at least some time talking individually with their provider while being treated for depression. Preserving this "one-on-one" time was viewed as important because as one depressed older man told us, "*... some of the things that I talked about was personal.*" This might also give providers a chance to query men about topics they would prefer not to discuss in the presence of family members.

"When the family is angry": navigating family tensions

Strained family relationships may make it difficult to engage and work effectively with family members in treatment. Sharing his reluctance to involve family members, one provider said: *"There might be a lot of family issues and problems because of like maybe even a family you know is almost you know there's maybe there's a lot of arguments and a lot of issues."* Older men discussed how strained relationships might make family involvement difficult. Referring to his wife, one man said: *"It scares me sometimes because we'll get on it about something like that right there, and she turns everything around that it's my fault."* Speaking about the possibility of having his brother participate in his depression care another man said: *"Yeah because like for me, me and my brother it would be a bad thing for him to be around where I can look at him and it'd be it'd be just a big fight. All I do is close my mind down."* Some marital relationship may be so frayed that the partner is not willing to help, as described by a social worker: *"So what levels of you know 'Screw you I, I don't really care about you anymore, I've stopped loving you a long time ago. Now you want my help?' You know so um there's that like what level of investment does the family have in helping this person who they may have all this antipathy for?"*

While highlighting friction and tensions that might exist between men and family members, stakeholders also pointed to approaches that might help to overcome these challenges. One older man suggested "ground rules" to facilitate more constructive involvement of family: *"That would be everybody on an even ground. We already have it pre-limited to where there would be no yelling, no cussing, ground rules."* An important part of getting people on "even ground" is to establish a common understanding of what depression is and the nature of the treatment model. One of the depressed older men said: *"Maybe the family is angry at the person who is suffering and so there's issues there that need to be addressed, education-wise. And there is some tender and loving care that needs to be done there, from that perspective."* A family member emphasized that education might be empowering to family members because *"if you know more about depression you know how to handle it."* This man and several others highlighted the need to "educate" family members, either about the nature of depression, its treatment or about how the family might be more supportive to help men recover from their depression. As a social worker told us, *"I wonder if family members had some basic motivational interviewing techniques, could they use that to support the family member maybe in moving a little closer to education, moving a little closer to behavioral activation and other treatment interventions. So sometimes their approach is a bit abrasive and it's purely in my opinion lack of education."* Thus, stakeholders voiced their opinion that a successful intervention would require anticipating and managing potential or emerging family conflict, as well as educating family members.

Discussion

There is a growing consensus that our health care system should be both person and family-centered to address the pressing needs of older adults who suffer from chronic health problems, including depression and other mental health conditions [33]. This study adds to our understanding of the types of challenges to involving family in depression care and how these challenges might be addressed in the development and implementation of a family-centered treatment model for depression. Through in-depth qualitative interviews with those who have the most at stake in a family-centered intervention model – depressed older men, family members, and providers - we identified four themes that represent core challenges as well as strategies to address them that are relevant for for both clinical reseach and primary care practice.

The core themes identified in this study are consistent with a growing literature on men, mental health and masculinity [34]. Men may be reluctant to seek help for depression or to accept the diagnosis because depression carries a "double-stigma" [1], threatening both men's masculine self-identity and their sense of normality (i.e. stigma of "craziness" or severe mental illness). The value men place on self-sufficiency and control, for example, reflect traditional maculine norms, such as stoicism, that may inhibit both the expression of distress and formal help-seeking [3]. In addition, the importance of privacy for older men may reflect concerns about appearing "weak" or "vulnerable" in the presence of family members, situations that may evoke discomfort and even shame. Loss of control and feelings of shame are central to older men's experience of depression [35]. An important caveat is that there is considerable variability among men in their masculine self-image (i.e., multiple masculinities) potentially creating more openness among some men to both depression treatment and family involvement [36]. Finally, it is important to stress that men may value independence in some aspects of depression self-management (e.g. taking medications) which may also serve to affirm their masculinity and to preserve their autonomy.

Our findings are also consistent with prior studies highlighting the complexity of work with families in the context of both health and mental health problems [37]. Prior work has shown how family members may serve as both barriers and facilitators of depression care in primary care [4] and among Latinos in mental health treatment [38]. There is also a literature on families and depression highlighting how families may offer support to people who are depressed but can also be unsupportive or even trigger or worsen depression [39, 40]. It is worth noting that for older men their family helpers are most likely to be women (i.e. either wives or daughter/daughter-in-laws) and that these gender and generational differences may also influence the qualities and dynamics of provision of support. Together, these prior findings and ours strike a cautionary note about family involvement in depression care that underscores the need for better guidelines and models to inform clinical practice and intervention work. These guidelines might also be helpful more broadly for mental health professionals, many of whom have not received formal training on how and when to involve family members in depression treatments for older adults.

In their description of themes, stakeholders offered practical suggestions that may help guide clinicians and interventionists in overcoming potential challenges. In Table 3 we summarize the possible approaches that could be used by clinicians, drawing on the suggestions of stakeholders and extrapolating from these based on our own insights from our work in this area. In terms of the timing of approaching men about family involvement in their depression care, our study suggests that there is not a "one size fits all" approach. While for some men the right time may be at the start of treatment for others it may be the middle phase of treatment to allow more time to come to terms with their diagnosis and to build trust with their PCP. To preserve men's sense of autonomy and control, our findings highlight the importance of having discussions with men to assess their values and preferences, both in terms of whether to involve family but also how family is to be involved and whether there are any "off-limits" topics. These discussions might also include discussion about any concerns related to losing control over the treatment process, not having "private time" with the provider, escalation of family tensions or conflicts, and burdening family with emotional troubles. Jointly educating older men and their families about the nature and treatment of depression, laying ground-rules, agreeing on an agenda for each session, and focusing on concrete behavioral tasks may help diffuse existing family tensions. Finally, providers might benefit from education about obtaining authorization from the patient to include family members in treatment. Finally, clinicians should also consider and assess the impact of participation in older men's depression care on family members themselves; it is possible, for example, that in some cases older men may want to include family but this might not be in the best interests of the family member's health or well-being.

This study has several limitations. First, caution should be used in drawing any conclusions about the gender-specific nature of our findings. Our study was focused on depressed older men and we lack a comparison group of older women and their family members that would allow us to examine gender similarities and differences. In addition, our interviews with staff did not include queries about gender differences. Second, while a strength of our study is the inclusion of multiple stakeholder perspectives to provide a richer description of these themes, systematic comparison of the viewpoints of the three stakeholder groups is beyond scope of this study. In addition, our study was not designed to systematically compare the perspectives of Latinos and white non-Hispanics (or other ethnic/racial groups) but rather to identify themes that were broadly reflected in the sample and were relevant to development and implementation of a common intervention. Finally, our sample is unique in certain ways (i.e. safety net clinic, men age 60–70, high representation of Latinos) and caution should be used in generalizing to other populations.

Conclusion

As our healthcare system moves toward more patient- and family-centered care, we need to understand how family members can most effectively be engaged to support care for depression and other chronic conditions in primary care and other treatment settings. To our knowledge, this is the first study to identify these four core challenges to family-centered depression treatment delivered in primary are settings and to provide practical suggestions on how these challenges might be addressed.

Table 3 Summary of core challenges to engaging family in men's depression treatment and possible strategies to overcome them

Challenge	Possible strategies
Engaging men at the right time	• Work with men to help them accept the diagnosis and need for treatment before involving family • Giving men time to "warm-up" to the idea of family involvement
Preserving men's sense of autonomy	• Communicate centrality of men's preferences and values in treatment • Assess men's preferences for family role in specific aspects of treatment
Managing privacy concerns	• Educate clinicians about guidelines for involving family members (e.g. HIPAA guidelines) [41] • Allow men to specify topics that are "off-limits" in discussions with family • Allow flexibility for care manager to meet individually with patient • Address men's concerns about burdening family members
Navigating family tensions	• Set ground rules for joint sessions • Educate family about the nature of depression • Focus on specific behavioral tasks that can be shared with family • Develop a jointly agreed upon agenda for each treatment session

This study, including the challenges we experienced in recruiting participants, demonstrates that engaging family in the delivery of mental health services is not always straightforward or easy and requires careful assessment of the preferences, concerns, and needs of patients and family members. To advance the field, we now need to apply knowledge from this and other observational studies to develop and test family-enhanced depression interventions in real-world settings.

Acknowledgements
Yesi Avelar B.A. assisted with data acquisition and management. Eduardo Delgadillo Alfaro assisted with data management. We are grateful to Dr. Andrew Smith for assistance in coordinating patient and staff recruitment.

Funding
This study was supported with funding from the National Institute of Mental Health (R34 MH099296).

Authors' contributions
LH was involved in all aspects of the study, including conceptual design of the study, obtaining grant funding to support the study, supervision of data collection, data analysis and interpretation, writing of the manuscript and integrating comments from co-authors. AS was involved in data collection, data analysis and interpretation, writing sections of the manuscript and critically reviewing drafts of the manuscript. CAV, JU and RK contributed to the conceptual design of the study, interpretation of the data and critically reviewing drafts of this manuscript. EE assisted with data acquisition, data management and interpretation, writing sections of the manuscript, and critically reviewing drafts. All authors read and approved the final manuscript.

Consent for publication
All authors have given their consent for publication.

Competing interests
The authors declare that they have no competing interests.

Author details
[1]Department of Psychiatry and Behavioral Sciences, University of California Davis, 2230 Stockton Blvd., Sacramento, CA 95618, USA. [2]Department of Psychiatry, University of California Davis, 2230 Stockton Blvd., Sacramento, CA 95618, USA. [3]Department of Psychiatry and Behavioral Sciences, 1959 NE Pacific Street, Seattle, WA 98195, USA. [4]Department of Biology, San Francisco State University, 1600 Holloway Avenue, San Francisco, CA 94132, USA. [5]Division of General Internal Medicine, University of California Davis, 4150 V Street, Sacramento, CA 95817, USA. [6]Betty Irene School of Nursing, University of California Davis, 4610 X Street, Sacramento, CA 95817, USA.

References
1. Hinton L, et al. Gender disparities in the treatment of late-life depresion: qualitative and quantitative findings from the IMPACT trial. Am J Geriatr Psychiatr. 2006;14(10):884–92.
2. Rochlen AB, Hoyer WD. Marketing mental health to men: theoretical and practical considerations. J Clin Psychol. 2005;61(6):675–84.
3. Seidler ZE, et al. The role of masculinity in men's help-seeking for depression: A systematic review. Clin Psychol Rev. 2016;49:106–18.
4. Hinton L, et al. A descriptive qualitative study of the roles of family members in older men's depression treatment from the perspectives of older men and primary care providers. Int J Geriatr Psychiatry. 2015;30(5):514–22.
5. Apesoa-Varano EC, et al. Clinician approaches and strategies for engaging older men in depression care. Am J Geriatr Psychiatr. 2010;18(7):586–95.
6. Dwight-Johnson M, et al. Depression treatment preferences of older white and Mexican origin men. Gen Hosp Psychiatry. 2013;35:59–65.
7. Compton MT, Esterberg ML. Treatment delay in first-episode nonaffective psychosis: a pilot study with African American family members and the theory of planned behavior. Compr Psychiatry. 2005;46(4):291–5.
8. Maly RC, et al. Racial/ethnic group differences in treatment decision-making and treatment received among older breast carcinoma patients. Cancer. 2006;106:957–65.
9. US-Administration-on-Aging, America's families care: A report on the needs of America's family caregivers. 2000.
10. Dettinger E, Clarkberg M. Informal caregiving and retirement timing among men and women: Gender and caregiving relationships in late midlife. J Fam Issues. 2002;23(7):857–79.
11. Lima JC, et al. Spousal caregiving in late midlife versus older ages: implications of work and family obligations. J Gerontol B Psychol Sci Soc Sci. 2008;63:229–38.
12. Sayers SL, et al. Family involvement in the care of healthy medical outpatients. Fam Pract. 2006;23(3):317–24.
13. Wolff JL, Roter DL. Hidden in plain sight: Medical visit companions as a resource for vulnerable older adults. Arch Intern Med. 2008;168(13):1409–15.
14. Cabassa LJ. Latino immigrant men's perceptions of depression and attitudes toward help seeking. Hisp J Behav Sci. 2007;29(4):492–509.
15. Murray J, et al. Primary care professionals' perceptions of depression in older people: a qualitative study. Soc Sci Med. 2006;63:1363–73.
16. Owens C, et al. A qualitative study of help seeking and primary care consultation prior to suicide. Br J Gen Pract. 2005;55(516):503–9.
17. Martire LM, et al. Is it beneficial to involve a family member? A meta-analysis of psychosocial interventions for chronic illness. Health Psychol. 2004;23(6):559–611.
18. Rosland AM, Heisler M, Piette JD. The impact of family behaviors and communication patterns on chronic illness outcomes: a systematic review. J Behav Med. 2012;35(2):221–39.
19. Jenkins JH, Karno M. The meaning of expressed emotion: theoretical Issues raised. Am J Psychiatry. 1992;149(1):9–21.
20. Sarkisian CA, Hays RD, Mangione CM. Do older adults expect to age successfully? The association between expecatations regarding aging and beliefs regarding healthcare seeking among older adults. J Am Geriatr Soc. 2002;50:1837–43.
21. Bogner HR, Dobransky LN, Wittink MN. Patient ethnicity and perceptions of families and friends regarding depression treatment. Ethn Health. 2008;13(5):465–78.
22. Burg M, Seeman T. Families and health: the negative side of social ties. Ann Behav Med. 1994;16:109–15.
23. Switzer JF, et al. "Pull yourself up by your bootstraps": a response to depression in older adults. Qual Health Res. 2006;16:1207–16.
24. Zivin K, Kales HC. Adherence to depression treatment in older adults: A narrative review. Drugs Aging. 2008;25(7):559–71.
25. Sirey J, Bruce ML, Alexopoulos GS. The treatment initiation program: an intervention to improve depression outcomes in older adults. Am J Psychiatr. 2005;162:184–6.
26. Moriarty AS, et al. Screening and case finding for major depressive disorder using the Patient Health Questionnaire (PHQ-9): a meta-analysis. Gen Hosp Psychiatry. 2015;37(6):567–76.
27. Chenail RJ. How to conduct clinical qualitative research on the patient's experience. Qual Rep. 2011;16(4):1173–90.
28. Sandelowski M. Focus on research methods: whatever happened to the qualitative description. Res Nurs Health. 2000;23:334–40.
29. Merriam SB. Qualitative research: a guide to design and implementation. San Francisco, CA: Jossey-Bass; 2009.
30. Neergaard MA, et al. Qualitative description - the poor cousin of health research? BMC Med Res Methodol. 2009;9:52.
31. Colorafi KJ, Evans B. Qualitative Descriptive Methods in Health Science Research. Herd. 2016;9(4):16–25.
32. Morse JM. "Data were saturated. .. ". Qual Health Res. 2015;25(5):587–588.
33. Schulz R, Eden J, editors. Families Caring for an Aging America. Washington, DC: The National Academies of Sciences, Engineering, Medicine; 2016.

34. Addis ME, Mahalik JR. Men, masculinity, and the contexts of help seeking. Am Psychol. 2003;58(1):5–14.
35. Apesoa-Varano EC, Barker JC, Hinton L. Shards of sorrow: Older men's accounts of their depression experience. Soc Sci Med. 2015;124:1–8.
36. Evans JF, Frank B, Oliffe JL, Gregory D. Health, illness, men and masculinities (HIMM): a theoretical framework for understanding men and their health. Journal of Men's Health. 2011;8(1):7–15.
37. Martire LM, Schulz R. Involving Family in Psychosocial: Interventions for Chronic Illness. Curr Dir Psychol Sci. 2007;16(2):90–4.
38. Martinez I, Interian A, Guarnaccia PJ. Antidepressant adherence among Latinos: the role of the family. Qual Res Psychol. 2013;10:63–85.
39. Fernandez y Garcia E, et al. Feeling labeled, judged, lectured, and rejected by family and friends over depression: Cautionary results for primary care clinicians from a multi-centered, qualitative study. BMC Family Practice. 2012;13(1):64.
40. Griffiths KM, et al. Seeking help for depression from family and friends: a qualitative analysis of perceived advantages and disadvantages. BMC Psychiatry. 2011;11:196
41. Mitnick S, Leffler C, Hood VL. Family Caregivers, Patients and Physicians: Ethical Guidance to Optimize Relationships. J Gen Intern Med. 2010;25(3):255–60.

13

Moderate mental illness as a predictor of chronic disease prevention and screening

Ginetta Salvalaggio*, Christopher Meaney, Rahim Moineddin, Eva Grunfeld and Donna Manca

Abstract

Background: Primary care plays a pivotal role in the provision of both mental health care and chronic disease prevention and screening (CDPS). Unfortunately, moderate mental illness (MMI) is associated with poorer general health outcomes. Part of this burden of illness may be due to reduced CDPS uptake. The Building on the Existing Tools to Improve Chronic Disease Prevention in Primary Care (BETTER) trial recruited 777 participants ages 40–65 from 32 family practice panels, of whom 135 (18.2%) had elevated GAD scores, 118 (16.4%) had elevated PHQ scores, and 264 (34.0%) had electronic medical record (EMR)-documented MMI. We hypothesized that patients with screen-positive or chart-documented MMI are 1) eligible for more CDPS actions, and 2) able to complete a lower proportion of CDPS actions than patients unaffected by MMI.

Methods: This study was a secondary analysis of data from the BETTER trial. Participants were stratified by both EMR-documented MMI and screen-positive evidence of MMI (using the General Anxiety Disorders (GAD-7) and Patient Health Questionnaire (PHQ-9) instruments for anxiety and depression screening, respectively). The primary outcome was the proportion of CDPS actions for which the patient was eligible completed at follow-up, using a composite index.

Results: After adjusting for age, gender, and social support, patients with evidence of MMI had a lower composite index than patients without evidence of MMI ($p < 0.05$). The lower composite index is primarily due to higher eligibility for CDPS at baseline; ability to complete CDPS was not statistically different.

Conclusions: Patients affected by MMI are eligible for more CDPS actions than their unaffected counterparts. Although they are able to complete a similar number of CDPS actions, they are not able to eliminate their baseline CDPS gap. Primary care teams need to be aware of this increased CDPS eligibility for patients with MMI and ensure best practices in CDPS supports are available to this patient population. Further study is needed to determine the ideal suite of targeted supports.

Keywords: Primary care, Family practice, Chronic disease prevention, Screening, Depression, Anxiety

Background

Primary care plays a significant role in the provision of mental health care [1]. Often, family physicians are the initial point of contact for moderate mental illness (MMI) such as anxiety and depression [2]. In addition, treatment of these mental health concerns is usually provided without the assistance of a specialist provider [3–5]. Primary care physicians are also responsible for the management of chronic nonpsychiatric illness and preventive health; it can be difficult to address all chronic medical issues and preventive health actions in traditional family practice visits [6–9]. MMI is commonly associated with higher social complexity, including reduced health literacy, lack of child care or transportation, low income, and unstable or unsafe living environments [10–12]. These factors can impede patients' ability to complete labwork or eat and exercise according to preventive care guidelines [11–13]. Often, the most pressing issues during any visit to a primary care team are managed, and other issues may be delayed until a subsequent appointment. Issues delayed to another appointment may never be adequately addressed and chronic disease prevention and screening (CDPS) can easily be lost among these other priorities [8, 9, 14].

* Correspondence: ginetta@ualberta.ca
Ginetta Salvalaggio, University of Alberta, Edmonton, Canada

Literature suggests that adherence to guideline based CDPS actions is not equal among different populations. Patients living with low socioeconomic position, addiction, and/or mental illness are disadvantaged with respect to CDPS, completing a lower number of screening actions compared to the general population [15, 16]. It could also be hypothesized that poorer health outcomes in these groups may be accounted for in part by reduced CDPS. Clinical practice guidelines for specific diseases acknowledge the association between mental and physical illness and encourage clinicians to screen for MMI in the presence of other chronic conditions [17]; however they do not address the converse (screening for chronic conditions in the presence of MMI). Few tools exist to support CDPS uptake for patients with MMI, and no rigorously studied interventions to improve CDPS uptake in this population have been published.

MMI is not uncommon in the primary care setting; a recent report from the World Health Organization found the prevalence of depression in primary care in various countries ranged from 5–20% and anxiety ranged from 4–15% [1]. In Canada, one study estimated that 1 in 5 Canadians are affected annually by MMI [18] and another identified that 14% of primary care patients had a diagnosis of depression [19]. Given the prevalence of MMI in primary care populations, it is particularly important to explore potential differences in CDPS uptake in these patients compared to those without MMI. The purpose of this study was to explore the relationship between eligibility for - and completion of CDPS - actions and MMI. Specifically, we investigated whether those patients with screen-positive or chart-documented MMI are eligible for more not-yet-completed CDPS actions compared to individuals without MMI. Further, we investigated whether those with MMI are able to accomplish CDPS actions for which they are eligible at a similar rate as their unaffected counterparts.

Methods

Design, setting and patients

To investigate differences in CDPS between patients with versus without MMI, this study used a subset of data from the Building on the Existing Tools to Improve Chronic Disease Prevention in Primary Care (BETTER) trial [20]. The BETTER trial was a pragmatic factorial randomized controlled trial conducted in eight primary care team practices in two Canadian cities (Toronto, Ontario and Edmonton, Alberta). Within each of the participating primary care teams were four primary care physicians. In total, 32 primary care physicians (and their patients) participated in the BETTER trial (16 from Toronto and 16 from Edmonton). Patients in the BETTER trial were limited to actively rostered patients between the ages of 40–65 (as most CDPS actions target individuals in this age range). The BETTER trial recruited patients based on information derived from the patients' electronic medical record. Patients were stratified into one of two groups: 1) without MMI and 2) with MMI. MMI was defined by attendance for a MMI diagnosis in the previous 12 months and documentation of 1) depression, anxiety, or pyschosomatic illness in two different places in the chart, 2) two different MMI diagnoses in the same charting field, or 3) one MMI diagnosis and one prescription for psychiatric medication. Forty-five randomly selected patients—25 without chart-documented MMI, and 20 with chart-documented MMI—from each physician practice were invited to participate. Patients documented as unstable or with more severe mental illnesses such as schizophrenia and bipolar affective disorder were excluded from the study.

The survey that patients completed at baseline included the Generalized Anxiety Disorder 7-item scale (GAD-7) and the Patient Health Questionnaire (PHQ-9). Moderate anxiety is more likely with a GAD score greater or equal to 10 [21, 22]; moderate depression is more likely with a PHQ score greater or equal to 10 [23, 24]. Our research team considered the likelihood that a) some patients *with* chart-documented MMI ("detected") may screen *negative* on both the GAD and PHQ ("inactive symptoms") as a result of disease remission, and b) some patients *without* chart-documented MMI ("not detected") may screen *positive* on either the GAD or PHQ ("active symptoms") due to undetected illness or lack of documentation. In theory, patients with clinically active symptoms would have the highest burden of illness, hence those with both chart-documented and screen-positive MMI would be the most affected by their condition and least able to carry out recommended CDPS actions, followed by patients with chart-documented MMI only, with screen-positive but undiagnosed patients least affected of these three groups and most able to achieve CDPS actions. Thus, for the purposes of this analysis, we stratified BETTER trial participants into four groups: 1) detected / active symptoms; 2) detected / inactive symptoms; 3) not detected / active symptoms; and 4) not detected / inactive symptoms ("unaffected").

Outcome measures

The primary outcome of the BETTER trial was a composite endpoint of the proportion of eligible CDPS actions for which patients were eligible at baseline (denominator), achieved at follow-up (numerator). This outcome, a composite index, was modeled after the Summary QUality InDex (SQUID) introduced by Nietert [25]. The 28 items in the composite related to primary prevention and screening for diabetes, cardiovascular disease and cancer, as well as the promotion of a healthy lifestyle (diet, exercise, weight management, smoking, alcohol), supported by clinical practice guidelines [17].

Table 1 Stratification of patients by screen-positive and chart-documented evidence of MMI

	Active Symptoms	Inactive Symptoms	
Detected	13%(99) EMR + / Screen +	21%(161) EMR + / Screen -	34%(260) Detected
Not Detected	10%(75) EMR - / Screen +	56%(425) EMR - / Screen -	66%(500) Not Detected
	23%(174) Active	77%(586) Inactive	100%(760) Total

Precise operational definitions of each of the 28 components of the composite endpoint can be found in the article describing the BETTER trial outcomes [20]. At baseline, each patient was assessed to determine (through use of a patient self-report survey and the patient's electronic medical record (EMR)) their eligibility for each of the 28 components under consideration. Patients were followed prospectively from baseline for six months, at which time actual completion of each action was reassessed.

Statistical analysis

Descriptive summaries of the data are presented as means and standard deviations for continuous variables; counts and percentages for categorical variables.

We compared our composite index outcome across discrete groups (i.e. the mental health indicator), using a non-parametric Kruskal-Wallis test; we also used generalized estimating equation (GEE) models to adjust for the design effect of patients being clustered within physicians. We present two variations of the GEE model;

Table 2 Characteristics of patients by baseline screen-positive (GAD-7/PHQ-9) and chart-documented MMI[a]

	Composite Covariate (GAD, PHQ, BETTER MMI)				
	Not Detected / Inactive Symptoms (Unaffected, *N* = 425)	Detected / Inactive Symptoms (*N* = 161)	Not Detected / Active Symptoms (*N* = 75)	Detected / Active Symptoms (*N* = 99)	*P*-value
Age (years)	53.4 (6.9)	53.9 (6.6)	51.3 (6.6)	51.8 (6.4)	0.006
Female sex	282 (66.4)	128 (79.5)	56 (74.7)	80 (80.8)	0.002
Minority race or ethnic group	49 (11.9)	13 (8.2)	10 (13.9)	13 (13.5)	0.47
≥1 yr. post-secondary education	377 (89.1)	130 (80.8)	65 (87.8)	77 (77.8)	0.006
Full or Part-time Employment	334 (79.0)	124 (77.0)	60 (81.1)	54 (55.7)	<0.0001
Married/common-law	350 (82.6)	116 (72.1)	52 (71.2)	57 (58.2)	<0.0001
Total Household Income					
≥ 100,000 CAD	236 (58.4)	76 (47.8)	32 (43.8)	28 (29.8)	<0.0001
60,000–99,999 CAD	109 (27.0)	48 (30.2)	20 (27.4)	29 (30.9)	
0–59,999 CAD	59 (14.6)	35 (22.0)	21 (28.8)	37 (39.3)	
Current smoker	26 (6.1)	12 (7.5)	8 (10.7)	33 (33.3)	<0.0001
Current alcohol consumption					
< 4× per month	260 (61.3)	105 (65.2)	52 (71.2)	72 (73.4)	0.04
≥ 4× per month and <2× per week	111 (26.2)	29 (18.0)	12 (16.4)	13 (13.3)	
≥ 2× per week	53 (12.5)	27 (16.8)	9 (12.4)	13 (13.3)	
Exercise status					
Extremely active	82 (19.3)	29 (18.2)	7 (9.6)	16 (16.3)	0.24
≤ Mildly active	342 (80.6)	130 (81.8)	66 (90.4)	82 (83.7)	
Body-mass index	24.9 (4.9)	25.3 (5.2)	26.5 (5.5)	26.8 (5.8)	0.004
Obese	58 (14.1)	27 (16.9)	16 (22.2)	29 (29.3)	0.003
MOS Social Support Score	83.4 (18.3)	75.2 (23.3)	60.7 (27.1)	55.4 (28.6)	<0.0001

[a] Continuous variables presented as means (SD) and categorical variables presented as N (%). Kruskal Wallis tests are used for continuous variables, and Person's chi-squared tests or Fisher's exact tests are used for categorical variables
CAD: Canadian dollars
MOS Social Support Questionnaire: Scores for the 22 items range from 0 to 100, higher scores indicate higher level of self-perceived support

the first, a bivariate GEE model using only the categorical grouping variable under consideration (i.e. the MMI indicator); and the second, a multivariate GEE model estimating the impact of the same categorical grouping variable on the composite index after adjusting for age, gender, and social support.

We considered individual components of the composite index related to smoking and alcohol as these behaviours are known to be more prevalent in populations affected by MMI [26–30]. As this analysis is exploratory, we only present counts and proportions corresponding to the number of patients eligible and achieving actions in each of the MMI groups.

All statistical analyses were conducted in SAS version 9.3 (Cary, North Carolina).

Research ethics and trial registration

The trial was approved by the Ontario Cancer Research Ethics Board (REB), University of Alberta REB, and all relevant REBs in each province and at each primary care team site. The registration number of the original RCT BETTER trial was ISRCTN07170460.

Results

The BETTER trial enrolled 789 patients. Twelve patients withdrew from the trial prior to completion and 777 patients were included in the analysis. Patients enrolled in the BETTER trial were ages 40–65, predominantly female, Caucasian, and well educated. A more detailed description of the trial participants can be found in Grunfeld et al. [20].

Of the patients with available scores, 18.2% (135/742) had elevated GAD scores, 16.4% (118/720) had elevated PHQ scores, and 34.0% (264/777) had chart-documented MMI, with significant overlap between those patients identified via screening and those identified through the medical record (Table 1). Of the 500 patients with available GAD and/or PHQ scores and without chart-documented MMI, a total of 15.0% (75/500) screened positive for MMI as determined by the GAD and the PHQ, with 12.0% (60/500) screening positive on the GAD and 8.2% (41/500) screening positive on the PHQ.

Table 2 summarizes demographic and behavioural characteristics across each of the screen-defined and chart-documented MMI strata. MMI was associated with female gender, lower levels of employment and income, and fewer social supports. Additionally, MMI was associated with higher levels of smoking, more frequent alcohol consumption, and higher levels of obesity.

Patients with the most active MMI accomplished the same number of, but were eligible for more, actions than their less affected counterparts (Table 3). The "detected/active symptoms" group (N = 99, composite index = 36.0%, SD = 27.5%) had a statistically lower mean composite index than each of the other three groups ($p < 0.05$). The mean composite indices for "detected/inactive symptoms" (N = 161, composite index = 41.7%, SD = 27.9), "not detected/active symptoms" (N = 75, composite index = 41.1%, SD = 27.9), and "unaffected" (N = 425, composite index = 45.3%, SD = 27.8) groups were not statistically different from one another.

We additionally examined the six alcohol / tobacco screening, monitoring and referral components of the composite index, in terms of both eligibility for these actions (E, Table 4) and meeting these actions (M, Table 5). The presence of MMI was associated with increased

Table 3 Estimates of Composite Index by baseline screen-positive (GAD-7/PHQ-9) and chart-documented MMI

	Composite Covariate (GAD, PHQ, BETTER MMI)				
	Not Detected / Inactive Symptoms (Unaffected, N = 425)	Detected / Inactive Symptoms (N = 161)	Not Detected / Active Symptoms (N = 75)	Detected / Active Symptoms (N = 99)	P-value
Total Composite					
Unadjusted Means	45.3 (42.6, 48.0)	41.7 (37.4, 46.1)	41.1 (34.7, 47.6)	36.0 (30.5, 41.5)	0.02
Bivariate GEE[a]	43.2 (36.5, 49.9)	40.6 (33.9, 47.3)	40.2 (32.3, 48.0)	32.8 (25.7, 39.9)	0.02
Multivariate GEE[b]	43.1 (36.4, 49.9)	41.2 (34.4, 48.0)	41.1 (33.1, 49.1)	34.2 (26.9, 41.5)	0.03
Eligible (E)					
Unadjusted Means	8.8 (8.5, 9.0)	9.1 (8.6, 9.6)	9.1 (8.4, 9.8)	10.3 (9.6, 10.9)	0.0003
Bivariate GEE[a]	8.7 (8.3, 9.1)	9.2 (8.6, 9.7)	9.1 (8.4, 9.9)	10.1 (9.4, 10.9)	0.06
Multivariate GEE[b]	8.7 (8.3, 9.1)	9.1 (8.6, 9.6)	9.2 (8.6, 9.9)	10.2 (9.5, 11.0)	0.048
Met (M)					
Unadjusted Means	3.9 (3.6, 4.2)	3.8 (3.4, 4.3)	3.9 (3.3, 4.6)	3.8 (3.2, 4.4)	0.87
Bivariate GEE[a]	3.7 (3.2, 4.3)	3.8 (3.2, 4.6)	3.9 (3.1, 4.9)	3.4 (2.7, 4.3)	0.45
Multivariate GEE[b]	3.7 (3.2, 4.3)	3.8 (3.2, 4.6)	4.1 (3.3, 5.1)	3.6 (2.9, 4.5)	0.51

[a]adjusting for clustering effect in design and single main effect
[b]adjusting for clustering effect in design as well as age, gender and social support

Table 4 Unadjusted Eligible (E) table for smoking and alcohol actions

	Composite Covariate (GAD, PHQ, BETTER MMI)				
	Not Detected / Inactive Symptoms (Unaffected, N = 425)	Detected / Inactive Symptoms (N = 161)	Not Detected / Active Symptoms (N = 75)	Detected / Active Symptoms (N = 99)	P-value
Smoking – Screening	92 (21.7)	33 (20.5)	18 (24.0)	18 (18.2)	0.76
Smoking – Monitoring	38 (8.9)	14 (8.7)	10 (13.3)	35 (35.4)	0.02
Smoking – Referral	38 (8.9)	14 (8.7)	10 (13.3)	35 (35.4)	0.02
Alcohol – Screening	129 (30.4)	49 (30.4)	26 (34.7)	23 (23.2)	0.23
Alcohol – Monitoring	75 (19.5)	36 (24.8)	13 (20.0)	26 (32.5)	0.06
Alcohol – Referral	75 (19.5)	36 (24.8)	13 (20.0)	26 (32.5)	0.06

eligibility for most smoking and alcohol monitoring and referral actions. A significant difference was not observed with respect to screening actions; nor were clear differences noted with respect to meeting any actions for which patients were eligible.

Discussion

The purpose of this study was to assess potential differences in eligibility for, and adherence to, guideline based CDPS actions in patients with and without MMI. Patients with screen-positive and chart-documented MMI are eligible for more CDPS actions than their unaffected counterparts and complete a similar number of actions [20]. This suggests that the nature of MMI places patients at a health promotion disadvantage.

Of the 500 patients with available GAD and/or PHQ scores and without chart-documented MMI, 15% (75/500) scored positive on the PHQ and/or GAD, supporting Craven's findings that primary care detection rates for MMI may be low [2]. However, screen positive patients without chart-documented MMI ("not detected/active symptoms") had similar composite indices to unaffected patients. This finding fails to support more universal primary care *screening* for MMI as a means to improve CDPS uptake.

In contrast, patients with chart-documented MMI who screened positive on the PHQ and/or GAD ("detected/active symptoms") had lower composite indices than unaffected patients, whereas patients with chart-documented MMI who screened negative ("detected/inactive symptoms") had similar composite indices to unaffected patients. This suggests that *treatment* of clinically significant MMI may have a potential impact on CDPS uptake; however, MMI treatment has yet to be confirmed in a prospective trial setting as an effective intervention for CDPS uptake.

For those patients with the highest burden of illness (detected and with active symptoms of MMI), there is increasing evidence of the cost effectiveness of interventions to promote the physical health of people with MMI [31]. Patients with MMI may particularly benefit from individualized patient-level support from a care team member, perhaps with special emphasis on health navigation and motivational interviewing as demonstrated by the BETTER trial [20]. Although screening asymptomatic patients may not be justified, we propose that primary care teams be vigilant for signs of MMI and maintain awareness of its impact on CDPS.

Our findings that MMI was associated with female gender, lower levels of employment and income, and fewer social supports are consistent with the literature [11]. Also, there is a known increased prevalence of smoking and excessive alcohol intake among patients with MMI, and vice versa [26–30]; smoking and alcohol-related CDPS uptake may be particularly affected by MMI. Teams would do well to address potential socioeconomic barriers to carrying out CDPS actions. Targeted CDPS interventions, designed with MMI-associated CDPS barriers in

Table 5 Unadjusted Met (M) table for smoking and alcohol actions[a]

	Composite Covariate (GAD, PHQ, BETTER MMI)				
	Unaffected	Detected / Inactive Symptoms	Not Detected / Active Symptoms	Detected / Active Symptoms	P-value
Smoking – Screening	60/92 (65.2)	21/33 (63.6)	12/18 (66.7)	12/18 (66.7)	0.61
Smoking – Monitoring	22/38 (57.9)	3/14 (21.4)	4/10 (40.0)	9/35 (25.7)	0.046
Smoking – Referral	8/38 (21.1)	4/14 (28.6)	5/10 (50.0)	11/35 (31.4)	0.21
Alcohol – Screening	72/129 (55.8)	29/49 (59.2)	9/26 (34.6)	12/23 (52.2)	0.23
Alcohol – Monitoring	44/75 (59.5)	23/36 (74.2)	7/13 (58.3)	17/26 (70.8)	0.27
Alcohol – Referral	8/75 (10.7)	5/36 (13.9)	4/13 (30.8)	6/26 (23.1)	0.33

[a]Where denominator for each cell = those participants eligible (E) for each action (see Table 4)

mind, are needed, but require evaluation of their effectiveness and relative cost prior to large scale implementation.

There exist potential limitations that should be considered when interpreting results from this study. First, as a pragmatic trial the BETTER trial employed minimal inclusion/exclusion criteria, and the demographics of the participating patients are not entirely representative of the general urban Canadian population, thus will have limited generalizability to rural, non-Caucasian, or socio-economically disadvantaged settings. That said, the characteristics of the MMI-affected patients enrolled in this study are similar to those reported in similar literature.

Secondly, the GAD-7 and PHQ-9 are not sufficient information to confirm the diagnosis of a MMI, and rely on self-report by participants. Use of these proxies without confirmation via clinician assessment may not necessarily be the most accurate reflection of patients who are living with untreated illness.

Lastly, the study was not designed with sufficient power to demonstrate a difference in CDPS uptake on the basis of whether or not patients with evidence of MMI symptoms had come to the attention of a physician. Similarly, although trends for increased need for smoking and alcohol CDPS were seen, we were unable to confirm any clear pattern on the basis of MMI status.

Conclusions

Compared to patients unaffected by MMI, patients with documented MMI and active symptoms complete a smaller proportion of CDPS actions for which they are eligible, and are eligible for more CDPS actions overall. Primary care teams should be aware of this CDPS gap and remain vigilant for patients with active MMI in need of CDPS support. Further research is required to better understand effective approaches to CDPS in patients with MMI, and if diagnosis and treatment of MMI can improve CDPS in primary care.

Abbreviations

BETTER: Building on the existing tools to improve chronic disease prevention in family practice; CAD: Canadian dollars; CDPS: Chronic disease prevention and screening; E: Eligible actions; EMR: Electronic medical record; GAD: Generalized anxiety disorder; GEE: Generalized estimating eq.; M: Met actions; MMI: Moderate mental illness; PHQ: Patient health questionnaire; REB: Research ethics board

Acknowledgements

The authors wish to thank the BETTER trial investigative team and prevention practitioners who administered the intervention and collected data used for this study. Thank you also to Carolina Aguilar for her assistance in preparing this manuscript for publication.

Funding

This research was made possible through a financial contribution from the Canadian Partnership Against Cancer and Health Canada and supported by the Heart and Stroke Foundation of Ontario Grant No. PG 10–0479. Dr. Grunfeld is supported by a clinician scientist award from the Ontario Institute for Cancer Research (OICR) with funds from the Ontario Ministry of Research and Innovation (MRI). The opinions, results, and conclusions reported are those of the authors and are independent from the funding sources and no endorsement by OICR or MRI is intended or should be inferred.

Authors' contributions

All authors have read and approved of the final manuscript. GS oversaw the design and interpretation of this secondary analysis and oversaw manuscript writing. CM conducted all statistical analyses, prepared all data for inclusion in the manuscript, and provided manuscript edits. RM contributed to statistical analyses and provided manuscript edits. EG assisted with interpretation of this secondary analysis and provided manuscript edits. DM assisted with the design and interpretation of this secondary analysis and provided substantive edits to the manuscript.

Authors' information

GS is an Associate Professor with the University of Alberta Department of Family Medicine, and a member of the Clinical Working Group for the BETTER trial investigative group.
CM is a biostatistician with the University of Toronto Department of Family and Community Medicine and the BETTER trial investigative group.
RM is a senior biostatistician with the University of Toronto Department of Family and Community Medicine and the BETTER trial investigative group.
EG is a Professor with the University of Toronto Department of Family and Community Medicine, and is a co-principal investigator for the BETTER trial investigative group.
DM is an Associate Professor with the University of Alberta Department of Family Medicine, and is a co-principal investigator for the BETTER trial investigative group.

Competing interests

The authors declare that they have no competing interests.

Consent for publication

Not applicable.

References

1. World Health Organization., World Organisation of National Colleges Academies and Academic Associations of General Practitioners/Family Physicians. Integrating mental health into primary care: a global perspective. Geneva, Switzerland, London: World Health Organization; Wonca; 2008.
2. Craven MA, Bland R. Depression in primary care: current and future challenges. Can J Psychiatry. 2013;58(8):442–8.
3. Katz SJ, Kessler RC, Lin E, Wells KB. Medication management of depression in the United States and Ontario. J Gen Intern Med. 1998;13(2):77–85.
4. Williams JW Jr, Rost K, Dietrich AJ, Ciotti MC, Zyzanski SJ, Cornell J. Primary care physicians' approach to depressive disorders. Effects of physician specialty and practice structure. Arch Fam Med. 1999;8(1):58–67.
5. Houle J, Beaulieu MD, Lesperance F, Frasure-Smith N, Lambert J. Inequities in Medical Follow-Up for Depression: A Population-Based Study in Montreal. Psychiatr Serv. 2010;61(3):258–63.
6. Ostbye T, Yarnall KS, Krause KM, Pollak KI, Gradison M, Michener JL. Is there time for management of patients with chronic diseases in primary care? Ann Fam Med. 2005;3(3):209–14.
7. Yarnall KS, Pollak KI, Ostbye T, Krause KM, Michener JL. Primary care: is there enough time for prevention? Am J Public Health. 2003;93(4):635–41.
8. Linzer M, Bitton A, Tu SP, Plews-Ogan M, Horowitz KR, Schwartz MD. Association of C, Leaders in General Internal Medicine Writing G, Poplau S, Paranjape A *et al*: The End of the 15-20 Minute Primary Care Visit. J Gen Intern Med. 2015;30(11):1584–6.
9. Raffoul M, Moore M, Kamerow D, Bazemore A. A Primary Care Panel Size of 2500 Is neither Accurate nor Reasonable. J Am Board Fam Med. 2016;29(4):496–9.
10. Health FPaTACoP. Toward a healthy future: second report on the health of Canadians. Ottawa, ON: Minister of Public Works and Government Services Canada; 1999.
11. Allen J, Balfour R, Bell R, Marmot M. Social determinants of mental health. Int Rev Psychiatry. 2014;26(4):392–407.

12. Canadian Medical Association. Health care in Canada: what makes us sick?. 2013. Available at https://www.cma.ca/Assets/assets-library/document/fr/advocacy/What-makes-us-sick_en.pdf .
13. Zgibor JC, Songer TJ. External Barriers to Diabetes Care: Addressing Personal and Health Systems Issues. Diabetes Spectrum. 2001;14(1):23–8.
14. Burack RC. Barriers to clinical preventive medicine. Prim Care. 1989;16(1):245–50.
15. Druss BG, Rosenheck RA, Desai MM, Perlin JB. Quality of preventive medical care for patients with mental disorders. Med Care. 2002;40(2):129–36.
16. Egede LE, Grubaugh AL, Ellis C. The effect of major depression on preventive care and quality of life among adults with diabetes. Gen Hosp Psychiatry. 2010;32(6):563–9.
17. Campbell-Scherer D, Rogers J, Manca D, Lang-Robertson K, Bell S, Salvalaggio G, et al. Guideline harmonization and implementation plan for the BETTER trial: Building on Existing Tools to Improve Chronic Disease Prevention and Screening in Family Practice. CMAJ open. 2014;2(1):E1–E10.
18. Smetanin P, Briante C, Stiff D, Ahmad S, Khan M, Mental Health Commission of Canada, RiskAnalytica (Firm). The life and economic impact of major mental illnesses in Canada. 2011. Available at http://www.mentalhealthcommission.ca/sites/default/files/MHCC_Report_Base_Case_FINAL_ENG_0_0.pdf.
19. Wong ST, Manca D, Barber D, Morkem R, Khan S, Kotecha J, et al. The diagnosis of depression and its treatment in Canadian primary care practices: an epidemiological study. CMAJ Open. 2014;2(4):E337–42.
20. Grunfeld E, Manca D, Moineddin R, Thorpe KE, Hoch JS, Campbell-Scherer D, et al. Improving chronic disease prevention and screening in primary care: results of the BETTER pragmatic cluster randomized controlled trial. BMC Fam Pract. 2013;14(1):175.
21. Spitzer RL, Kroenke K, Williams JB, Lowe B. A brief measure for assessing generalized anxiety disorder: the GAD-7. Arch Intern Med. 2006;166(10):1092–7.
22. Herr NR, Williams JW Jr, Benjamin S, McDuffie J. Does this patient have generalized anxiety or panic disorder?: The rational clinical examination systematic review. JAMA. 2014;312(1):78–84.
23. Manea L, Gilbody S, McMillan D. Optimal cut-off score for diagnosing depression with the Patient Health Questionnaire (PHQ-9): a meta-analysis. CMAJ. 2012;184(3):E191–6.
24. Kroenke K, Spitzer RL, Williams JB. The PHQ-9: validity of a brief depression severity measure. J Gen Intern Med. 2001;16(9):606–13.
25. Nietert PJ, Wessell AM, Jenkins RG, Feifer C, Nemeth LS, Ornstein SM. Using a summary measure for multiple quality indicators in primary care: the Summary QUality InDex (SQUID). Implement Sci. 2007;2:11.
26. Hasin DS, Goodwin RD, Stinson FS, Grant BF. Epidemiology of major depressive disorder: results from the National Epidemiologic Survey on Alcoholism and Related Conditions. Arch Gen Psychiatry. 2005;62(10):1097–106.
27. Dierker LC, Avenevoli S, Stolar M, Merikangas KR. Smoking and depression: an examination of mechanisms of comorbidity. Am J Psychiatry. 2002;159(6):947–53.
28. Sullivan LE, Goulet JL, Justice AC, Fiellin DA. Alcohol consumption and depressive symptoms over time: A longitudinal study of patients with and without HIV infection. Drug Alcohol Depend. 2011;117(2–3):158–63.
29. Fuehrlein BS, Mota N, Arias AJ, Trevisan LA, Kachadourian LK, Krystal JH, et al. The burden of alcohol use disorders in US military veterans: results from the National Health and Resilience in Veterans Study. Addiction. 2016; 111(10):1786–94.
30. Lawrence D, et al. Smoking, mental illness and socioeconomic disadvantage: analysis of the Australian National Survey of Mental Health and Wellbeing. BMC Public Health. 2013;13:462. doi:10.1186/1471-2458-13-462.
31. Park AL, McDaid D, Weiser P, Von Gottberg C, Becker T, Kilian R, et al. Examining the cost effectiveness of interventions to promote the physical health of people with mental health problems: a systematic review. BMC Public Health. 2013;13:787.

14

Using self-reported data on the social determinants of health in primary care to identify cancer screening disparities: opportunities and challenges

A.K. Lofters[1,2,3,4,7*], A. Schuler[1,3], M. Slater[1], N.N. Baxter[4,5], N. Persaud[1,2,3], A.D. Pinto[1,2,3,4], E. Kucharski[6], S. Davie[1], R. Nisenbaum[3,4] and T. Kiran[1,2,3,7]

Abstract

Background: Data on the social determinants of health can help primary care practices target improvement efforts, yet relevant data are rarely available. Our family practice located in Toronto, Ontario routinely collects patient-level sociodemographic data via a pilot-tested survey developed by a multi-organizational steering committee. We sought to use these data to assess the relationship between the social determinants and colorectal, cervical and breast cancer screening, and to describe the opportunities and challenges of using data on social determinants from a self-administered patient survey.

Methods: Patients of the family practice eligible for at least one of the three cancer screening types, based on age and screening guidelines as of June 30, 2015 and who had answered at least one question on a socio-demographic survey were included in the study. We linked self-reported data from the sociodemographic survey conducted in the waiting room with patients' electronic medical record data and cancer screening records. We created an individual-level income variable (low-income cut-off) that defined a poverty threshold and took household size into account. The sociodemographic characteristics of patients who were overdue for screening were compared to those who were up-to-date for screening for each cancer type using chi-squared tests.

Results: We analysed data for 5766 patients for whom we had survey data. Survey participants had significantly higher screening rates (72.9, 78.7, 74.4% for colorectal, cervical and breast cancer screening respectively) than the 13, 036 patients for whom we did not have survey data (59.2, 65.3, 58.9% respectively). Foreign-born patients were significantly more likely to be up-to-date on colorectal screening than their Canadian-born peers but showed no significant differences in breast or cervical cancer screening. We found a significant association between the low-income cut-off variable and cancer screening; neighbourhood income quintile was not significantly associated with cancer screening. Housing status was also significantly associated with colorectal, cervical and breast cancer screening. There was a large amount of missing data for the low-income cut-off variable, approximately 25% across the three cohorts.

Conclusion: While we were able to show that neighbourhood income might under-estimate income-related disparities in screening, individual-level income was also the most challenging variable to collect. Future work in this area should target the income disparity in cancer screening and simultaneously explore how best to collect measures of poverty.

Keywords: Screening, Cervical cancer, Colorectal cancer, Breast cancer, Social determinants of health

* Correspondence: aisha.lofters@utoronto.ca
[1]Department of Family & Community Medicine, St. Michael's Hospital, 30 Bond Street, Toronto, ON M5B 1W8, Canada
[2]Department of Family & Community Medicine, University of Toronto, 500 University Avenue, 5th Floor, Toronto, ON M5G 1V7, Canada
Full list of author information is available at the end of the article

Background

The social determinants of health (SDOH), such as income, race/ethnicity, education, and working and living conditions, are responsible for substantial morbidity and mortality worldwide, with income being perhaps the most important determinant [1–8]. The World Health Organization defines the SDOH as "the conditions in which people are born, grow, work, live and age, and the wider set of forces and systems shaping the conditions of daily life" [9]. The SDOH influence one's health-related behaviours, health literacy levels, sense of self-control and self-efficacy, and access to societal resources including access to healthcare [8, 10]. The Institute of Medicine is moving to capture SDOH in electronic medical records, due to increased recognition that data on the SDOH can provide crucial information useful for treatment choices, health care system design and targeted innovations [11].

Quality primary care has been associated with an attenuation of the health effects of income inequalities [12, 13], making primary care a highly appropriate healthcare setting in which to measure and intervene on the SDOH, especially with the expansion of multidisciplinary patient-centred teams [14, 15]. However, individual-level data and practice-level data on the SDOH are rarely available within the primary care context and the best way to systematically collect and use these data in the primary care setting is not yet clear. Improving colorectal, cervical and breast cancer screening uptake for patients is an example of an area in primary care where data on the SDOH could be valuable, as disparities in cancer screening at the population level are well established, particularly related to income and foreign-born status [16–27].

In our large urban primary care practice in Ontario, Canada, we now routinely collect data on the SDOH from our patients using a self-completed survey in the waiting room. These data allow us to identify potential gaps in care related to SDOH and target our quality improvement efforts [28]. In this study, we aimed to understand: i) the relationship between the SDOH, particularly income, and colorectal, cervical and breast cancer screening, and ii) challenges and opportunities of using SDOH data from a self-administered patient survey.

Methods

Study setting

Our study was conducted in a large Family Health Team, a common medical home model in Ontario, Canada [29]. Our Family Health Team is comprised of six clinics, approximately 70 physicians, and 60 other health professionals serving over 35,000 patients. Our practice is situated in downtown Toronto, Canada's most populous and sociodemographically diverse city with approximately 2.6 million people.

In the province of Ontario, cancer screening is covered through the universal provincial healthcare plan. Ontario has organized screening programs for colorectal, cervical and breast cancers, which include invitations, information about test results, and reminders for when it is time to repeat screening sent directly to residents of the province who are screen-eligible [30–32]. However, cancer screening is still fundamentally embedded in primary care.

Collection of patient-level SDOH data

Since 2014, our practice has been routinely collecting individual-level data from our patients through a voluntary sociodemographic survey (See Additional File 1), completed in the waiting room at routine office visits. Details on survey development are published elsewhere [28]. Briefly, the survey was developed by a multi-organizational steering committee, refined by an iterative process, and pilot tested with 400 patients.

The survey is completed either on an electronic tablet or on paper and then transferred to the electronic medical record (EMR) by clerical staff. For both methods, responses to the survey questions are stored directly in the patient's EMR and are immediately available for viewing. The survey is available in Canada's two official languages, English and French. Participants are able to select "prefer not to answer" or "do not know" for all questions, and no questions are mandatory. As of June 30, 2015, approximately 30% of patients had participated in the survey. We used the survey to obtain individual-level data on the SDOH, specifically, immigrant status, ethnicity, household income and number of people in the household, sexual orientation, preferred language of communication, and housing status.

Study participants

We included all patients of the family practice who were eligible for at least one of the three cancer screening types, based on age and screening guidelines [33–35] as of June 30, 2015 and who had answered at least one question on the sociodemographic survey. Adults were eligible for colorectal cancer screening if they were 50 – 74 years of age, and women were eligible for cervical and breast cancer screening if they were 21 – 69 years or 50 – 74 years respectively. We obtained data on cancer screening eligibility from a monthly cancer screening report provided to Ontario family physicians by the provincial cancer agency. The monthly report provides information to physicians on which of their patients are eligible for and due for each of the three types of cancer screening based on provincial guidelines [36]. Screening data are obtained from diagnostic and fee codes billed throughout the province. On the monthly screening report, patients who have a personal history of one of the three cancers are excluded from eligibility for that particular screening modality, and men and women with a history of a colectomy are excluded from colorectal cancer screening. Women with a history of total hysterectomy are excluded from eligibility for cervical cancer screening, and those with a history of a mastectomy or enrolment in the Ontario Breast Screening Program's High Risk Screening Program are excluded from eligibility for breast cancer screening.

Outcome definition

We used data provided on the provincial cancer agency's monthly report to determine the screening status for patients eligible for colorectal and breast cancer screening. In our setting, most Pap tests were processed in a hospital laboratory and thus excluded from the provincial report, so to determine cervical cancer screening we combined data from the provincial agency with data from our practice's EMR. Study participants were categorized as being up-to-date for screening (binary variable: yes/no) for each of the three cancers of interest. Screening status was defined as of June 30, 2015. For the three outcome variables, up-to-date was defined as at least one documented faecal occult blood test in the last two years, flexible sigmoidoscopy in the last five years, or colonoscopy in the last ten years (colorectal cancer screening), at least one Pap test in the last three years (cervical cancer screening) and at least one mammogram in the last two years (breast cancer screening).

Survey variables

To identify individual-level income, we used responses from the sociodemographic survey to create an adapted version of the Low-Income Cutoff Before Taxes (LICO-BT) used by Statistics Canada [37]. The LICO-BT is the income threshold below which an affected family would be expected to spend at least 20% more of its household income on necessities (food, shelter, clothing) than the average family [37]. Cut-offs vary by family size and by area of residence to reflect differences in cost of living. To create an adapted LICO-BT variable, we used the responses from two survey questions: i) What was your total family income before taxes last year? (where response categories were in $30,000 increments), and ii) How many people does your income support? (see Additional file 1, questions 7 and 8). We correlated responses with the 2014 LICO-BT calculations for a Census Metropolitan Area of 500,000 inhabitants or more available from Statistics Canada. If participants reported a total family income before taxes of $0 to $29,999 and reported that their income supported two people or less they were considered below the LICO-BT. Similarly, if participants reported a total family income before taxes of $0 to $29,999 or $30,000 to $59,999 and reported their income supported between 3 to 6 people they were considered to be below the LICO-BT.

The survey includes a question on housing status with nine categories excluding "prefer not to answer" and "do not know" (see Additional file 1, question 11). We created a three-level variable for housing status (homeowners, renters, and other). Respondents in the "other" housing category reported that they lived in a boarding home, correctional facility, group home, shelter, hostel, supportive housing, on the street, or selected "other".

The sociodemographic survey includes one question on race/ethnicity that provides sixteen potential responses, excluding "prefer not to answer" and "do not know" (see Additional file 1, question 3). Potential responses included "First Nations", "Indigenous/Aboriginal" and "Metis", all of which refer to Canada's indigenous peoples. As the survey was not developed using Ownership, Control, Access and Possession principles, we chose to include data for these respondents with respondents who selected other. These principles enable self-determination over all research concerning Canada's indigenous peoples, and include "the right to make decisions about what, why, how and by whom information is collected, as well as how it will be used and shared" [38].

Additional study variables

Other variables collected from the EMR and monthly report included age, sex, and postal code. In addition to individual-level income, we determined neighbourhood income quintile. Patients' postal codes were categorized into neighbourhood income quintiles using the Statistics Canada Postal Code Conversion File and data from the 2006 Census (the last Census for which accurate data are available).

Data analysis

We used descriptive statistics to describe study participants for each variable of interest noted above, and used chi-squared tests to compare screening uptake, age, sex (for colorectal cancer screening only), and neighbourhood income quintile amongst study participants to the rest of the patient population eligible for screening for each cancer type. We compared the characteristics of patients who were overdue for screening to those who were up-to-date for screening for each cancer type using chi-squared tests. Age was characterized as both a continuous variable and a categorical variable using the following categories: 20–29 years, 30–39 years, 40–49 years, 50–59 years, 60–69 years, and 70 plus years. We compared the age of patients who were overdue for screening to those who were up-to-date for screening using both independent samples t-tests (continuous variable) and chi-squared tests (categorical variable). Participants with missing data or who had selected "prefer not to answer" or "do not know" were excluded from bivariate analyses. In bivariate analyses, ethnicity was collapsed to White versus all other ethnicities because of the small numbers in the latter category. A two-tailed test was used and a p-value of less than 0.05 was considered statistically significant. All statistical analyses were conducted using SPSS 20.0 [39].

Results

We analysed data for 5766 patients who answered at least one question on the sociodemographic survey (Fig. 1). Table 1 describes the sociodemographic characteristics of the study participants, including missing data, as well as the proportion of patients up-to-date on the three screening types by sociodemographic subgroup. These categories were not mutually exclusive; 1207 women were eligible for all three screening types. There was a large amount of missing data for the LICO-BT variable, approximately 25% across the three cohorts.

Patients who completed the sociodemographic survey were significantly more likely to be up-to-date on colorectal, cervical and breast cancer screening than those who did not complete the sociodemographic survey (Fig. 2). Study participants were most likely to be up-to-date on cervical cancer screening (78.7%) and least likely for CRC screening (72.9%), which also held true for the general practice population. No significant differences were observed for any of the screening modalities based on age or neighbourhood income quintile (data not shown) between participants who completed the sociodemographic survey and those who did not complete the sociodemographic survey. Among those eligible for colorectal cancer screening,

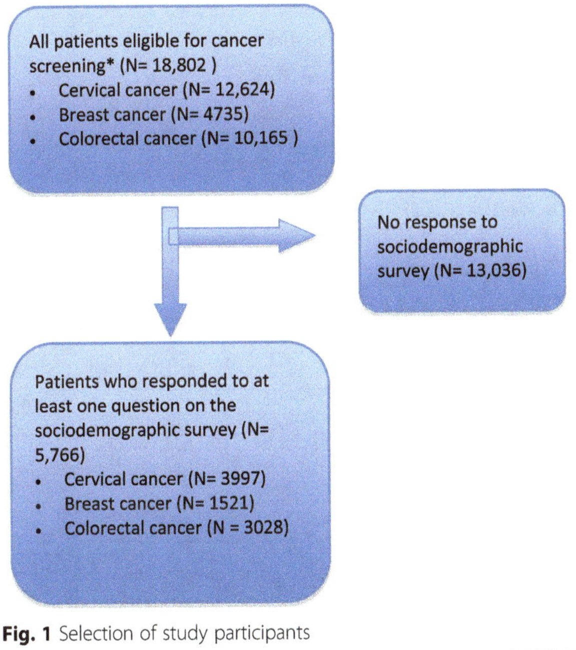

Fig. 1 Selection of study participants

female patients were more likely to complete the sociodemographic survey than male patients.

In bivariate analyses (Table 2), age, immigrant status, income and housing showed statistically significant associations with cancer screening. Patients who were up-to-date with colorectal cancer screening were significantly older than those were overdue, whereas those who were up-to-date with cervical cancer screening were significantly younger than those were overdue. Foreign-born patients were more likely to be up-to-date on colorectal screening than their Canadian-born peers but showed no significant differences in breast or cervical cancer screening. Although there were no significant differences for any of the screening modalities based on neighbourhood income quintile, the derived LICO-BT variable was associated with all three screening types. People living below the LICO-BT were less likely to be up-to-date on screening for all screening types and this difference was most marked for breast cancer screening. Housing status was also associated with all three cancer screening types. Screening was less common among patients who rented a home and those who reported their housing as "other" than among those who owned a home. There were differences in breast and cervical cancer screening between heterosexual and non-heterosexual women but these were not statistically significant.

We did not conduct multivariable analyses because of the large amount of missing data for income (approximately 25%), which was our main variable of interest. It was not possible to use neighbourhood income as a proxy in multivariable analysis because there was not a high level of agreement between neighbourhood income and the LICO. For example, 50.9% of participants in the lowest income quintile and 65.5% of participants in the second lowest income quintile lived above the LICO.

To better understand our results, we looked at the relationship between housing status and LICO-BT status. Of those who were homeowners, the vast majority lived above the LICO-BT (90.1% for the CRC screening cohort, 90.9% for cervical cohort, 89.4% for breast cohort). Similarly, of those who lived in "other" housing i.e. were neither homeowners nor renters, most were below the LICO-BT (81.1% for CRC cohort, 76.2% for cervical cohort, 76.6% for breast cohort).

Discussion

We used self-reported SDOH data within the primary care setting to describe the association between the SDOH and clinical outcomes: colorectal, cervical and breast cancer screening. We found that participants living below a low-income threshold indicative of poverty and people who did not own their homes were significantly less likely to be screened for cancers than their more advantaged peers. However, we also found that patients who responded to

Table 1 Subset of patients with survey data available[a]

	Colorectal cancer		Cervical cancer		Breast cancer	
	Eligible for screening, N	Receiving Screening, row %	Eligible for screening, N	Receiving Screening, row %	Eligible for screening, N	Receiving Screening, row %
TOTAL	3028	72.9	3997	78.7	1521	74.4
Age categories						
20–29	--	--	618	76.7	--	--
30–39	--	--	1149	81.4	--	--
40–49	--	--	960	82.9	--	--
50–59	1588	67.3	760	77.9	797	72.8
60–69	1091	78.5	510	68.0	540	77.4
70+ years	349	81.1	--	--	184	72.8
Sex						
Male	1433	72.6	--	--	--	--
Female	1595	73.2	3997	78.7	1521	74.4
Immigrant status						
Foreign-born	1203	75.8	1604	77.7	654	76.0
Canadian-born	1722	71.4	2317	79.5	817	73.6
Prefer not to answer/Do not know/Missing	103	64.1	76	73.7	50	68.0
Ethnicity						
White-North American	1173	73.1	1325	80.1	564	74.3
White-European	724	73.5	773	78.1	334	73.4
Asian - East (e.g., Chinese, Japanese, Korean)	144	79.2	255	81.6	82	82.9
Asian - South East (e.g., Malaysian, Filipino, Vietnamese)	126	73.0	203	77.8	92	84.8
Asian - South (e.g., Indian, Pakistani, Sri Lankan)	124	74.2	299	76.6	64	78.1
Black - African (e.g., Ghanaian, Kenyan, Somali)	73	80.8	204	78.9	47	70.2
Black - Caribbean (e.g., Barbadian, Jamaican)	87	75.9	169	77.5	59	72.9
Black - North American (e.g., Canadian, American)	17	64.7	29	72.4	8	75.0
Indian - Caribbean (e.g., Guyanese with origins in India)	40	57.5	43	81.4	24	70.8
Latin American (e.g., Argentinean, Chilean, Salvadorian)	86	73.3	129	76.7	35	80.0
Middle Eastern (e.g., Egyptian, Iranian, Lebanese)	40	70.0	67	68.7	13	84.6
Mixed heritage (e.g., Black- African and White-North American	25	64.0	93	76.3	11	72.7
Other (including First Nations/Indigenous/Aboriginal not included elsewhere/Inuit/Métis)	113	69.0	154	84.4	55	56.4
Prefer not to answer/Do not know/Missing	256	68.8	254	74.8	133	71.4
Neighbourhood income quintile						
Q1	714	73.2	949	76.4	337	70.0
Q2	447	72.9	633	79.5	230	73.0
Q3	451	71.8	612	78.1	251	74.1
Q4	477	73.2	600	79.0	261	75.9
Q5	738	75.5	826	82.1	353	77.6
Missing	201	63.7	377	75.9	89	78.7
Low-income cut-off, before taxes (LICO-BT)[b]						
Below low-income cut-off	710	68.6	836	76.4	312	64.7
Above low-income cut-off	1529	74.9	2130	80.9	769	79.8
Prefer not to answer/Do not know/Missing	789	72.9	1031	75.6	440	71.8

Table 1 Subset of patients with survey data available[a] *(Continued)*

Sexual orientation						
Heterosexual	2305	72.8	3395	79.3	1300	74.6
Gay/Bisexual/Lesbian/Queer/Two-Spirit/Other	463	72.4	277	75.1	71	66.2
Prefer not to answer/Do not know/Missing	260	74.6	325	75.1	150	76.7
Language						
What language would you feel most comfortable speaking in with your healthcare provider?						
English	2875	72.9	3732	78.6	1437	74.4
Other Language	136	72.1	252	79.4	77	77.9
Prefer not to answer/Do not know/Missing	17	76.5	13	76.9	7	42.9
In what language would you prefer to read healthcare information?						
English	2750	73.1	3656	78.7	1379	74.3
Other language	115	67.8	211	79.1	61	73.8
Prefer not to answer/Do not know/Missing	163	72.4	130	76.9	81	77.8
Housing						
Own Home	1508	75.5	1744	81.9	805	79.0
Renting Home	942	71.3	1697	76.6	442	73.8
Other	325	65.5	284	74.3	147	59.2
Prefer not to answer/Do not know/Missing	253	72.3	272	75.0	127	65.4

[a]Screening rates are reported as row percentages
[b]LICO-BT derived from 2014 Statistics Canada LICO-BT calculations with the following modifications:
i) if participants reported a total family income before taxes of $0 to $29,999 (question #7) and reported that their income supported ≤ 2 people (question #8) they were below the LICO-BT
ii) if participants reported a total family income before taxes of $0 to $29,999 or $30,000 to $59,999 (question #7) and reported their income supported between 3 to 6 people (question #8) they were below the LICO-BT
iii) if participants reported a total family income before taxes of $0 to $29,999 or $30,000 to $59,999 or $60,000 to $89,999 (question #7) and reported their income supported seven or more people (question #8) they were below the LICO-BT

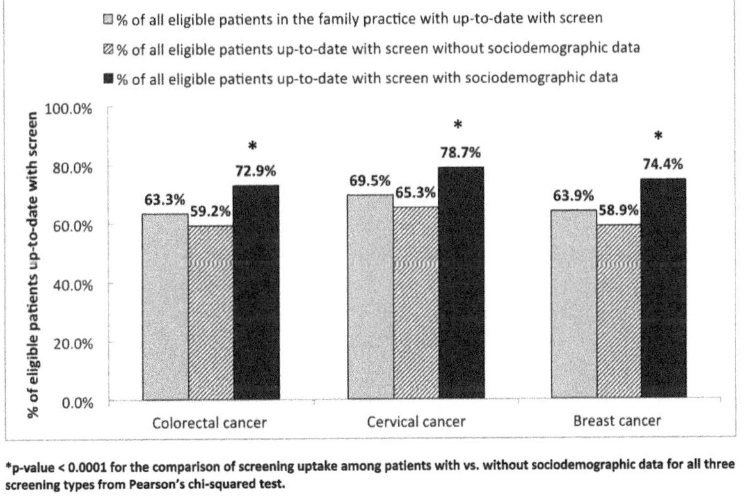

Fig. 2 Colorectal, cervical, and breast cancer screening rates for all eligible patients and eligible patients with survey data. *p-value < 0.0001 for the comparison of screening uptake among patients with vs. without sociodemographic data for all three screening types from Pearson's chi-squared test

Table 2 Bivariate results for screening rates among patients with survey data[a]

	Colorectal cancer			Cervical cancer			Breast cancer		
	Overdue for colorectal screening, %	Up-to-date for colorectal screening, %	*p*-value	Overdue for cervical cancer screening, %	Up-to-date for cervical cancer screening, %	*p*-value	Overdue for breast cancer screening, %	Up-to-date for breast cancer screening, %	*p*-value
TOTAL	821	2207		853	3144		389	1132	
Age categories									
20–29	– –	– –	**<0.0001**	16.9	15.1	**<0.0001**	– –	– –	0.141
30–39	– –	– –		25.1	29.7		– –	– –	
40–49	– –	– –		19.2	25.3		– –	– –	
50–59	63.3	48.4		19.7	18.8		55.8	51.2	
60–69	28.6	38.8		19.1	11.0		31.4	36.9	
70+ years	8.0	12.8		– –	– –		12.9	11.8	
Age, mean (SD)	57.8(6.7)	60.6(6.8)	**<0.0001**	44.5(13.8)	42.7(12.1)	**<0.0001**	59.3(7.3)	60.1(6.7)	0.06
Sex									
Male	47.9	47.1	0.715	– –	– –	– –	– –	– –	– –
Female	52.1	52.9		100.0	100.0		100.0	100.0	
Immigrant status									
Foreign-born	37.1	42.6	**0.008**	43.0	40.3	0.171	42.1	45.3	0.287
Canadian-born	62.9	57.4		57.0	59.7		57.9	54.7	
Ethnicity									
White	68.6	68.4	0.934	54.9	56.4	0.455	66.7	64.0	0.372
Other ethnicity	31.4	31.6		45.1	43.6		33.3	36.0	
Neighbourhood income quintile									
Q1	23.3	23.7	0.692	26.3	23.1	0.062	26.0	20.8	0.219
Q2	14.7	14.8		15.2	16.0		15.9	14.8	
Q3	15.5	14.7		15.7	15.2		16.7	16.4	
Q4	15.6	15.8		14.8	15.1		16.2	17.5	
Q5	22.0	25.2		17.4	21.6		20.3	24.2	
Low-income cut-off, before taxes (LICO-BT)									
Below low-income cut-off	36.7	29.8	**0.002**	32.7	27.0	**0.006**	41.5	24.8	**<0.0001**
Above low-income cut-off	63.3	70.2		67.3	73.0		58.5	75.2	
Sexual orientation									
Heterosexual	83.0	83.4	0.845	91.1	92.8	0.099	93.2	95.4	0.115
Gay/Bisexual/ Lesbian/Queer/ Two-Spirit/Other	17.0	16.6		8.9	7.2		6.8	4.6	
What language would you feel most comfortable speaking in with your healthcare provider?									
English	95.3	95.5	0.828	93.9	93.6	0.779	95.6	94.7	0.488
Other Language	4.7	4.5		6.1	6.4		4.4	5.3	
Housing									
Own Home	49.1	56.3	**<0.0001**	40.1	48.6	**<0.0001**	49.0	60.6	**<0.0001**
Renting Home	36.0	33.2		50.6	44.2		33.6	31.1	
Other	14.9	10.5		9.3	7.2		17.4	8.3	

[a]Screening rates reported as column percentages
Statistically significant *p*-values were bolded

the sociodemographic survey were not typical of all patients in the practice, with higher cancer screening rates than patients who did not respond to the survey. Although we were able to use survey data to formulate a low-income cut-off based on the Statistics Canada definition, there was a large amount of missing income information, approximately 25% across the three cancer screening cohorts, precluding us from conducting multivariable analyses. It is possible that income was on the causal pathway of the relationship we observed between housing status and screening. Other variables (e.g. age) may have also confounded the relationships we observed between income and screening and housing and screening or acted as intermediate factors.

Our study highlights opportunities in the use of self-reported SDOH data in primary care. We found a significant association between the low-income cut-off variable and cancer screening despite the high amount of missing income data, and despite neighbourhood income quintile not being associated with cancer screening. Most studies on income inequities in health use neighbourhood income as a proxy for individual income, as the latter is often not available [19, 23, 25, 27, 40–44]. Our results demonstrate that neighbourhood income may under-represent income-related inequalities and were not in high agreement with the individual-level LICO. This may be especially true in urban centres like Toronto where the demographics of neighbourhoods are changing rapidly and faster than a quinquennial census can accurately track [45].

We also found intriguing results based on housing status. We found no other studies that examined the relationship between housing status and cancer screening. However, housing status has been associated with other aspects of cancer care in the international literature. A recent U.S. study showed that both renters and people in unstable housing had delays in the time to diagnostic resolution after a cancer screening abnormality when compared to homeowners, potentially due to barriers such as coordination and scheduling, transportation, childcare and low literacy [46]. Hagedoorn et al. found that home ownership (versus tenancy) provided a beneficial effect on lung cancer mortality in Belgium [47]. Housing status may simply be a marker of income, but it may also be a marker of wealth or social stability. Future research should further explore the causal pathway that lies between housing and cancer screening, taking into account sociodemographic variables that have been previously found to be associated with cancer screening, such as age, income, immigrant status, and co-morbidities, and that could serve as confounders for observed associations [19, 23, 26, 27, 48, 49].

Our results also highlight several challenges in collecting individual-level income status using self-reported data. One-quarter of participating patients did not provide a household income; missing data for other social determinants were otherwise less than 10%. Our findings of missing income are in line with previous literature. Kirst et al. found that 67% of Ontario residents were uncomfortable with disclosing household income and there was a general lack of awareness of the importance of collecting sociodemographic data [50]. Similarly, a national survey conducted in 2009 found that 65% of Canadian respondents were uncomfortable with the collection of household income in healthcare settings [51]. Respondents were most comfortable with sociodemographic data being directly collected by their family physician and certain groups were more comfortable with the collection of income, such as visible minorities and males [51].

It is possible that asking about socioeconomic status in different ways might have been more acceptable to our survey participants and might have led to less missing data. The question "Do you have difficulty making ends meet at the end of the month?" has been found to be a good predictor in a Canadian primary care population of being below the low-income cut-off, with a sensitivity of 98% and specificity of 40%, with the caveat that non-English speakers may not understand this colloquial term [52]. Future research could test such questions for their acceptability and validity in our setting [15]. Interestingly, in the pilot testing of our sociodemographic survey, only 10.1% of patients did not answer the income question [28], stressing the importance of ongoing post-implementation surveillance of such initiatives.

We also experienced several other challenges with collecting and using SDOH data. First, although there were a large number of categories for ethnicity in the survey, many of these categories had quite small cell sizes. We also had data on indigenous persons that we did not feel comfortable using due to a lack of adherence to Ownership, Control, Access and Possession principles [38]. We ultimately collapsed these categories into White vs. non-White for bivariate analyses. However, different categorizations might have led to more meaningful ethnicity-based screening results. How to best categorize ethnicity while maximizing both sample size and granularity needs to be further explored. Second, our survey was only available in English or French, which may explain the low proportion of patients in our survey who reported their preferred language as one other than English. This may have dissuaded some foreign-born patients from participating in the survey, and may partially explain why we saw no disparities based on immigrant status. Third, study participants were not representative of all patients in the practice, as noted by their higher screening rates. Participants were all willing to answer a waiting room survey, so it is plausible that they may have been more likely to come in for visits than other patients and that they may also have been more likely to be intrinsically motivated to participate in prevention and screening manoeuvres. These latter two points may partially explain why we found no disparities in screening for foreign-born patients despite well-documented disparities at the provincial level [23, 26, 44]. Fourth, although a sizeable proportion of our patients have completed the survey, detecting differences in care among some patient groups (e.g. non-heterosexual patients, certain ethnic groups) would likely require a larger sample. Fifth, the survey did not include a question on education, another known social determinant of health. Prior research demonstrates that higher education levels are positively associated with colorectal, cervical cancer, and breast cancer screening adherence [53–55]. Sixth, we were unable to track family history of cancer, which has been shown to be a motivator for cancer screening [56–59]. Seventh, younger participants in our study had less opportunity for cancer screening, which may at least partially explain our findings on age and colorectal cancer screening. Finally, it is plausible that the missing data encountered in all questions was non-random and potentially biased our findings.

Conclusions

Our experiences highlight key considerations for primary care providers and researchers interested in collecting and intervening on SDOH in primary care. While we were able to show that neighbourhood income might under-estimate income-related disparities in screening, individual-level income was also the most challenging variable to collect. Future work in this area should focus on targeted interventions that reduce income-related disparities in cancer screening [60] and simultaneously continue to explore how best to collect socioeconomic data, particularly measures of poverty. Further research is also needed to understand whether housing is an independent risk factor for under-screening.

Abbreviations

EMR: Electronic medical record; LICO-BT: Low-Income Cutoff Before Taxes; SDOH: Social determinants of health

Acknowledgements

The authors thank Ms. Lisa Miller for her technical assistance.

Funding

This study was supported by a research grant from the St. Michael's Foundation Translational Innovation Fund. Dr. Lofters. Dr. Pinto, Dr. Persaud and Dr. Kiran are supported as Clinician Scientists by the University of Toronto Department of Family & Community Medicine. Dr. Lofters is supported by a Canadian Cancer Society Research Institute Career Development Award in Cancer Prevention. Dr. Kiran is supported by a Canadian Institutes of Health Research Embedded Clinician Researcher Award. Dr. Persaud is funded by a PSI Graham Farquharson Knowledge Translation Fellowship. The funders had no role in study design, data collection and analysis, decision to publish, or preparation of the manuscript.

Authors' contributions

AL and TK conceived of the study; AL, TK, and MS participated in the design of the study; AS analyzed the quantitative data; AL drafted the manuscript; TK, AS, MS, NB, NP, AP, EK, SK, and RN participated in the preparation of the manuscript by providing critical revisions of drafts; and all authors read and approved the final manuscript.

Competing interests

The authors declare that they have no competing interests.

Consent for publication

Not applicable.

Author details

[1]Department of Family & Community Medicine, St. Michael's Hospital, 30 Bond Street, Toronto, ON M5B 1W8, Canada. [2]Department of Family & Community Medicine, University of Toronto, 500 University Avenue, 5th Floor, Toronto, ON M5G 1V7, Canada. [3]Centre for Urban Health Solutions, Li Ka Shing Knowledge Institute, St. Michael's Hospital, 30 Bond Street, Toronto, ON M5B 1W8, Canada. [4]Dalla Lana School of Public Health, University of Toronto, Health Sciences Building, 155 College Street, 6th Floor, Toronto, ON M5T 3M7, Canada. [5]Department of Surgery, Li Ka Shing Knowledge Institute, St. Michael's Hospital, 30 Bond Street, Toronto, ON M5B 1W8, Canada. [6]Cancer Care Ontario, 620 University Avenue, Toronto, ON M5G 2L7, Canada. [7]Institute for Clinical Evaluative Sciences, 2075 Bayview Avenue, Toronto, Ontario M4N 3M5, Canada.

References

1. Determinants of Health: What Makes Canadians Healthy or Unhealthy? http://www.phac-aspc.gc.ca/ph-sp/determinants/determinants-eng.php#unhealthy. Accessed 17 Feb 2017.
2. Chandola T, Ferrie J, Sacker A, Marmot M. Social inequalities in self reported health in early old age: follow-up of prospective cohort study. BMJ. 2007;334(7601):990.
3. Commission on Social Determinants of Health. Closing the gap in a generation: health equity through action on the social determinants of health. In: Final report of the commission on social determinants of health. Geneva: World Health Organization; 2008.
4. Galobardes B, Davey Smith G, Jeffreys M, McCarron P. Childhood socioeconomic circumstances predict specific causes of death in adulthood: the Glasgow student cohort study. J Epidemiol Community Health. 2006;60(6):527–9.
5. Lofters A, Slater M, Kirst M, Shankardass K, Quinonez C. How do people attribute income-related inequalities in health? a cross-sectional study in Ontario, Canada. PLoS One. 2014;9(1):e85286.
6. Marmot M. Social determinants of health inequalities. Lancet. 2005; 365(9464):1099–104.
7. Marmot M, Friel S. Global health equity: evidence for action on the social determinants of health. J Epidemiol Community Health. 2008;62(12):1095–7.
8. Mikkonen J, Raphael D. Social determinants of health: the Canadian facts. Toronto: York University School of Health Policy and Management; 2010.
9. Social determinants of health. http://www.who.int/social_determinants/en/. Accessed 17 Feb 2017.
10. Bierman AS, Magari ES, Jette AM, Splaine M, Wasson JH. Assessing access as a first step toward improving the quality of care for very old adults. J Ambul Care Manage. 1998;21(3):17–26.
11. Institute of Medicine. Capturing social and behavioral domains in electronic health records: phase 1. Washington: National Academies Press; 2014.
12. Shi L, Starfield B. The effect of primary care physician supply and income inequality on mortality among blacks and whites in US metropolitan areas. Am J Public Health. 2001;91(8):1246–50.
13. Starfield B, Shi L, Macinko J. Contribution of primary care to health systems and health. Milbank Q. 2005;83(3):457–502.
14. DeVoe JE, Bazemore AW, Cottrell EK, Likumahuwa-Ackman S, Grandmont J, Spach N, Gold R. Perspectives in primary care: a conceptual framework and path for integrating social determinants of health into primary care practice. Ann Fam Med. 2016;14(2):104–8.

15. Gottlieb LM, Tirozzi KJ, Manchanda R, Burns AR, Sandel MT. Moving electronic medical records upstream: incorporating social determinants of health. Am J Prev Med. 2015;48(2):215–8.
16. Borkhoff CM, Saskin R, Rabeneck L, Baxter NN, Liu Y, Tinmouth J, Paszat LF. Disparities in receipt of screening tests for cancer, diabetes and high cholesterol in Ontario, Canada: a population-based study using area-based methods. Can J Public Health. 2013;104(4):e284–290.
17. Fernandes KA, Sutradhar R, Borkhoff CM, Baxter N, Lofters A, Rabeneck L, Tinmouth J, Paszat L, Ontario Cancer Screening Research N. Small-area variation in screening for cancer, glucose and cholesterol in Ontario: a cross-sectional study. CMAJ Open. 2015;3(4):E373–81.
18. Glazier RH, Creatore MI, Gozdyra P, Matheson FI, Steele LS, Boyle E, Moineddin R. Geographic methods for understanding and responding to disparities in mammography use in Toronto, Canada. J Gen Intern Med. 2004;19(9):952–61.
19. Guilcher SJ, Lofters A, Glazier RH, Jaglal SB, Voth J, Bayoumi AM. Level of disability, multi-morbidity and breast cancer screening: does severity matter? Prev Med. 2014;67:193–8.
20. Honein-AbouHaidar GN, Baxter NN, Moineddin R, Urbach DR, Rabeneck L, Bierman AS. Trends and inequities in colorectal cancer screening participation in Ontario, Canada, 2005–2011. Cancer Epidemiol. 2013;37(6):946–56.
21. Kiran T, Wilton AS, Moineddin R, Paszat L, Glazier RH. Effect of payment incentives on cancer screening in Ontario primary care. Ann Fam Med. 2014;12(4):317–23.
22. Lofters A, Guilcher S, Maulkhan N, Milligan J, Lee J. Patients living with disabilities: the need for high-quality primary care. Can Fam Physician. 2016;62(8):e457–464.
23. Lofters AK, Hwang SW, Moineddin R, Glazier RH. Cervical cancer screening among urban immigrants by region of origin: a population-based cohort study. Prev Med. 2010;51(6):509–16.
24. Lofters AK, Moineddin R, Hwang SW, Glazier RH. Low rates of cervical cancer screening among urban immigrants: a population-based study in Ontario, Canada. Med Care. 2010;48(7):611–8.
25. Lofters AK, Moineddin R, Hwang SW, Glazier RH. Predictors of low cervical cancer screening among immigrant women in Ontario, Canada. BMC Womens Health. 2011;11:20.
26. Lofters A, Ng R, Lobb R. Primary care physician characteristics associated with cancer screening: A retrospective cohort study in Ontario, Canada. Cancer Med. 2014. doi:10.1002/cam4.358.
27. Vahabi M, Lofters A, Kumar M, Glazier RH. Breast cancer screening disparities among urban immigrants: a population-based study in Ontario, Canada. BMC Public Health. 2015;15:679.
28. Pinto AD, Glattstein-Young G, Mohamed A, Bloch G, Leung FH, Glazier RH. Building a foundation to reduce health inequities: routine collection of sociodemographic data in primary care. J Am Board Fam Med. 2016;29(3):348–55.
29. Rosser WW, Colwill JM, Kasperski J, Wilson L. Patient-centered medical homes in Ontario. N Engl J Med. 2010;362(3):e7.
30. About the Ontario Breast Screening Program. https://www.cancercare.on.ca/pcs/screening/breastscreening/. Accessed 17 Feb 2017.
31. Cervical Screening - CCO. http://www.cancercare.on.ca/pcs/screening/cervscreening/. Accessed 17 Feb 2017.
32. Ontario Cancer Plan 2008–2011. http://ocp.cancercare.on.ca/cms/One.aspx?portalid=14464%pageid=14471. Accessed 17 Feb 2017.
33. Screening Guidelines - CCO. https://www.cancercare.on.ca/pcs/screening/breastscreening/breasthealth/. Accessed 17 Feb 2017.
34. Screening Guidelines - CCO. https://www.cancercare.on.ca/pcs/screening/cervscreening/screening_guidelines/. Accessed 17 Feb 2017.
35. Screening. http://www.cancercare.on.ca/pcs/screening/. Accessed 17 Feb 2017.
36. Screening Activity Report. http://www.cancercare.on.ca/pcs/primcare/sar/. Accessed 17 Feb 2017.
37. Low Income Cut-Offs. http://www.statcan.gc.ca/pub/75f0002m/2012002/lico-sfr-eng.htm. Accessed 17 Feb 2017.
38. First Nations Centre. OCAP: ownership, control, access and possession. In: Sanctioned by the first nations information governance committee, assembly of first nations. Ottawa: National Aboriginal Health Organization; 2007.
39. IBM Corp. IBM SPSS statistics for windows, version 20.0. Armonk: IBM Corp; 2011. Released.
40. Decker KM, Demers AA, Nugent Z, Biswanger N, Singh H. Reducing income-related inequities in colorectal cancer screening: lessons learned from a retrospective analysis of organised programme and non-programme screening delivery in Winnipeg, Manitoba. BMJ Open. 2016;6(2):e009470.
41. Elit L, Krzyzanowska M, Saskin R, Barbera L, Razzaq A, Lofters A, Yeritsyan N, Bierman A. Sociodemographic factors associated with cervical cancer screening and follow-up of abnormal results. Can Fam Physician. 2012;58(1):e22–31.
42. Kiran T, Kopp A, Moineddin R, Victor JC, Campbell RJ, Shah BR, Glazier RH. Unintended consequences of delisting routine eye exams on retinopathy screening for people with diabetes in Ontario, Canada. CMAJ. 2013; 185(3):E167–173.
43. Sholzberg M, Gomes T, Juurlink DN, Yao Z, Mamdani MM, Laupacis A. The influence of socioeconomic status on selection of anticoagulation for atrial fibrillation. PLoS One. 2016;11(2):e0149142.
44. Vahabi M, Lofters A, Kumar M, Glazier RH. Breast cancer screening disparities among immigrant women by world region of origin: a population-based study in Ontario, Canada. Cancer Med. 2016;5(7):1670–86.
45. Toronto Community Health Profiles. http://www.torontohealthprofiles.ca/. Accessed 17 Feb 2017.
46. Rodday AM, Parsons SK, Snyder F, Simon MA, Llanos AA, Warren-Mears V, Dudley D, Lee JH, Patierno SR, Markossian TW, et al. Impact of patient navigation in eliminating economic disparities in cancer care. Cancer. 2015;121(22):4025–34.
47. Hagedoorn P, Vandenheede H, Willaert D, Vanthomme K, Gadeyne S. Regional inequalities in lung cancer mortality in Belgium at the beginning of the 21st century: the contribution of individual and area-level socioeconomic status and industrial exposure. PLoS One. 2016;11(1):e0147099.
48. Tilbrook D, Polsky J, Lofters A. Are women with psychosis receiving adequate cervical cancer screening? Can Fam Physician. 2010;56(4):358–63.
49. Lofters A, Guilcher S, Glazier R, Jaglal S, Voth J, Bayoumi A. Screening for cervical cancer in women with disability and multimorbidity: A retrospective cohort study in Ontario, Canada. CMAJ Open. 2014;2(4):E240-7. doi:10.9778/cmajo.20140003.
50. Kirst M, Shankardass K, Bomze S, Lofters A, Quinonez C. Sociodemographic data collection for health equity measurement: a mixed methods study examining public opinions. Int J Equity Health. 2013;12(1):75.
51. Lofters AK, Shankardass K, Kirst M, Quinonez C. Sociodemographic data collection in healthcare settings: an examination of public opinions. Med Care. 2011;49(2):193–9.
52. Brcic V, Eberdt C, Kaczorowski J. Development of a tool to identify poverty in a family practice setting: a pilot study. Int J Family Med. 2011;2011:812182.
53. Limmer K, LoBiondo-Wood G, Dains J. Predictors of cervical cancer screening adherence in the United States: a systematic review. J Adv Pract Oncol. 2014;5(1):31–41.
54. Wools A, Dapper EA, de Leeuw JR. Colorectal cancer screening participation: a systematic review. Eur J Public Health. 2016;26(1):158–68.
55. Schueler KM, Chu PW, Smith-Bindman R. Factors associated with mammography utilization: a systematic quantitative review of the literature. J Womens Health (Larchmt). 2008;17(9):1477–98.
56. Bellinger JD, Brandt HM, Hardin JW, Bynum SA, Sharpe PA, Jackson D. The role of family history of cancer on cervical cancer screening behavior in a population-based survey of women in the Southeastern United States. Womens Health Issues. 2013;23(4):e197–204.
57. Laiyemo AO, Thompson N, Williams CD, Idowu KA, Bull-Henry K, Sherif ZA, Lee EL, Brim H, Ashktorab H, Platz EA, et al. Race and colorectal cancer screening compliance among persons with a family history of cancer. World J Gastrointest Endosc. 2015;7(18):1300–5.
58. Williams KP, Reiter P, Mabiso A, Maurer J, Paskett E. Family history of cancer predicts papanicolaou screening behavior for African american and white women. Cancer. 2009;115(1):179–89.
59. Ramsey SD, Yoon P, Moonesinghe R, Khoury MJ. Population-based study of the prevalence of family history of cancer: implications for cancer screening and prevention. Genet Med. 2006;8(9):571–5.
60. Berkowitz SA, Percac-Lima S, Ashburner JM, Chang Y, Zai AH, He W, Grant RW, Atlas SJ. Building equity improvement into quality improvement: reducing socioeconomic disparities in colorectal cancer screening as part of population health management. J Gen Intern Med. 2015;30(7):942–9.

15

Development and use of an index for measuring implementation of a weight management program in children in primary care clinics in Texas

Meliha Salahuddin[1,2,3*], Sarah E. Barlow[4,5], Stephen J. Pont[6], Nancy F. Butte[7] and Deanna M. Hoelscher[1]

Abstract

Background: The Texas Childhood Obesity Research Demonstration study was an integrated, systems-oriented intervention that incorporated primary and secondary obesity prevention approaches targeting multiple sectors, including primary care clinics, to address childhood obesity. The primary care clinic component included the American Academy of Pediatrics' *Next Steps* weight management counseling materials that support brief healthy lifestyle-focused visits. The current study describes the methodology and assesses the implementation of the *Next Steps* program in the participating primary care clinics, as well as the association of implementation with enrollment of children with overweight and obesity in the secondary prevention intervention.

Methods: The study used a serial cross-sectional study design to collect data from 11 primary care clinics in Houston ($n = 5$) and Austin ($n = 6$), Texas, in 2013–2014. Responses of primary care providers on 42 self-reported survey questions assessing acceptability, adoption, appropriateness, and feasibility of the program were utilized to create a mean standardized clinic implementation index score. Provider scores were aggregated to represent *Next Steps* implementation scores at the clinic level. A mixed effects logistic regression test was conducted to determine the association between program implementation and the enrollment of children in the secondary prevention.

Results: Mean implementation index score was lower at Year 2 of implementation (2014) than Year 1 (2013) although the decrease was not significant [63.2% (12.2%) in 2013 vs. 55.3% (16.5%) in 2014]. There were no significant associations between levels of implementation of *Next Steps* and enrollment into TX CORD secondary prevention study.

Conclusions: The development of an index using process evaluation measures can be used to assess the implementation and evaluation of provider-based obesity prevention tools in primary care clinics.

Keywords: Next steps, Weight management, Primary care clinics, Implementation index, Process evaluation, Children with overweight/obesity, TX CORD

* Correspondence: msalahuddin@utsystem.edu; meliha.salahuddin@gmail.com
[1]Michael & Susan Dell Center for Healthy Living, University of Texas Health Science Center at Houston (UTHealth) School of Public Health in Austin, Austin, TX, USA
[2]University of Texas Health Science Center at Tyler, Tyler, TX, USA
Full list of author information is available at the end of the article

Introduction

Over one-third of children in the United States have overweight or obesity, with more Hispanic, non-Hispanic black, and children from low socioeconomic conditions being affected than non-Hispanic white children [1, 2]. Primary care providers (PCP) are tasked with a periodic screening of children's health and growth, and thus play a critical role in recognizing and addressing childhood obesity, a condition associated with heavy health and economic burdens [3–5]. However, at present, there is low active participation from PCPs in assessing or managing children with overweight or obesity in the primary care clinics [5], even though pediatricians can easily identify children with obesity [6]. Thus, it is essential to equip PCPs with effective prevention and treatment tools to address childhood obesity that they can easily implement.

Implementation research focuses on the processes and factors associated with successful integration of evidence-based programs within a particular setting, e.g., healthcare settings [7]. Many studies have implemented and assessed the effectiveness of different weight management programs in healthcare settings [8]; however, none, to the best of our knowledge, have developed and/or assessed the level of implementation of an intervention specific to weight management in healthcare settings using a composite score. Composite indicators are widely used in healthcare settings to measure and track provider performance as well as for external and internal benchmarking against other providers or institutions for quality improvement [9]. Developing a similar indicator or index for weight management interventions in primary healthcare settings will not only help to evaluate the fidelity of the intervention but also help to compare how the different primary care clinics perform.

The overall goal of this study was to describe the methodology and development of an index that can assess the implementation of the *Next Steps* program component of the Texas Childhood Research Demonstration (TX CORD) primary prevention study. The *Next Steps* program, which comprises weight management counseling materials [10], was pilot tested in the TX CORD study. The materials support brief counseling during busy office visits, with a goal of encouraging healthcare providers' attention to obesity. Thus, it served as an engagement tool in study recruitment for the TX CORD primary prevention study and was also utilized in the comparison arm for the TX CORD secondary prevention study [11]. As a result, in our study, as a secondary objective, we examined the association of the implementation index of *Next Steps* with the enrollment of children with overweight and obesity in the TX CORD secondary prevention study.

Method

Study setting

The Texas childhood research demonstration (TX CORD) study

The TX CORD study was an integrated, systems-oriented model that incorporated primary and secondary obesity prevention approaches at multiple levels and sectors including primary care clinics in Houston and Austin, Texas, 2012–2014. The target population was low-income, underserved predominantly Hispanic and non-Hispanic black children aged 2–12 years [12, 13]. The primary prevention component was a quasi-experimental pre- and post-test community trial focused on improving healthy eating and physical activity in different settings, including primary care clinics.

Primary care clinic component of the TX CORD primary prevention study

Primary care clinics that served majority Medicaid, Children's Health Insurance Program (CHIP), and uninsured population in the TX CORD catchment areas were invited to participate. The primary prevention component of the TX CORD study engaged five and seven primary care clinics from Houston and Austin, respectively. One Austin clinic was closed for remodeling during process data collection, and so this evaluation used data from the 11 participating primary care clinics.

All clinics received a set of coordinated counseling materials known as *Next Steps*, which were adapted for TX CORD and translated into Spanish. In Houston, an electronic health record (EHR) alert system was adapted from Taveras et al., (2014) and implemented to flag children with body mass index (BMI) ≥ 85th percentile, and to provide additional tools for the evaluation of comorbidities of obesity, obesity-related diagnostic codes, orders, and referrals [14]. Because Austin clinics were part of three different federally qualified health centers, with different EHR systems, the modifications were not implemented in the Austin EHRs. The providers received brief training in the use of the *Next Steps* materials, EHR changes (if applicable), and had a brief introduction to motivational interviewing techniques.

Measures

Description of the next steps program

Next Steps is a set of coordinated weight management counseling materials for pediatric PCPs. These materials were created through a partnership with the National Initiative for Children's Healthcare Quality, the Barbara Bush Children's Hospital at Maine Medical Center, and the Maine Chapter of American Academy of Pediatrics (AAP) [10]. The materials included a menu of different healthy lifestyle themes, presented via poster and a desktop flip chart with a patient facing page and a provider-facing page with counseling tips. The TX CORD team also developed a patient home-based activity book, as a reinforcement tool for each theme that they gave to families at their discretion. Materials were available in both English and Spanish. Providers attended an in-person or webinar orientation to the material at the start of the project in 2012 and also received informal office visits from project staff two or three times per year between 2012 and early 2014, to ask questions and provide feedback.

Process evaluation survey

Providers, including those with MD, DO, nurse practitioner or physician assistant degrees, in the clinics, received a survey about the *Next Steps* material once in fall 2013 (Year 1 of implementation), approximately one year after the project started, and in fall 2014 (Year 2 of implementation). The *Next Steps* survey included data on provider characteristics, as well as different implementation measures [15], including acceptability, adoption, appropriateness, and feasibility of *Next Steps* program materials across the primary care clinics. These measures of implementation are in alignment with some of the measures for Diffusion of Innovation [16] and RE-AIM (Reach, Effectiveness, Adoption, Implementation, and Maintenance) [17, 18] implementation frameworks, which are further detailed below.

Provider characteristics

Data included provider gender, age, race/ethnicity, years of experience in the current position, medical field, working with pediatric patients after completion of medical training, and any prior training in the management of children with overweight and obesity.

Acceptability of using the next steps program materials

The acceptability construct included 3 items measuring providers' ease of learning to use the materials and 6 items measuring their satisfaction with the materials. These were measured on a 5-point Likert scale from strongly disagree to disagree to neither agree nor disagree to agree to strongly agree. They were adapted from the *Next Steps* Guide: Feedback Survey [10]. This construct is supported by Roger's "complexity" framework in the Diffusion of Innovation theory [15, 16].

Adoption of the next steps program materials

The adoption construct measured the frequency of use of the *Next Steps* program materials on a 5-point Likert scale ranging from less than 10% to 10–25% to 25–50% to 50–75% to 75–100%. The 5 items were developed by the TX CORD research team, and supported by the "adoption" framework from RE-AIM [17, 18] and Roger's "trialability" framework from Diffusion of Innovation theories [15, 16].

Appropriateness of the next steps program materials

This construct measured providers' perception of the effectiveness of the *Next Steps* program materials in treating children with overweight and obesity. These were measured on a 5-point Likert scale as well (strongly disagree to strongly agree). This construct also included whether the providers wanted any modification in any of the *Next Steps* healthy lifestyle themes encompassing three categories: Category A: Setting the foundation ($n = 1$ theme), Category B: Introduce concepts that are important to cover early for success ($n = 5$ themes), and Category C: Focus on other important concepts ($n = 13$ themes). Examples included understanding health, meaning of healthy food, home environment, themes around physical activity, body image, screen time, meal patterns and so on. The response options were on a 5-point Likert scale, ranging from "remove: theme not useful-remove from guide" to "reprioritize: like theme but it needs lower priority" to "edit: I like the theme, but content need revising" to "keep as is: I like theme as is" to "not applicable: I have not used this theme". These were operationalized as binary variables, "keep as is" versus collapsing the rest of the groups. These items were adapted from the *Next Steps* Guide: Feedback Survey [10]. This construct is supported by Roger's "compatibility" framework from Diffusion of Innovation theory [15, 16].

Feasibility of the next steps program materials

This construct included 4 items and measured whether the different *Next Steps* program components were made available to the providers by the TX CORD research team. They were developed by the TX CORD research team. This construct is supported by Roger's "trialability" and "compatibility" framework from Diffusion of Innovation theory [15, 16].

Study design and sample

The study utilized a serial cross-sectional study design. Process evaluation data were collected from 11 primary care clinics in Houston and Austin, Texas, respectively, in 2013 and 2014. These 11 primary care clinics were the participant recruitment source for the TX CORD secondary prevention study, which was a 12-month randomized controlled trial comparing intensive weight management programs among children with BMI ≥ 85th percentile and aged 2–12 years. Participant recruitment for the TX CORD secondary prevention study occurred between the end of 2012 and the beginning of 2014 [11].

Informed consents were obtained from healthcare personnel before survey administration. The Institutional Review Boards of University of Texas Health

Science Center at Houston (UTHealth) and Baylor College of Medicine approved all protocols and procedures for the study (HSC-SPH-11–0513).

Statistical analysis

All analyses were conducted by year of implementation (Year 1 or Year 2). We report frequencies with proportions to describe the characteristics of the providers. Mean scores with standard deviations for continuous variables and frequencies with proportions for categorical variables across the 42 survey items were computed. Mean scores were also reported for constructs with similar items.

Development of the implementation index

We computed an implementation index score from the 42 *Next Steps* items for each primary care clinic aggregated from the respective provider scores. A summative score was computed for items with similar constructs (four constructs: acceptability, adoption, appropriateness, and feasibility) at the provider level. Each of these summative scores was then converted to a percent score [percent score = (summative score)/(maximum potential score)]. For example, the summative score for feasibility construct was 'x' at a provider level. The maximum potential score for this construct was 4 (sum of the score of the 4 underlying binary items). The percent score for feasibility at the provider level would be [(100*x)/4]. The provider construct percent scores were then aggregated to the clinic level. We computed the implementation index score at the clinic level by taking the average of the construct percent scores. Only the surveys with ≥80% reported items were included in the score calculation ($n = 5$ surveys excluded). Cronbach's alpha for the survey scales was calculated at both years.

Examination of implementation index score

We examined the mean implementation index scores with standard deviation (SD) for each year of implementation (Years 1 or 2). Mann-Whitney U-test was conducted to compare the mean implementation index score between the two years due to the small sample size.

Examination of association of implementation index levels with the enrollment of children with overweight and obesity in the TX CORD secondary prevention study

The 1957 referred patients from 11 primary care clinics were categorized as enrolled or not enrolled in the TX CORD secondary prevention study. The implementation index scores for the primary care clinics were converted into categorical variables with quartile splits collapsed into three categories: (a) relatively high level of implementation (upper quartile of the index), (b) medium level of implementation (middle two quartiles), and (c) relatively low level of implementation (lower quartile of the index). We then conducted a mixed effects logistic regression test with a random intercept term for primary care clinics to examine the association between implementation index levels and enrollment of children with overweight and obesity into the TX CORD secondary prevention study, separately for each year. Similar regression models were also used to examine the associations of underlying constructs, including acceptability, adoption, appropriateness, and feasibility with the enrollment of children into the TX CORD secondary prevention study. Significance was set at P value< 0.05. STATA software version 14.0 (College Station, TX) was used for data analysis.

Results

Provider characteristics

Table 1 presents the description of the PCPs by Years 1 and 2 of TX CORD clinic implementation. A total of 30 PCPs in Year 1 of implementation and 34 PCPs in Year 2 of implementation completed the survey across the 11 participating primary care clinics.

Next steps process evaluation data

Table 2 presents the descriptive information for the individual *Next Steps* items, separately for Year 1 and Year 2 of implementation. Overall, the providers felt the materials were acceptable, appropriate and feasible to use in treating patients with childhood overweight and obesity. However, they reported low to moderate adoption of the *Next Steps* program materials.

Implementation index score

Based on provider report, the implementation score for the *Next Steps* material was 63.2 (12.2)% at Year 1 and 55.3 (16.5)% at Year 2 across all clinics. The scores in Year 1 and Year 2 were not statistically different (P value = 0.375).

Figure 1 shows the range of implementation index scores across the primary care clinics, by years of implementation. The scores ranged from 45.9–84.4% in Year 1, compared to 18.0–78.5% in Year 2 of implementation. Cronbach's alpha for the survey scales, including the individual constructs was high at both years (> 0.80).

Implementation index levels and TX CORD secondary prevention enrollment

Implementation scores were categorized into three levels based on observed groupings at each year. Relatively low implementation was defined as scores in the lowest quartile (three clinics with score range in Year 1: 45.9–52.5% and Year 2: 18.0–42.4%). Relatively high implementation was defined as scores in the highest quartile

Table 1 Sociodemographic characteristics of primary care providers by year of implementation in the TX CORD study, 2013–2014

	Year 1 of implementation (2013), 30 (%)	Year 2 of implementation (2014), 34 (%)	*P* value
Female	25 (83.3)	26 (76.5)	0.496
At least 40 years of age	16 (53.3)	18 (52.9)	0.983
Race/ethnicity			
Non-Hispanic white	12 (40.0)	9 (26.5)	0.418
Non-Hispanic black	5 (16.7)	6 (17.7)	
Hispanic	4 (13.3)	10 (29.4)	
Others	8 (26.7)	9 (26.5)	
At least 6 years of employment in the current position	17 (56.7)	19 (55.9)	0.950
At least 6 years of experience in the medical field	25 (83.3)	26 (76.5)	0.348
At least 6 years of experience working with pediatric patients after completing medical training	25 (83.3)	26 (76.5)	0.496
More than 10 hours of prior training on how to manage childhood overweight or obesity	14 (46.7)	16 (47.1)	0.560

TX CORD Texas Childhood Obesity Research Demonstration
Missing data for all variables of interest was around 10%, thus, not reported in the table

(two clinics with score range in Year 1: 76.6–84.4% and Year 2: 74.3–78.5%).

Table 3 reports the frequency and proportions of children with overweight and obesity seen, referred, and enrolled from each clinic into the TX CORD secondary prevention study. Of the children with overweight and obesity seen at the 11 clinics ($n = 6198$), study referral rates by the individual clinics ranged from 8.5–66.8%. Of those referred ($n = 1957$), enrollment into TX CORD secondary prevention study from the individual clinics ranged from 18.3–50.0% [mean = 30.6 (11.7)%].

Table 4 presents the results for the associations between clinic implementation index levels and enrollment of children with overweight and obesity into the TX CORD secondary prevention study. No significant relation was observed between implementation and enrollment into TX CORD secondary prevention study. Associations between underlying constructs of the implementation index and enrollment are also presented in Table 4.

Discussion

Our study examined the acceptability, adoption, appropriateness, and feasibility of the *Next Steps* program materials, which were pilot tested in primary care clinics that participated in the primary prevention component of the TX CORD study over two years of implementation. Implementation scores were lower in Year 2 than Year 1, though not statistically significant. There were no significant associations between levels of implementation of *Next Steps* and enrollment into TX CORD secondary prevention study.

We used a novel methodology to develop an index using process evaluation measures that assessed the implementation of weight management programs to improve the health of children with overweight and obesity in primary care clinics. Indices to assess implementation of child weight management programs in healthcare clinical settings are lacking; thus, our study is the first to develop such an index. Multiple studies have assessed the different components of a weight management program implementation such as reach, effectiveness, adoption, climate, cost, etc., in different settings [11, 19–21], although none has comprehensively assessed the implementation of the program with a single index score. The clinic index we developed was reliable (Cronbach's alpha> 0.80) in assessing the underlying constructs; however, it warrants further psychometric analysis to include both measures of reliability and validity.

Although the providers in the current study perceived the *Next Steps* materials to be acceptable, appropriate and feasible, the frequency of use was around 10–50% of the time. The relatively low adoption of *Next Steps* material in the current study indicates that other factors led to a lower utilization of the materials during a clinic visit, such as limited time during a clinic visit, lack of training and retraining of providers, parental disengagement, providers' preference for other obesity prevention approaches, lack of clinic administrative support for this protocol, or something as simple as materials being misplaced [11]. Future studies can assess the reasons for low adoption and then examine ways to increase providers' use and accessibility to these materials [22].

The results of our study demonstrated some degree of fidelity of the *Next Steps* program materials across the primary care clinics, particularly during Year 1. Given that primary care clinics in this study primarily serve low-income populations, and since many factors

Table 2 Descriptive statistics of individual items included in the primary care clinic implementation index by year of implementation in the TX CORD study, 2013–2014

	Year 1 of implementation (2013)	Year 2 of implementation (2014)
Acceptability, mean (SD)		
Ease of learning to use the *Next Steps* materials		
I learned to use it quickly	2.8 (1.0)	2.6 (1.2)
I easily remember how to use it	2.6 (1.0)	2.5 (1.2)
The training I received was adequate	2.8 (0.8)	2.6 (1.1)
Satisfaction with *Next Steps* materials		
With overweight or obese kids, I am likely to use *Next Steps* during well child visits	2.8 (1.2)	2.2 (1.3)
With overweight or obese kids, I am likely to use *Next Steps* during acute care visits	1.7 (1.1)	1.5 (1.1)
With overweight or obese kids, I am likely to use *Next Steps* during obesity-specific visits	3.2 (1.1)	2.8 (1.2)
I am likely to use *Next Steps* with non- overweight/obese kids	1.8 (0.9)	1.7 (1.0)
Patients/families refer to the *Next Steps* poster	2.0 (0.9)	1.7 (1.0)
I refer to the *Next Steps* poster when I talk with patients/families	2.2 (1.0)	1.8 (1.0)
Mean score (SD) of the acceptability items at clinic provider level	2.5 (0.6)	19.4 (7.9)
Adoption, mean (SD)		
Frequency of use of *Next Steps* materials for counseling with patients who are overweight or obese?	1.7 (1.4)	1.4 (1.4)
How often do you use each of the following with patients who are overweight or obese?		
Next Steps poster	1.4 (1.3)	0.9 (1.2)
Next Steps flip chart	1.7 (1.4)	1.2 (1.4)
Next Steps activity books for home	0.9 (1.1)	0.6 (1.2)
List of community resources that support a healthy lifestyle	1.8 (1.3)	1.9 (1.7)
Mean score (SD) of the adoption items at clinic provider level	1.5 (1.0)	1.2 (1.1)
Appropriateness, mean (SD)		
When I talk with patients and families about obesity, the *Next Steps*		
Materials overall helps me be more effective	2.8 (0.9)	2.8 (1.1)
Poster helps me be more effective	2.3 (0.9)	2.4 (1.0)
Flip chart helps me be more effective	2.7 (1.0)	2.6 (1.1)
Patient activity book helps me be more effective	2.2 (1.0)	2.2 (0.9)
Materials fits into my patient/office flow	2.3 (1.0)	2.2 (1.1)
Mean score (SD) of the appropriateness items at clinic provider level	2.4 (0.7)	2.4 (0.9)
Appropriateness, mean (SD)		
Applicability of the themed visits, n (%)		
Category A: Setting the foundation		
Understanding health (set a foundation for good health) was applicable	17 (56.7)	22 (64.7)
Category B: Introduce concepts that are important to cover early for success		
Understanding healthy food was applicable	20 (66.7)	24 (70.6)
Home environment was applicable	17 (56.7)	20 (58.8)
Eating and your emotions was applicable	16 (53.3)	23 (67.7)
Portion sizes was applicable	20 (66.7)	25 (73.5)
Healthy drinks was applicable	21 (70.0)	24 (70.6)
Category C: Focus on other important concepts		
Physical activity was applicable	18 (60.0)	23 (67.7)
Feeling good about yourself was applicable	15 (50.0)	20 (58.8)

Table 2 Descriptive statistics of individual items included in the primary care clinic implementation index by year of implementation in the TX CORD study, 2013–2014 *(Continued)*

	Year 1 of implementation (2013)	Year 2 of implementation (2014)
Reading food labels was applicable	16 (53.3)	21 (61.8)
Screen time and sleep was applicable	20 (66.7)	24 (70.6)
Meal patterns and snacks was applicable	18 (60.0)	24 (70.6)
Holidays/Special occasions was applicable	14 (46.7)	23 (67.7)
Eating away from home was applicable	17 (56.7)	22 (64.7)
Parenting was applicable	17 (56.7)	18 (52.9)
Community partners was applicable	10 (33.3)	21 (61.8)
Healthy family was applicable	17 (56.7)	22 (64.7)
Bullying and teasing was applicable	14 (46.7)	19 (55.9)
Goal setting was applicable	18 (60.0)	21 (61.8)
Unintentional disruptions was applicable	10 (33.3)	17 (50.0)
Mean score (SD) of the appropriateness items at clinic provider level	0.7 (0.4)	0.7 (0.4)
Feasibility, mean (SD)		
Access to the following materials provided by the CORD team, n (%)		
Next Steps poster was accessible	25 (83.3)	26 (76.5)
Next Steps flip chart was accessible	25 (83.3)	28 (82.4)
Next Steps activity books for home was accessible	23 (76.7)	20 (58.8)
List of community resources that support a healthy lifestyle was accessible	24 (80.0)	24 (70.6)
Mean score (SD) of the feasibility items at clinic provider level	0.9 (0.3)	0.7 (0.3)

SD Standard deviation, *TX CORD* Texas Childhood Obesity Research Demonstration
Acceptability scale: Strongly disagree (0), disagree (1), neither agree nor disagree (2), agree (3), and strongly agree (4)
Adoption scale: Less than 10% (0), 10–25% (1), 25–50% (2), 50–75% (3), and 75–100% (4)
Appropriateness scale measuring the effectiveness of *Next Steps* materials: Strongly disagree (0), disagree (1), neither agree nor disagree (2), agree (3), and strongly agree (4)
Appropriateness scale measuring the acceptability of themed visits: Keep as is/Rest of the groups
Feasibility Scale: Yes/No

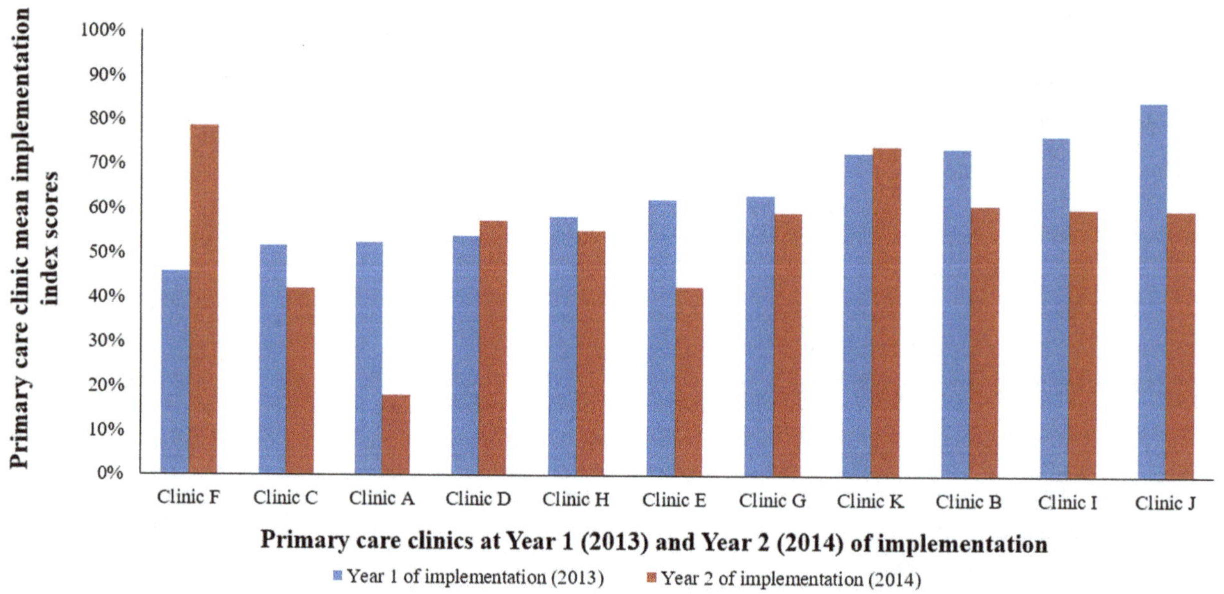

Fig. 1 Primary care clinic implementation index scores (constructs included acceptability, adoption, appropriateness, and feasibility), by year of implementation, TX CORD study

Table 3 Total number of children with overweight and obesity seen, referred, and enrolled into TX CORD secondary prevention study, 2013–2014

Clinics	Children with overweight and obesity seen ($n = 6198$)	Referred ($n = 1957$)	Enrolled ($n = 533$)	% referred (out of total seen)	% enrolled (out of total seen)	% enrolled (out of total referred)
Clinic I	1364	116	26	8.5%	1.9%	22.4%
Clinic C	436	82	15	18.8%	3.4%	18.3%
Clinic J	263	56	27	21.3%	10.3%	48.2%
Clinic D	677	171	61	25.3%	9.0%	35.7%
Clinic B	91	28	14	30.8%	15.4%	50.0%
Clinic F	540	194	34	35.9%	6.3%	17.5%
Clinic H	712	272	62	38.2%	8.7%	22.8%
Clinic K	716	293	77	40.9%	10.8%	26.3%
Clinic E	513	254	91	49.5%	17.7%	35.8%
Clinic G	684	356	74	52.0%	10.8%	20.8%
Clinic A	202	135	52	66.8%	25.7%	38.5%

TX CORD Texas Childhood Obesity Research Demonstration

influence these populations and their access to healthcare, implementing the *Next Steps* program 60% of the time in eight out of 11 clinics indicates the initial feasibility of the program in disadvantaged settings. Implementation scores were lower in Year 2 than Year 1, though not statistically significant. The providers received formal training in the *Next Steps* materials in 2012 when the primary care clinics were first recruited into TX CORD primary prevention study. During the Year 1 assessment of implementation, the research team was actively encouraging the providers to use the *Next Steps* tools with any potential patients that might benefit from them, as well as the recruiting tools for the TX CORD secondary prevention study. The second process evaluation data collection occurred 9–10 months after participant recruitment into TX CORD secondary prevention study had ended, when the research team was less visible in the clinics. Furthermore, 13.5% of the providers were in the primary care clinics for < 1 year in Year 2, and the new providers in Year 2 may not have been familiar with the material and study. These, along with the cross-sectional nature of the study and the perception of the TX CORD project as a study and not necessarily a program, might explain the decrease in the implementation of *Next Steps* materials between Year 1 and Year 2, and the inverse relationship observed between feasibility and enrollment in Year 2. Our results suggest the need for ways to increase engagement of providers such as repeat training of providers to increase the sustainability of *Next Steps* in primary care clinics [22].

There were no significant associations between levels of implementation of *Next Steps* and enrollment into TX CORD secondary prevention study. The potential effect of implementation of weight management materials on referral and enrollment of children into weight management programs is uncertain from this study as some of the largest clinics had a high implementation but low referral and enrollment, while the reverse was true in the

Table 4 Odds of enrollment of children with overweight and obesity into TX CORD secondary prevention study by primary care clinic implementation index levels and by underlying constructs, 2013–2014

	Enrollment Year 1 (2013) OR (95% CI)	Enrollment Year 2 (2014) OR (95% CI)
Implementation index (reference: relatively low implementation)		
Medium implementation	1.32 (0.71–2.47)	0.96 (0.53–1.76)
Relatively high implementation	1.62 (0.71–3.72)	0.61 (0.29–1.29)
Underlying constructs		
Acceptability	1.04 (1.00–1.08)	1.00 (0.98–1.02)
Adoption	1.01 (1.00–1.02)	0.99 (0.97–1.00)
Appropriateness	1.01 (0.99–1.03)	1.00 (0.98–1.01)
Feasibility	1.00 (0.99–1.02)	0.99 (0.98–0.99)

CI Confidence interval, *OR* Odds ratio, *TX CORD* Texas Childhood Obesity Research Demonstration

small clinics (Table 3). The small number of clinics in this study limits the generalizability of the study, and the wide variation in percent of patients referred and enrolled in the TX CORD secondary prevention study, even within implementation level categories, delineates the need for future studies to understand the barriers and enablers to referral and enrollment to a weight management program both from provider and patient perspective [23]. For example, studies [24, 25] have reported that some of the provider-level barriers were lack of actual or perceived skill to discuss weight issues with patients and families and being ill-informed about existing services. At the patient-level [25–27], barriers included parents not perceiving the need for such programs for their children, parents not initiating the provider's recommended care, lack of motivation from both parent and children, personal health problems, and logistics (e.g., scheduling issues, weather, transportation). Furthermore, referral to the program may be an inadequate outcome measure of implementation; the PCPs may have been using the weight management materials without referral of the children to the program. A more appropriate indicator of the use of *Next Steps* could be an improvement in BMI rather than enrollment into TX CORD secondary prevention. Because the TX CORD secondary prevention study was an experimental study that compared two weight management programs where *Next Steps* was the comparison group, we limited our outcome to an immediate one, enrollment of children with overweight and obesity into a weight management program.

There were certain limitations to our study. The study design was serial cross-sectional, thus, the implementation index scores at Year 1 came from a somewhat different cohort than in Year 2. Surveys with < 80% completion were excluded from the analysis ($n = 5$). This might introduce selection bias to the study findings if the non-responses were due to non-adherence with the *Next Steps* program. The process measures were self-reported, thus subject to recall or social desirability bias. Additional objective measures such as direct observations may provide a deeper insight into implementation fidelity of programs, and comparison of implementation of programs from different perspectives. The process measures were reported by the PCPs, so future studies could also assess the implementation of these measures by other clinicians such as dietitians or health educators. Only 11 primary care clinics participated in the study, providing limited extrapolation of study findings to other weight management primary care clinics. The TX CORD study was the first to pilot test *Next Steps* as a weight management program in primary care clinics, and there were no comparison clinics. Future studies should evaluate and validate the implementation of the *Next Steps* program in healthcare settings in a more rigorous design.

Despite these limitations, our study had strengths. This is the first study to develop a simple methodology for assessing implementation of weight management programs in healthcare settings. Survey scales had good internal consistencies at both years of implementation. Additionally, the implementation levels at the different primary care clinics demonstrated face validity. The *Next Steps* program materials were available in Spanish, thus, tailored towards the target population (predominantly, Hispanic/Latino). Finally, the homogeneity of the targeted population (2–12-year-old children from low-income underserved areas in Houston and Austin, Texas) also reflected a fair comparison of implementation of *Next Steps* program materials across the different primary care clinics.

Conclusions

The results of our study highlight the importance of process evaluation and sustainability in primary care settings that are part of intervention programs. The implementation index scores created in this study provide an opportunity to assess how effective and comfortable the providers are at using the different weight-management tools in such settings. Using a standardized scoring procedure, we observed there was wide variability in the implementation levels across the primary care clinics that help to identify the best practices, barriers, and the need for modification of weight management tools tailored towards specific primary care clinics.

In conclusion, our study demonstrated an application of a novel implementation assessment technique to weight-management materials in primary care clinics in the TX CORD study.

Abbreviations

AAP: American Academy of Pediatrics; BMI: Body Mass Index; CHIP: Children's Health Insurance Program; EHR: Electronic Health Record; PCP: Primary Care Providers; SD: Standard Deviation; TX CORD: Texas Childhood Research Demonstration; UTHealth: University of Texas Health Science Center at Houston

Acknowledgements

Not applicable.

Funding

This research was supported by cooperative agreement RFA-DP-11-007 from the CDC. The content is solely the responsibility of the authors and does not necessarily represent the official views of the CDC. Additional support was provided by the Michael and Susan Dell Foundation through the Michael & Susan Dell Center for Healthy Living. This work is a publication of the USDA (USDA/ARS) Children's Nutrition Research Center, Department of Pediatrics, Baylor College of Medicine, Houston, Texas, and had been funded, in part, with federal funds from the USDA/ARS under Cooperative Agreement No. 58-6250-0-008. The contents of this publication do not necessarily reflect the views or policies of the USDA, nor does mention of trade names, commercial products, or organizations imply endorsement from the U.S. government.

Authors' contributions
MS contributed substantially to the conception, design, analysis, and interpretation of the data with critical guidance from the SEB, SJP, NFB, and DMH. All the authors (MS, SEB, SJP, NFB, and DMH) have revised the manuscript critically for intellectual content. All authors (MS, SEB, SJP, NFB, and DMH) have seen and approved the final content, and agreed to be accountable for all aspects of the work.

Consent for publication
Not applicable.

Competing interests
The authors declare that they have no competing interests.

Author details
[1]Michael & Susan Dell Center for Healthy Living, University of Texas Health Science Center at Houston (UTHealth) School of Public Health in Austin, Austin, TX, USA. [2]University of Texas Health Science Center at Tyler, Tyler, TX, USA. [3]Population Health, Office of Health Affairs, University of Texas System, Austin, TX, USA. [4]Texas Children's Hospital, Baylor College of Medicine, Houston, TX, USA. [5]UT Southwestern Medical Center, Dallas, TX, USA. [6]Texas Center for the Prevention and Treatment of Childhood Obesity, Dell Children's Medical Center, University of Texas at Austin Dell Medical School, Houston, TX, USA. [7]USDA/ARS Children's Nutrition Research Center; Department of Pediatrics, Baylor College of Medicine, Houston, TX, USA.

References
1. Barriuso L, Miqueleiz E, Albaladejo R, Villanueva R, Santos JM, Regidor E. Socioeconomic position and childhood-adolescent weight status in rich countries: a systematic review, 1990–2013. BMC Pediatr. 2015;15(1):1–15. https://doi.org/10.1186/s12887-015-0443-3.
2. Ogden CL, Carroll MD, Lawman HG, et al. Trends in obesity prevalence among children and adolescents in the United States, 1988-1994 through 2013-2014. JAMA. 2016;315(21):2292–9. https://doi.org/10.1001/jama.2016.6361.
3. Bass R, Eneli I. Severe childhood obesity: an under-recognised and growing health problem. Postgrad Med J. 2015;91(1081):639–45. https://doi.org/10.1136/postgradmedj-2014-133033.
4. Finkelstein EA, Khavjou OA, Thompson H, et al. Obesity and severe obesity forecasts through 2030. Am J Prev Med. 2012;42(6):563–70 https://doi.org/10.1016/j.amepre.2011.10.026.
5. Huang TTK, Borowski LA, Liu B, et al. Pediatricians' and family Physicians' weight-related Care of Children in the U.S. Am J Prev Med. 2011;41(1):24–32 https://doi.org/10.1016/j.amepre.2011.03.016.
6. Barlow SE, Bobra SR, Elliott MB, Brownson RC, Haire-Joshu D. Recognition of childhood overweight during health supervision visits: does BMI help pediatricians? Obesity. 2007;15(1):225. https://doi.org/10.1038/oby.2007.535.
7. Rabin BA, Brownson RC, Haire-Joshu D, Kreuter MW, Weaver NL. A glossary for dissemination and implementation research in health. Journal of public health management and practice : JPHMP. 2008;14(2):117–23. https://doi.org/10.1097/01.PHH.0000311888.06252.bb.
8. Oud[illegible] et al. Cochrane review: interventions for treating obesity in children. Evidence-Based Child Health: A Cochrane Review Journal. 2009;4(4):1571–729. https://doi.org/10.1002/ebch.462.
9. Profit J, Typpo KV, Hysong SJ, Woodard LD, Kallen MA, Petersen LA. Improving benchmarking by using an explicit framework for the development of composite indicators: an example using pediatric quality of care. Implement Sci. 2010;5(1):13. https://doi.org/10.1186/1748-5908-5-13.
10. National Initiative for Children's Health Care Quality. Next Steps: A Practitioner's Guide For Themed Follow-up Visits For Their Patients to Achieve a Healthy Weight. American Academy of Pediatrics Elk Grove Village, IL. 2013. https://shop.aap.org/next-steps-a-practitioners-guide-for-themed-follow-up-visits-for-their-patients-to-achieve-a-heal/. Accessed March 8 2017.
11. Barlow SE, Butte NF, Hoelscher DM, Salahuddin M, Pont SJ. Strategies to recruit a diverse low-income population to child weight management programs from primary care practices. Prev Chronic Dis. 2017;14:170301. https://doi.org/10.5888/pcd14.170301.
12. Hoelscher DM, Butte NF, Barlow SE, et al. Incorporating primary and secondary prevention approaches to address childhood obesity prevention and treatment in a low-income, ethnically diverse population: study design and demographic data from the Texas childhood obesity research demonstration (TX CORD) study. Childhood Obesity. 2015;11(1):71–91.
13. Oluyomi AO, Byars A, Byrd-Williams C, et al. The utility of geographical information systems (GIS) in systems-oriented obesity intervention projects: the selection of comparable study sites for a quasi-experimental intervention design—TX CORD. Childhood Obesity. 2015;11(1):58–70. https://doi.org/10.1089/chi.2014.0054.
14. Taveras EM, Marshall R, Horan CM, et al. Improving children's obesity-related health care quality: process outcomes of a cluster-randomized controlled trial. Obesity (Silver Spring). 2014;22(1):27–31. https://doi.org/10.1002/oby.20612.
15. Proctor E, Silmere H, Raghavan R, et al. Outcomes for implementation research: conceptual distinctions, measurement challenges, and research agenda. Adm Policy Ment Health Ment Health Serv Res. 2011;38(2):65–76. https://doi.org/10.1007/s10488-010-0319-7.
16. Rogers EM. Diffusion of innovations. 4th ed. New York: The Free Press; 1995.
17. Glasgow RE. Translating Research to Practice. Lessons learned, areas for improvement, and future directions. 2003;26(8):2451–2456. https://doi.org/10.2337/diacare.26.8.2451.
18. Glasgow RE, Vogt TM, Boles SM. Evaluating the public health impact of health promotion interventions: the RE-AIM framework. Am J Public Health. 1999;89(9):1322–7. https://doi.org/10.2105/ajph.89.9.1322.
19. Estabrooks PA, Wilson KE, McGuire TJ, et al. A quasi-experiment to assess the impact of a scalable, community-based weight loss program: combining reach, effectiveness, and cost. J Gen Intern Med. 2017;32(1):24–31. https://doi.org/10.1007/s11606-016-3971-0.
20. Johnson SE. Pragmatic implementation trials: understanding the integrated research-practice partnership approach to lifestyle obesity management across a transforming health system: Virginia Tech; 2016.
21. Parcel GS, Perry CL, Kelder SH, et al. School climate and the institutionalization of the CATCH program. Health Educ Behav. 2003;30(4):489–502.
22. Chambers D, Simpson L, Neta G, et al. Proceedings from the 9th annual conference on the science of dissemination and implementation. Implement Sci. 2017;12(1):48. https://doi.org/10.1186/s13012-017-0575-y.
23. Perez AJ, Ball GDC. Helping children and families to enrol in weight management: what can stakeholders do? Paediatr Child Health 2018: pxy056-pxy. doi:https://doi.org/10.1093/pch/pxy056
24. Perez AJ, Kebbe M, Holt NL, et al. Parent recommendations to enhance enrollment in multidisciplinary clinical Care for Pediatric Weight Management. J Pediatr. 2018;192:122–9. https://doi.org/10.1016/j.jpeds.2017.09.025.
25. Perez A, Holt N, Gokiert R, et al. Why don't families initiate treatment? A qualitative multicentre study investigating parents' reasons for declining paediatric weight management. Paediatr Child Health. 2015;20(4):179–84.
26. Barlow SE, Ohlemeyer CL. Parent reasons for nonreturn to a pediatric weight management program. Clin Pediatr. 2006;45(4):355–60. https://doi.org/10.1177/000992280604500408.
27. Perez AJ, Avis JL, Holt NL, et al. Why do families enrol in paediatric weight management? A parental perspective of reasons and facilitators. Child Care Health Dev. 2016;42(2):278–87. https://doi.org/10.1111/cch.12311.

16

Does patient self-management education of primary care professionals improve patient outcomes

Andree Rochfort[1], Sinead Beirne[1], Gillian Doran[1], Patricia Patton[1], Jochen Gensichen[2], Ilkka Kunnamo[3], Susan Smith[4], Tina Eriksson[5] and Claire Collins[1*]

Abstract

Background: Patient self-management support is recognised as a key component of chronic care. Education and training for health professionals has been shown in the literature to be associated with better uptake, implementation and effectiveness of self-management programs, however, there is no clear evidence regarding whether this training results in improved health outcomes for patients with chronic conditions.

Methods: A systematic review was undertaken using the PRISMA guidelines using the Cochrane Library, PubMEd, ERIC, EMBASE, CINAHL, PsycINFO, Web searches, Hand searches and Bibliographies. Articles published from inception to September 1st, 2013 were included. Systematic reviews, Meta-analysis, Randomized controlled trials (RCTs), Controlled clinical trials, Interrupted time series and Controlled before and after studies, which reported on primary care health professionals' continuing education or evidence-based medicine/education on patient self-management for any chronic condition, were included. A minimum of two reviewers participated independently at each stage of review.

Results: From 7533 abstracts found, only two papers provided evidence on the effectiveness of self-management education for primary healthcare professionals in terms of measured outcomes in patients. These two articles show improvement in patient outcomes for chronic back pain and diabetes based on RCTs. The educational interventions with health professionals spanned a range of techniques and modalities but both RCTs included a motivational interviewing component.

Conclusions: Before and up to 2 years after the incorporation of patient empowerment for self-management into the WONCA Europe definition of general practice, there was a scarcity of high quality evidence showing improved outcomes for patients as a result of educating health professionals in patient self-management of chronic conditions.

Keywords: Self-management, Patient empowerment, Primary care, Chronic conditions

Key messages

Despite a vast literature on the topic of patient self-management, evidence on the association between training of health professionals in patient self-management with measured patient health outcomes was rare prior to and up to 2 years after its incorporation into the WONCA Europe definition of general practice.

However, the limited available evidence suggests that specific training programmes for primary care health professionals (a) may improve and support patient competencies for self-management and (b) may improve quality of life for patients with chronic conditions.

Background

The European Definition of General Practice by the World Organization of National Colleges, Academies and Academic Associations of General Practitioners/Family Physicians (WONCA) in the European Region, lists 12 characteristics within six core competencies to define the activities of general practice / family medicine (GP/FM) [1]. The twelfth characteristic of general practice *"Promotion of patient empowerment and self-management"* was officially approved in 2011 [1]. It follows therefore, that

* Correspondence: claire.collins@icgp.ie
[1]Irish College of General Practitioners, 4-5 Lincoln Place, Dublin 2, Ireland
Full list of author information is available at the end of the article

European family physicians agree that among the various disciplines of medicine, GP/FM has a key role in harnessing patient autonomy to develop their expertise in managing their own health and wellness [2].

Promoting patient self-management (PSM) in the European definition of General Practice is listed under the core competency of "Patient-centered care", in keeping with scientific evidence on patient empowerment within general practice [3]. The concept of patient empowerment for patient self-management in chronic conditions has been further explored by the European Society for Quality and Safety in General Practice (EQuiP) [4].

The World Health Organisation (WHO) defines chronic conditions as those that encompass disability and disease that people 'live with' for extended periods of time [5]. They include non-communicable diseases (NCD), such as cardiovascular diseases, cancers, respiratory diseases and diabetes, and are associated with lifestyle factors and patient behaviours and account for 70% of deaths globally (40 million deaths) in 2017 [6]. By 2030, the total annual number of NCD deaths is projected to increase to 52 million per year [6]. This escalation of the prevalence of chronic conditions is a significant factor in the increasingly heavy workload in family medicine internationally, which is also increasing in complexity as people live longer often with multiple co-existing chronic conditions.

By definition, chronic disease is not reversible or curable [6]. The Chronic Care Model (CCM) [7] is an internationally accepted model for the management of NCD and specifies self-management support as a key component. Patient self-management can be described as *"a set of tasks and processes that are used by a patient to maintain wellness in the presence of an ongoing illness* [8] *and it may also encompass prevention..."* [9]. In addition to knowledge of the disease and treatment options, patient self-management *"involves active involvement in decision making, coping with signs and symptoms of disease, making lifestyle changes and managing the impact of the disease on life"* [10].

The benefits of supporting patients to implement and maintain self-management skills have been shown to improve patients' self-care and more appropriate utilisation of health services [11–13]. Improved patient self-management can also reduce health care costs through fewer outpatient visits [14–17] and fewer hospital admissions [18–20]. Lifestyle interventions by patients have been shown to have clinical benefit in a wide range of conditions such as diabetes, coronary heart disease, heart failure, and rheumatoid arthritis [21].

In the Chronic Care Model, achieving optimum outcomes for patients requires a productive interaction between "an informed activated patient and a prepared proactive practice team" [22]. Many studies focus on the role of *patient education* in self-management, yet no systematic reviews are published on whether *clinician education* to improve patient self-management has an effect on patient outcomes. A preliminary literature review [23] indicated that effective patient self-management support would require specific training of primary care health professionals. Education and training have been identified as a potential way of engaging primary care clinicians in patient self-management support [24]. However, though existing studies suggest that health professional training is associated with better uptake and implementation of patient self-management programs [9, 14, 25, 26], it is not clear which type of professional training this might involve, or whether it actually improved patient outcomes.

The primary aim of this systematic review was to examine the effectiveness of educational interventions for primary care professionals that are designed to improve their support for patient self-management of chronic conditions and improve patient outcomes. The timeframe was specifically chosen in order to establish if this evidence was available prior to and up to 2 years after the concept of patient empowerment for self-management was introduced into the WONCA Europe definition of general practice. Furthermore, this systematic review was used to inform the subsequent project work packages, which included the creation of an online educational module and its evaluation.

Methods

A systematic review was undertaken using the PRISMA guidelines [27] and follows the methodology outlined in the PROSPERO registered protocol (Database registration number: CRD42013004418) [28].

Sourcing information

Two specialist subject librarians assisted in the development of the search strategy designed to identify internationally recognised terminology in peer-reviewed journals. Full details of this strategy are available in the published protocol [28]. Six databases were searched - Cochrane Library, PubMed, ERIC, EMBASE, CINAHL and PsycINFO - in addition to Web searches, Hand searches and Bibliographies. Articles published in advance of September 1st, 2013 were included in the review, with the search conducted by GD and PP. The full search terms and sample search are shown in 'Additional file 1'. The timeframe was deliberately chosen in order to coincide with the inclusion of the concept of patient empowerment in WONCA Europe's definition of general practice. It was also the first work package of a larger project. It is intended to repeat the systematic review in 2018.

Selection criteria

Studies with the following designs were included: systematic reviews, randomized controlled trials (RCTs), controlled clinical trials, interrupted time series, and controlled before and after studies.

Participants were physicians in primary care settings, other clinicians in primary care settings and patients 18 + years with chronic conditions in primary care settings. Included interventions had an educational focus designed to train primary care clinicians to support patient self-management. This review was concerned with all chronic conditions as they occur generically in the primary care setting, rather than focusing on any one specific chronic condition. Only articles including reference to patient outcomes, measured using validated measurement scales, were included. The primary patient outcome was change in patients' self-management behaviours; the secondary outcomes were changes in physical health measures, health behaviours including medical adherence and compliance, service utilisation, psychological health, psycho-social function (e.g. Quality of Life, SF36, SF12) physical functioning and knowledge.

The eligibility of studies was determined using the inclusion and exclusion criteria listed in the registered proposal and shown in Table 1.

Data extraction

All abstracts were reviewed using the RefWorks package to categorise the abstracts identified by the search. The initial review of abstracts was undertaken by SB with 10% of same re-checked by AR. The full text articles of all those considered to be of possible relevance to the systematic review were read independently by SB, JG and CC and categorised using the same exclusion reasons. Disagreements were reviewed by AR. The final list of full text articles were then reviewed by JG to confirm relevance. The quality assessment and extraction of thematic content of the final list of articles applicable to the systematic review question were considered by CC and AR.

Quality assessment

We assessed risk of bias and overall quality of individual studies using the Quality of Assessment Tool for Quantitative Studies [29] (Tables 2, 3 and 4). For each study, reviewers rated six components (selection bias, study design, confounders, blinding, data collection methods, and withdrawals and dropouts) leading to an overall methodological quality rating for each study of strong, moderate, or weak, with strong quality indicating a low risk of bias. Reviewers resolved rating disagreements through discussion.

Data synthesis

We performed a narrative data synthesis as the clinical heterogeneity and differences in outcomes in the two studies meant meta-analysis would have been inappropriate.

Results

Study review and selection

Overall 7533 abstracts were reviewed following removal of duplicates from the database and hand/web searches; of these, 43 full text articles were retrieved and read

Table 1 Inclusion and exclusion criteria

Inclusion Criteria	Exclusion Criteria	Exclusion code
English papers	Non- English papers	Eng
Adults (18+)	Study population < 18	Age
Primary Care/Community	Secondary Care/Hospital	Not PC
Chronic conditions, chronic illness, chronic disease, non-communicable disease (NCD)	Acute conditions	Acute
Study Type- Systematic reviews, meta- analysis, RCTs, controlled clinical trials, interrupted time series. Controlled before and after studies	Study Type- Qualitative studies, populations studies, surveys, cross sectional, uncontrolled before and after studies (cohort)	Study
Education and training of primary care Health Professionals for patient education in promoting change, behaviour change, lifestyle change, patient engagement, patient empowerment, motivational skills, patient collaboration, patient adherence and compliance, Patient self-management, decision making, patient problem- solving	Not education/training of health care professionals	Int
	Not primary care health professionals	Pop
	Primary outcome measures not included	Out
	Direct patient education only	Edu
Continuing education / CME / Lifelong learning / Evidence based medicine	Guideline adherence, clinical performance	Guid
All studies published to September 2013	Organisational interventions	Org
	Financial changes and incentives	Fi
	Regulatory interventions	Reg

Table 2 Risk of bias

Bias	Becker et al. [30]	Rubak et al. [31]
Random sequence generation (selection bias)	Low - Selection by central permuted block randomisation	Low - Selection by drawing lots
Allocation Concealment (selection bias)	Low	Unclear-Insufficient information provided
Blinding of participants and personnel (performance bias)	High – Blinding of participants and personnel was not possible	High – Blinding of participants and personnel was not possible
Blinding of outcome assessment (detection bias)	High – Self-reported outcomes	High – Self-reported outcomes
Incomplete outcome data (attrition bias)	Low – Clear participant flow reported	Low – Clear participant flow reported
Selective reporting (reporting bias)	Low – The published report includes all expected outcomes	Low – The published report includes all expected outcomes
Other bias	Unclear – but unlikely. Insufficient information to assess whether another important risk of bias exists	Unclear – but possible; no baseline data. Insufficient information to assess whether another important risk of bias exists

(Fig. 1). Following this second stage review, only two articles that reported patient outcomes were included in the systematic review.

The two papers were both RCTs of educational interventions in primary care health professionals and examined their impact on patient outcome measures (Table 5).

The primary outcome of this review is the effectiveness of educational interventions in terms of patient outcomes. Our results show that education and skills training of primary care health professionals may improve patient performance of self-management activities, improve patient lifestyle behaviours, and patient self-efficacy in making behaviour changes. These changes were associated with improved perception of quality of life.

Becker et al. [30] compared outcomes of three groups of patients with low back pain from one control group of several practices and two intervention groups. The control group comprised of 43 practices with 410 patients and received printed educational information alone. One intervention group received education on guideline implementation (GI) alone (37 practices, 479 patients) and the other intervention group received GI plus training in motivational interviewing techniques (MIT) (38 practices, 70 practice nurses, 489 patients). Both intervention group patients showed significant improvements in functional capacity at six months though there was no difference at 12 months. Patients of the clinicians in the motivational interviewing group showed significant improvement in functional capacity after six months with a greater number of patients reporting pain free days (less permanent pain) after six months and after 12 months. These same patients also demonstrated a significant improvement in quality of life scale, having received one session from a practice nurse trained in motivational interviewing. The control group demonstrated no improvement in functional capacity, no perceived improvement in quality of life and they reported greater levels of permanent pain compared to both intervention groups.

Rubak et al. [31] included 65 GPs from 48 practices and all GPs attended a half day course on intensive treatment of type-2 diabetes. Practices were then randomised into control and intervention groups and the intervention group had an additional one and a half day residential course for 29 GPs from 21 practices (137 patients) on motivational interviewing techniques. The intervention practices also had a half day follow up course on MIT, twice during the following one year. The patients of the intervention group clinicians were shown to be more motivated to change behaviours and significantly more autonomous in their choice of actions leading to behavioural changes than patients of the control clinicians. The patients of the intervention clinicians also reported having received significantly more specific advice from their GP regarding diet, exercise and self-control of diabetes, and they also reported receiving significantly more counselling re smoking cessation. Intervention group patients reported an increase in their awareness of the importance of taking control of their own specific risk factors for diabetes. This study also reported a significant improvement in self-efficacy between pre-training and post training for all primary care health professionals undergoing motivational interviewing training.

Discussion

Main findings

The key finding of this systematic review is the scarcity of studies that assess the impact on patient outcomes of training primary care clinicians in patient self-management of chronic conditions. This was surprising given that patient

Table 3 Quality assessment using EPHPP tool

Component	Becker et al. [30]	Rubak et al. [31]
Selection Bias 1. Are the individuals selected to participate likely to be representative of the target populations?	Can't tell = 4	Can't tell = 4
Selection Bias 2. What percentage of the selected individuals agreed to participate?	Less than 60% agreement = 3	Can't tell = 5
SELECTION BIAS RATING	WEAK	WEAK
Study design	Randomized control trial = 1	Randomized control trial = 1
Was the study described as randomized?	Yes	Yes
Was the method of randomization described?	Yes	Yes
Was the randomization process appropriate?	Yes	Yes
Study design rating	Strong	Strong
Were there important differences between groups prior to the intervention?	No = 2	No = 2
What percentage of relevant confounders were controlled?	N/A	N/A
Confounders rating	Strong	Strong
Were the outcome assessors aware of the intervention status of participants?	Can't tell = 3	Can't tell = 3
Were the participants aware of the research question?	No = 2	No = 2
Blinding rating	Moderate	Moderate
Were data collection tools shown to be valid?	Yes = 1	Yes = 1
Were data collections tools shown to be reliable?	Yes = 1	Yes = 1
Data collection rating	Strong	Strong
Were withdrawals and drop-outs reported in terms of numbers/reasons?	Yes = 1	Yes = 1
Percentage of participants completing the study	80 = − 100% = 1	80 = −100% = 1
Withdrawals and drop outs rating	Strong	Strong
Intervention Integrity: What percentage of participants received the allocated intervention?	80 = −100% = 1	80 = − 100% = 1
Was the consistency of the intervention measured	Can't tell = 3	Can't tell = 3
Is it likely that subjects received an unintended intervention that may influence results?	No = 5	No = 5
Analyses: Unit of allocation	Practice	Practice
Unit of analysis	Individual	Individual
Are the statistical methods appropriate for the study design?	Yes = 1	Yes = 1
Is the analysis performed by intervention allocation status (ITT) rather than actual intervention received?	Yes = 1	Yes = 1

Table 4 Summary of Global rating for Quality using EPHPP Quality Assessment tool

Component	Becker et al. [30]	Rubak et al. [31]
Selection Bias	Weak	Weak
Study Design	Strong	Strong
Confounders	Strong	Strong
Blinding	Moderate	Moderate
Data Collection Methods	Strong	Strong
Withdrawals and Dropouts	Strong	Strong
Global rating	Moderate	Moderate

Criteria for global rating; 1. Strong = no weak ratings 2. Moderate = one weak rating, 3. Weak = two or more weak ratings

self-management is a core element of person-centered healthcare in family practice and given the volume of published material on patient self-management.

This review shows that when health professionals undergo training in empowering patients for self-management of chronic conditions, it is possible to achieve improvement in patients' self-efficacy, autonomy and motivation to change, functional capacity, pain free days and quality of life.

One study [30] demonstrated improvement in functional capacity, quality of life scale and a greater number of pain free days reported by patients after six months and after 12 months among those whose primary care

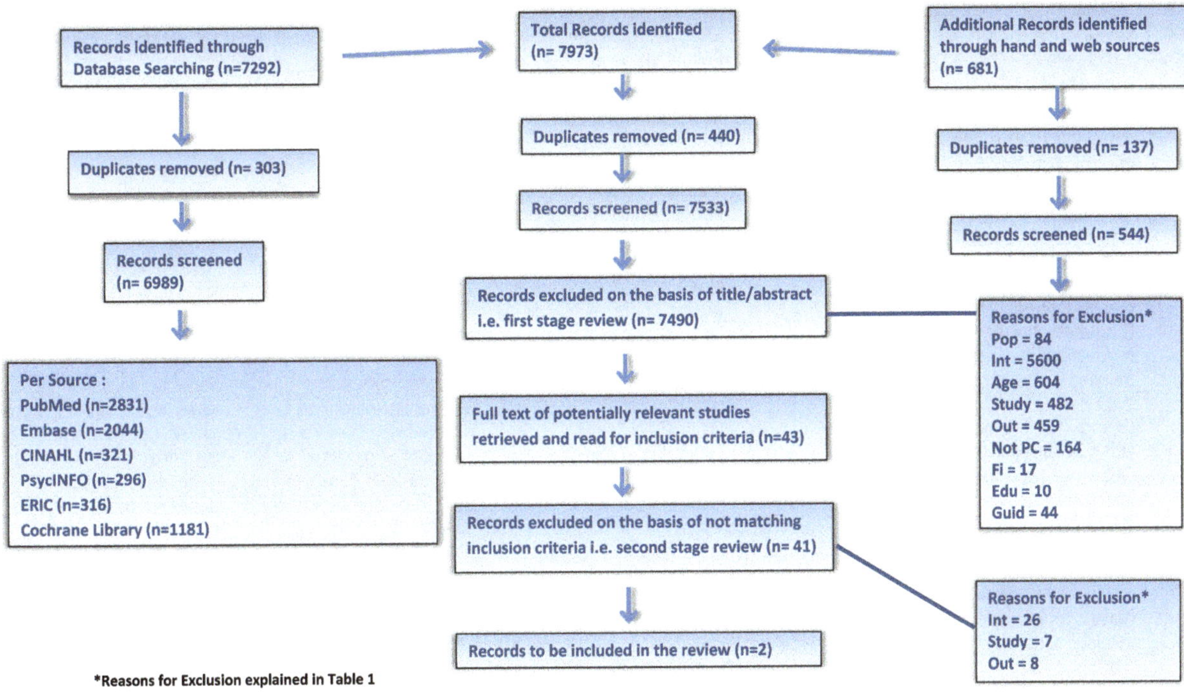

Fig. 1 Summary of Systematic Review Process

clinicians had been given training in motivational interviewing techniques. A second study [31] showed that patients of the health professionals who participated in specific training programmes were more motivated to change behaviours and were more autonomous in their choice of behavioural changes compared to a control group. These patients were significantly more aware of the importance of controlling their diabetes for specific factors, and had a higher level of perception of having received specific advice from their GP on healthy behaviour changes.

Limitations of the review

Despite much literature on patient self-management in chronic disease, focussing on whether training health professionals regarding patient self-management improves patient outcomes, resulted in only two articles being eligible for inclusion in this systematic review. We are aware that some additional studies have been published more recently on self-management that were outside the chosen search period of this review. We plan to update this review in 2018. However, we feel it is important to publish the findings of this first phase review to highlight that, despite a vast volume of literature on one topic, evidence of impact on patient outcomes is largely lacking during the study period despite the publicity and interest in patient empowerment for self-management in the years leading up to its official inclusion in the European definition in 2011.

The small number of studies included and the range of outcome measures therein made concrete conclusions impossible, both papers describe positive outcomes from teaching motivational interviewing skills to clinicians, but we do not yet know if other approaches would be equally or more effective. The two studies did not report effect sizes, further complicating the interpretation of results. A further limitation is that only articles in English were included, based on available resources.

A total of 1643 patients, 191 clinicians and 164 practices were involved in these studies in two European countries, however further research on this topic is also needed to clarify if other factors are effective in improving patient outcomes other than those involving time constrained clinicians in general practice.

Interpretation of findings in the context of existing evidence

This review has given us concrete evidence of the lack of studies in the English language on improving patient outcomes through training primary care clinicians in patient self-management. Previous studies focus on patient education, group discussion among patients, shared experiences and unstructured acquisition of knowledge during clinical encounters or through leaflets and brochures [16, 25, 32, 33] rather than on assessing the specific effect of specific clinician training on patient outcomes in this setting. Primary care professionals have a longitudinal relationship with patients in the patient's

Table 5 Study Description

Author Country Year	Design/Intervention	Analysis (unit of analysis/power calculation)	Objective measurement/ Follow-up period	Successful Educational Aspects	Limitations
Becker et al. Germany 2008 [30]	Cluster RCT with 2 intervention arms and 1 control arm. Control arm guidelines only (C). Two intervention groups - both received a multifaceted general practitioner education and GI one additionally received motivational counselling training for practice nurses (MC) GI and MC trained in using LBP guideline for the DEGAM – 4 modules: 3 interaction seminars; information given on local facilities; 2 individual educational visits by study nurses. In MC group, 2 nurses per practice received 2 full day workshops and 1–3 supervision sessions and study coordinators contacted the nurses regularly.	Unit of analysis is the patient. Power calculation for small effects. Drop out analyses included.	Main Outcome: Hannover Functional Ability Questionnaire for Measuring Back Pain Related Functional Limitations. Secondary outcomes: Freiburg Questionnaire on Physical Ability; Korffs severity of chronic pain scale; Euro Quality of life questionnaire; Fear Avoidance Beliefs questionnaire; Days of sick leave. Follow-up: 6 and 12 months.	After 6 months: functional capacity improvement more pronounced in intervention groups and significantly so for adjusted differed between MC and C groups; both GI and MC patients significantly less days in pain during previous 6 months and less patients in intervention groups indicated suffering permanent pain than C patients. 12 months: more pronounced reduction in days in pain in GI and MC compared to C group. Patients in MC group showed significant improvement in quality of life. Clinical guidelines improve outcome; physician education has a little benefit, motivational interviewing adds slightly more benefit but probably only useful for some patients.	Inclusion rate 44% which might be due to selection bias. Patient sample had wide representation of pain qualities and quantities as well as different motivational stages for behaviour change, so individual differences in effects of interventions may be masked. Included patients may have had lower levels of pain, higher physical activity and readiness for change than general LBP patients in general – may reduce external validity of the study. Validity of the FQPA for a primary care sample with low disability may be insufficient and may limit its discriminative power. Insufficient counselling sessions to draw conclusions.
Rubak et al. Denmark 2009 [31]	One year follow up of an RCT/1.5 day residential MI course for GPs and a half day follow up twice during first year. Both I and C groups had half day course on intensive treatment of type 2 diabetes.	Unit of analysis is the patient. Sample size determined by power analysis.	Health Care Climates Questionnaire; Treatment Self-regulation Questionnaire; Diabetes Illness Representation Questionnaire; Summary of Diabetes self-care activities. Follow-up: 12 months.	Patients in I group significantly more autonomous in their choice of action towards behavioural changes and more motivated to change behaviours; also significantly more aware of the importance of controlling their diabetes for specific factors.	Not blinded at randomization. No baseline data; Patients were newly diagnosed so there was no change behaviour and no statements regarding diabetes at baseline. No blinding of behavioural changes –Hawthorne effect may exist; but if so, existed in both groups. Involvement in study may have influenced and diminished effect of MI.

own community, are accessible to patients, and though contacts are intermittent, there is coordination and continuity of care. This review suggests that teaching motivational interviewing skills to health professionals in primary care may improve self-efficacy and quality of life in their patients, compared to those patients of clinicians who did not participate in this training. It suggests that the addition of motivational interviewing techniques to usual care may have added benefit for patients over usual care in the primary care setting, however further research is needed to identify if other educational interventions or skills are useful.

Implications for further research

Further research is needed to distil the specific techniques to empower patients for self-management [34]; to explore and define the various aspects of the concept of patient empowerment [35]; and the variety of approaches that can be taken by primary care physicians to support patients to self monitor and make decisions about their chronic condition. We also need to identify and address potential barriers for self-management in patients [36].

Patients with chronic conditions interact over time with many professionals in primary and secondary care. There are many other interventions that may help to improve patient self-management, (for example group education, health coaching, telemedicine, e-health, media led interventions, voluntary associations, sports organisations and community group activities). Additional factors having a potential impact on successful outcomes include patient preferences for individual or group interventions, and patients' values, goals, level of education and literacy. Patients have increasingly easy and direct access to online resources. We need research to guide both clinicians and patients to know which methods are best used in which settings [37], and which methods are not suited to particular settings. Careful designs and methods need to be used in future studies to assess the impact of such factors on measuring the outcomes of patient self-management including the Hawthorne effect and language bias. Appropriate assessment tools are required taking account of the integrative model of change appropriate in different settings [38].

Studies are also needed on evidence for the feasibility of training health professionals in patient self-management approaches including efficient use of resources such as time, people and finance, as research into the value and effectiveness of the various methods that can be used to "empower patients" is still in its infancy [37].

We also need to promote the inclusion of validated scales and instruments in future research for measurement and comparison of patient outcomes in chronic conditions.

Conclusions

Effective training for healthcare staff in patient self-management support is important in the context of patient centred care, patient outcomes, health care economics, strategy and delivery of healthcare on a global perspective.

This review suggests that primary care health professionals can help to harness patients' capacity to contribute to improvement of their own health outcomes. Despite increasing literature on patient self-management and on health professional training on this topic, the evidence is very limited on measured patient health outcomes up to two years after patient self-management was incorporated into the WONCA definition of general practice. We plan to undertake a follow-up systematic review to establish if this changes over time or if further research is needed to assure health professionals and policy makers that patient self-management is a worthwhile and effective aspect of general practice.

Abbreviations

CCM: Chronic care model; EQUIP: European Society for Quality and Safety in General Practice / Family Medicine; GI: Guideline implementation; GP/FM: General Practitioner/ Family Physician; MIT: Motivational interviewing techniques; NCD: Non-communicable disease; PSM: Patient self-management; RCT: Randomised controlled trial; WHO: World Health Organisation; WONCA: World Organization of National Colleges, Academies and Academic Associations of General Practitioners/Family Physicians

Acknowledgements

We acknowledge the contributions of Dr. Ernesto Mola (Scientific Interdisciplinary Association of Both Family and Community Medicine (ASSIMEFAC), Lecce, Italy) and Associate Professor John Litt (Flinders University, Adelaide, Australia and Deputy Chair of National Quality Committee RACGP) on the theories and concepts of patient empowerment for self-management which encouraged EQuiP to conduct this research.

Funding

Funding for this project was provided by WONCA Europe through its 20th Anniversary Fund and supplemented by the authors' institutions. The WONCA Europe Executive Board had no role in the design of the study, data collection, analysis, interpretation of data or in writing the manuscript.

Authors' contributions

AR participated in the original protocol, review of articles, the write up of the paper and the steering group and reviewed the final version of the paper. SB participated in the original protocol, review of articles and reviewed the final version of the paper. GD participated in the original protocol, the literature search, and reviewed the final version of the paper. PP participated in the original protocol, the literature search, and reviewed the final version of the paper. JG participated in the review of articles, and the steering group and reviewed the final version of the paper. IK participated in the steering group and reviewed the final version of the paper. SS participated in the steering group and reviewed the final version of the paper. TE participated in the steering group and reviewed the final version of the paper. CC participated in the original protocol, review of articles, the write up of the paper, the steering group and reviewed the final version of the paper. All authors read and approved the final manuscript.

Consent for publication

Not applicable as this is a systematic review with no primary data collection.

Competing interests

The authors declare that they have no competing interests.

Author details

[1]Irish College of General Practitioners, 4-5 Lincoln Place, Dublin 2, Ireland. [2]Institute of General Practice and Family Medicine, University Hospital, LMU, Munich, Germany. [3]University of Helsinki, EBM Guidelines, Duodecim Medical Publications Ltd, Helsinki, Finland. [4]Royal College of Surgeons in Ireland, Dublin, Ireland. [5]GP Copenhagen, Copenhagen, Denmark.

References

1. WONCA Europe. The European Definition of General Practice/Family Medicine WONCA Europe 2011 Edition. Available at: http://www.wonca europe.org/sites/default/files/documents/Definition%203rd%20ed%20 2011%20with%20revised%20wonca%20tree.pdf. Accessed 31 Jan 2018.
2. Grüninger U, Kissling B. Die Hausarztmedizin als eigene Disziplin und als Spezialgebiet (family medicine - a specialty of its own). Primary Care. 2005; 5(11):269–71.
3. Mola E, De Bonis JA, Giancane R. Integrating patient empowerment as an essential characteristic of the discipline of general practice/family medicine. Eur J Gen Pract. 2008;14(2):89–94.
4. Patient Empowerment in Chronic Conditions – Wonca Europe (PECC-WE). The WONCA Anniversary Research Fund 2012–2015 project. Available at: http://equip.woncaeurope.org/tools/pecc-we-patient-empowerment/ patient-empowerment Accessed 13 Sept 2016.
5. World Health Organization. Innovative care for chronic diseases. Building blocks for action. Global Report. Geneva: WHO; 2002. Available at: http://www.who.int/ chp/knowledge/publications/icccglobalreport.pdf. Accessed 11 Nov 2015.
6. World Health Organization. Global status report on Non-Communicable Diseases 2014. Geneva: WHO; 2014. Available at: http://www.who.int/nmh/ publications/ncd-status-report-2014/en/. Accessed 11 Nov 2015.

7. Wagner E, Austin B, Von Korff M. Organising care for patients with chronic illness. Millbank Quarterly. 1996;74(4):511–44.
8. Lorig KR, Holman H. Self-management education: history, definition, outcomes, and mechanisms. Ann Behav Med. 2003;26(1):1–7.
9. Battersby M, Lawn S. Capabilities for supporting prevention and chronic condition self-management: a resource for educators of primary health care professionals. Flinders University, Adelaide: Australian Government Department of Health and Ageing; 2009.
10. Gruman J, Von Korff M. Indexed bibliography on self-management for people with chronic diseases. Washington, DC: Center for Advancement in Health; 1996.
11. Parlour R, Slater PF. An evaluation of the effectiveness of a self-management Programme. Office of the Nursing and Midwifery Services Director, Health Service Executive: Dublin; 2011.
12. Bradley PM, Lindsay B. Care delivery and self-management strategies for adults with epilepsy. Cochrane Database of Syst Rev. 2008;23(1):CD006244.
13. Deakin T, McShane CE, Cade JE, Williams RD. Group based training for self-management strategies in people with type 2 diabetes mellitus. Cochrane Database of Syst Rev. 2005;18(2):CD003417.
14. Holman H, Lorig K. Patient self-management: a key to effectiveness and efficiency in care of chronic disease. Public Health Rep. 2004;119(3):239–43.
15. Ofman JJ, Badamgarav E, Henning JM, Knight K, Gano AD Jr, Levan RK, et al. Does disease management improve clinical and economic outcomes in patients with chronic diseases? A systematic review. Am J Med. 2004;117(3):182–92.
16. Marks R, Allegrante JP, Lorig K. A review and synthesis of research evidence for self-efficacy-enhancing interventions for reducing chronic disability: implications for health education practice (part II). Health Promot Pract. 2005;6(2):148–56.
17. Du S, Yuan C. Evaluation of patient self-management outcomes in health care: a systematic review. Int Nurs Rev. 2010;57(2):159–67.
18. Lorig KR, Sobel DS, Stewart AL, Brown BW Jr, Bandura A, Ritter P, et al. Evidence suggesting that a chronic disease self-management program can improve health status while reducing hospitalization: a randomized trial. Med Care. 1999;37(1):5–14.
19. Bodenheimer T, Wagner EH, Grumbach K. Improving primary care for patients with chronic illness. JAMA. 2002;288(14):1775–9.
20. Muenchberger H, Kendall E. Predictors of preventable hospitalization in chronic disease: priorities for change. J Public Health Policy. 2010; 31(2):150–63.
21. Wagner EH, Austin BT, Davis C, Hindmarsh M, Schaefer J, Bonomi A. Improving chronic illness care: translating evidence into action. Health Aff (Millwood). 2001;20(6):64–78.
22. Bodenheimer T, Wagner EH, Grumbach K. Improving primary care for patients with chronic illness: the chronic care model, part 2. JAMA. 2002; 288(15):1909–14.
23. Litt J, Rochfort A, Collins C, O'Riordan M. Patient self-Management in Chronic Conditions. Dublin: Irish College of General Practitioners; 2011.
24. Dennis CL. Peer support within a health care context: a concept analysis. Int J Nurs Stud. 2003;40(3):321–32.
25. Lawn S, Schoo A. Supporting self-management of chronic health conditions: common approaches. Patient Educ Couns. 2010;80(2):205–11.
26. Jordan JE, Briggs AM, Brand CA, Osborne RH. Enhancing patient engagement in chronic disease self-management support initiatives in Australia: the need for an integrated approach. Med J Aust. 2008;189(10 Suppl):S9–S13.
27. Moher D, Liberati A, Tetzlaff J, Altman DG. Preferred reporting items for systematic reviews and meta-analyses: the PRISMA statement. Ann Intern Med. 2009;151(4):264–9.
28. Collins C, Rochfort A, Beirne S, Doran G, Patton P. The effectiveness of educational interventions for primary care health professionals designed to improve self-management in patients with chronic conditions. PROSPERO. 2013:CRD42013004418 http://www.crd.york.ac.uk/PROSPERO/display_record.asp?ID=CRD42013004418. Accessed 13 Nov 2015.
29. Thomas H. Quality assessment tool for quantitative studies. McMaster University, Toronto: Effective Public Health Practice Project; 2003.
30. Becker A, Leonhardt C, Kochen MM, Keller S, Wegscheider K, Baum E, et al. Effects of two guideline implementation strategies on patient outcomes in primary care: a cluster randomized controlled trial. Spine (Phila Pa 1976). 2008;33(5):473–80. https://doi.org/10.1097/BRS.0b013e3181657e0d.
31. Rubak S, Sandbaek A, Lauritzen T, Borch-Johnsen K, Christensen B. General practitioners trained in motivational interviewing can positively affect the attitude to behaviour change in people with type 2 diabetes. One year follow-up of an RCT, ADDITION Denmark. Scand J Prim Health Care. 2009; 27(3):172–9. https://doi.org/10.1080/02813430903072876.
32. Solberg HS, Steinsbekk A, Solbjør M, Granbo R, Garåsen H. Characteristics of a self-management support programme applicable in primary health care: a qualitative study of users' and health professionals' perceptions. BMC Health Serv Res. 2014;14:562.
33. NHS. Expert Patients Programme (EPP). 2014. Available at: http://www.nhs.uk/NHSEngland/AboutNHSservices/doctors/Pages/expert-patients-programme.aspx. Accessed 16 Nov 2015.
34. Lenzen SA, Daniëls R, van Bokhoven MA, van der Weijden T, Beurskens A. Setting goals in chronic care: Shared decision making as self-management support by the family physician. Eur J Gen Pract. 2015;21(2):138–44. https://doi.org/10.3109/13814788.2014.973844 Epub 2014 Dec 26.
35. Bravo P, Edwards A, Barr PJ, Scholl I, Elwyn G, Mc Allister M, Cochrane Healthcare Quality Research Group, Cardiff University. Conceptualising patient empowerment: a mixed methods study. BMC Health Serv Res. 2015; 15:252. https://doi.org/10.1186/s12913-015-0907-z.
36. Eikelenboom N, van Lieshout J, Jacobs A, Verhulst F, Lacroix J, van Halteren A, Klomp M, Smeele I, Wensing M. Effectiveness of personalised support fro self-management in primary care: a cluster randomised controlled trial. Br J Gen Pract. 2016;66(646):e354–61. https://doi.org/10.3399/bjgp16X684985 Epub 2016 Apr 14.
37. Grol R. Improving the quality of medical care: building bridges among professional pride, payer profit, and patient satisfaction. JAMA. 2001;286: 2578–85.
38. Prochaska JQ, DiClemente CC. Transtheoretical therapy: toward a more integrative model of change. Psychotherapy. 1982;20:161–73.

17

Targeted prevention in primary care aimed at lifestyle-related diseases

Lars Bruun Larsen[1*], Anders Larrabee Sonderlund[1], Jens Sondergaard[1], Janus Laust Thomsen[1], Anders Halling[2], Niels Christian Hvidt[1], Elisabeth Assing Hvidt[1], Troels Mønsted[3], Line Bjornskov Pedersen[1,4], Ewa M. Roos[5], Pia Vivian Pedersen[6] and Trine Thilsing[1]

Abstract

Background: The consequences of lifestyle-related disease represent a major burden for the individual as well as for society at large. Individual preventive health checks to the general population have been suggested as a mean to reduce the burden of lifestyle-related diseases, though with mixed evidence on effectiveness. Several systematic reviews, on the other hand, suggest that health checks targeting people at high risk of chronic lifestyle-related diseases may be more effective. The evidence is however very limited. To effectively target people at high risk of lifestyle-related disease, there is a substantial need to advance and implement evidence-based health strategies and interventions that facilitate the identification and management of people at high risk. This paper reports on a non-randomized pilot study carried out to test the acceptability, feasibility and short-term effects of a healthcare intervention in primary care designed to systematically identify persons at risk of developing lifestyle-related disease or who engage in health-risk behavior, and provide targeted and coherent preventive services to these individuals.

Methods: The intervention took place over a three-month period from September 2016 to December 2016. Taking a two-pronged approach, the design included both a joint and a targeted intervention. The former was directed at the entire population, while the latter specifically focused on patients at high risk of a lifestyle-related disease and/or who engage in health-risk behavior. The intervention was facilitated by a digital support system. The evaluation of the pilot will comprise both quantitative and qualitative research methods. All outcome measures are based on validated instruments and aim to provide results pertaining to intervention acceptability, feasibility, and short-term effects.

Discussion: This pilot study will provide a solid empirical base from which to plan and implement a full-scale randomized study with the central aim of determining the efficacy of a preventive health intervention.

Keywords: Targeted health checks, Primary care, Intersectoral collaboration

* Correspondence: lblarsen@health.sdu.dk
[1]Department of Public Health, Research Unit of General Practice, University of Southern Denmark, Odense, Denmark
Full list of author information is available at the end of the article

Background

In this paper we report on a non-randomized pilot study examining the efficacy of a preventive healthcare intervention. The intervention has been designed to systematically identify patients at high risk of developing lifestyle-related disease, and provide targeted and coherent preventive services to these individuals [1].

Lifestyle-related disease refers to health conditions that are predominantly caused by health-risk behaviors, such as poor diet, smoking, high consumption of alcohol, or lack of exercise. The consequences of lifestyle-related disease represent a major challenge for the individual as well as for society at large [2]. In Denmark, people who smoke tobacco, consume excessive amounts of alcohol, and have a sedentary lifestyle are nearly seven times as likely to die from lifestyle-related diseases than physically active non-smokers with a moderate intake of alcohol [3]. It is estimated that 80% of cardio-vascular disease (CVD), type 2-diabetes mellitus (T2DM), and chronic obstructive pulmonary disease (COPD), and 40% of all cancers may be averted by maintaining healthy dietary habits, regularly exercising, and refraining from smoking [4]. Indeed, preventable lifestyle-related diseases account for approximately 50 to 60% of all hospital admissions [5]. It is expected that increasing rates of obesity and physical inactivity will lead to a surge in the number of patients with lifestyle-related diseases in the decades to come [6–8]. In light of these trends, there is a substantial need to advance and implement evidence-based health strategies and interventions that facilitate the identification and management of people at risk of developing these diseases [9].

Disease prevention is a central task in general practice in Denmark and the Nordic countries [10]. Two recent systematic reviews of general practice health checks suggest that people at high risk of chronic disease may benefit from targeted preventive health checks [11, 12]. Indeed, targeted, or selective, preventive healthcare is a generally accepted and well-integrated part of healthcare systems worldwide (e.g. treatment of hypertension and hyperlipidemia). Other studies, however, suggest that systematic screening of the general population does not improve clinical endpoints above and beyond those associated with opportunistic screening. These studies indicate that, at a population level, systematic screening of the general population does more harm than good [13–15]. Overall, however, the evidence on targeted and systematic screening of chronic disease is very limited, possibly providing an explanation for the apparent contradictions in the literature. To this end, projects in the Netherlands and Great Britain are currently underway, testing different approaches to targeted and systematic intervention in general practice [16, 17].

There is an even greater lack of evidence when it comes to targeted preventive interventions that comprise both general practice and community health services. In such an approach the general practitioner (GP) targets patients at high risk for lifestyle-related diseases and engages in risk-management of biomarkers and disease with behavior change and pharmaceutical interventions when needed. Community health services, on the other hand, focus primarily on the prevention of health-risk behaviors - including tobacco use, poor diet, excessive alcohol consumption, and sedentary lifestyles - and provide behavior-change interventions such as smoking cessation assistance and dietary advice. Danish studies suggest a potential to enhance the collaboration and cohesiveness of the various components that comprise the preventive healthcare services in the Danish primary care system – especially between GPs and community health services [18, 19]. Outside of the Danish context, the benefits of a more unified and coherent healthcare service have also been advanced in peer-reviewed studies [20, 21]. However, effectiveness studies of a unified approach, such as that described above, seem to be lacking.

In 2012, we carried out a feasibility study, testing a novel approach to population-based risk stratification at four Danish GP clinics [22]. The intervention combined lifestyle survey data with health record information in order to identify presumably healthy individuals who nonetheless were at high risk of developing lifestyle-related diseases. These individuals were then offered a health check at their GP for a more definitive assessment of their general health as well as their risk of developing lifestyle-related diseases. Results indicated that this approach to preventive action was indeed feasible, and thus ultimately inspired the development of a large randomized study, the present TOF-project (TOF is a Danish acronym for Early Detection and Prevention). The principal aim of the upcoming TOF-project is to examine the efficacy of a preventive healthcare intervention that systematically identifies individuals at high risk of lifestyle-related disease, and provides targeted and coherent preventive services. We expect that significant changes in the targeting and systematization of disease prevention in the Danish primary care sector, including earlier detection and more coherent preventive services, will diminish the individual and societal burden of chronic disease. Due to the complexity of the TOF intervention, and the relatively high number of stakeholders, a pilot study needs to be conducted before full-scale implementation and evaluation [23]. The aim of the pilot study is to test the acceptability, feasibility, and short-term effects of a selective preventive program, designed to systematically help patients evaluate their individual risk of lifestyle-related disease. The program also offers targeted and coordinated preventive services in the primary healthcare sector.

Methods

The pilot study was designed as a population based non-randomized study in the Region of Southern Denmark, comprising 22 municipalities, 787 GPs, and a general population of 1,2 million. The Danish health care system is a tax-based system comprising three levels: A national level responsible for, among other things, public health, planning, and patient safety; a regional level responsible for the hospitals and the primary care sector; and a municipal level responsible for primary prevention, rehabilitation, and patient education. General practice and the municipalities have shared responsibility for preventive services aimed at the individual. Specifically, GPs assess patient health and implement disease-specific secondary prevention. The municipalities, however, are tasked with primary prevention such as smoking cessation, alcohol treatment, and other lifestyle related services. GPs are organized in clinics with an average of two GPs per clinic. While most clinics comprise a single GP, some have up to ten. Almost all Danish citizens (98%) are registered with a GP [24, 25]. Each GP has an average of 1600 registered patients.

Recruitment

The pilot study targets adults born between year 1957 and 1986. All 22 municipalities in the Region of Southern Denmark were invited to participate in TOF. Ten municipalities (Esbjerg, Haderslev, Varde, Sønderborg, Aabenraa, Middelfart, Kerteminde, Nyborg, Svendborg, Langeland) submitted expressions of interest to participate in the study, and were approved for participation by the Regional Council. Two of the municipalities (Haderslev and Varde) volunteered to participate in the pilot study.

The municipalities of Haderslev and Varde comprise 55,971 and 50,110 citizens, and 37 and 29 GPs, respectively. All GPs from each municipality were invited to an information meeting before being formally invited to participate in the pilot study. The invitation was followed up with telephone calls to the individual GP clinics. All patients were invited at baseline, and the intervention was taken up by the patients at their own convenience during the intervention period. See Additional file 1 for a more detailed project flow showing the recruitment, intervention and evaluation phases.

Organization and development of the intervention

The intervention was planned during a two-year combined effort involving all stakeholders. End users were involved in the design of the intervention, including patients, GPs, and municipal health professionals. A group of seven GPs developed the targeted intervention at a general practice level during five workshops. Similarly, a group of 10 municipal health workers, one from each of the participating municipalities, developed the targeted intervention at a municipal level during 10 workshops. The workshops lasted between 2 h and 2 days. A digital support system was created and tested by user populations, including patients, non-government patient organizations, GPs, and municipal health professionals.

A steering committee was established at the start of the project, consisting of managers or board members from the Region of Southern Denmark (project owner), The Organization of General Practitioners in Denmark (PLO), the 10 participating municipalities, the Research Unit for General Practice at the University of Southern Denmark (FEA), and the Danish Quality Unit for General Practice (DAK-E). The chair of the committee is the health director from the Region of Southern Denmark. A research committee with participation from the steering committee chair and the primary investigator has been established. A mission statement has been approved by the steering committee and an agreement of co-operation has been signed between the Region of Southern Denmark and the University of Southern Denmark. The agreement states that the University of Southern Denmark holds all rights, intellectual as well as judicial, to the research data, and that the Region of Southern Denmark has no right to oppose publication of results. The research committee approves all access to research data from affiliated researchers.

Prior to study commencement, all enrolled GPs, practice nurses (PN), and health professionals from the municipalities were invited to a joint three-hour training course (August 2016). The course focused on the assigned intervention activities and tasks both within the GP clinics and the municipality respectively, and between GPs and the municipality.

Invitation and consent

The source population received an invitation to participate, sent on behalf of the GP and the municipality to the individual's digital mailbox. All permanent residents in Denmark are obligated to have a digital mailbox, which is essentially a digital mail-system provided by the government for secure and direct communication between individuals and public authorities and other trusted organizations (e.g. banks and insurance companies) [26]. People may opt out of the digital mail system, citing low IT-literacy (usually elderly persons), cognitive impairment, or other complicating factors. To enroll in the study, individuals were asked to follow a link in the invitation to a digital support system protected by a two-phased NemID password [27]. NemID is a password system providing an exact identification of the user. This system is utilized by Danish public and non-public institutions to provide secure access to personal information, such as health and financial data. Through digital mail and NemID, we were able to reach and identify 97% of the target population. In April 2016, participants received an invitation with an embedded hyperlink to a digital consent form on a secure webpage in their digital mailbox. The consent form outlined study participation and disclosure of data from the GPs electronic patient record (EPR) and was supplemented with short videos describing the purpose of the study and the intervention. Participants were asked to read the information and electronically sign the consent form. Two reminders were sent after one and 2 weeks if participants failed to sign the form. Enrollment closed after 6 weeks. At this time, information on relevant diagnosis (International Classification of Primary Care (ICPC-2) codes) and prescribed medicine (Anatomical Therapeutic Chemical Classification (ATC) codes incl. Text fields with indication for treatment) were collected from the GPs EPR system (See Table 1 for the ICPC-2 codes and ATC codes that were accessed based on the consent). Five months after consent (September 2016), participants received another digital invitation in the digital mailbox, this time to fill in a questionnaire and access a personal health profile. Participants could opt-out at any time during the intervention period by clicking an "opt-out" button on the digital support system.

Intervention

The duration of the intervention was 3 months and took place between September 2016 and December 2016. The intervention comprised a two-pronged approach: [1] a joint intervention applied to the entire sample, regardless of whether the participants were healthy, at risk, or already in treatment for T2DM, COPD, CVD, hypercholesterolemia or hypertension [2] a targeted intervention that was offered only to participants who presumably would benefit from either further examinations at the GP (high risk), or from receiving community health services, such as smoking cessation, dietary advice, or physical activity (health-risk behavior).

The joint intervention consisted of:

- Stratification to one of four risk groups. Stratification to a specific risk group was determined by use of risk algorithms and EPR information
- A digital support system with user interfaces for all users, including the patient, the GP, and the municipal health professional
- An individual health profile

The targeted intervention consisted of:

- A focused clinical examination and a subsequent health dialogue with a GP (targeting patients at high risk), *and / or*
- A short telephone-based health dialogue with a municipal health professional. For patients with limited capability to care for their own health, this initial talk could be followed up with a subsequent face-to-face health dialogue (targeting patients with health-risk behavior)

For all present intents and purposes, the term *health dialogue* refers to a consultation that includes the elements of the 5As model (see Table 1) and the techniques used in motivational interviewing [28, 29].

The joint intervention

All participants gained access to the digital support system and were invited to fill in a questionnaire. The participant questionnaire contained 15 items on height, weight, self-perceived health status, family history of lifestyle-related diseases, COPD related symptoms, smoking status, leisure activity level, alcohol consumption, diet, and osteoarthritis risk factors. Questions about family history of diabetes and leisure activity level were taken from the Danish Diabetes Risk model [30]. Similarly, questions on COPD-related symptoms and smoking status were derived from the COPD-PS screener [31] and the Heartscore BMI score [32]. Items tapping dietary habits were from the Swedish National Guidelines on Disease Prevention [33]. The questionnaire took approximately 5 min to complete.

Based on the questionnaire and information from the individual EPR, participants were stratified into four distinct risk groups:

Group 1 – Participants with a pre-existing diagnosis and/or in current treatment for a lifestyle-related disease.
Group 2 – Participants at high risk of developing lifestyle-related disease, and thus eligible for the offer of a targeted intervention at the GP.

Table 1 The 5As model

Assess	Initial questionnaire-derived assessment of the patients' health / risk profile for the purpose of identifying patients in need of health-risk behavior change Subsequent health examination at the GP to confirm or disprove estimated risk of disease
Advice	Counseling, based on the patient's symptoms / risk profile. The patient's values and attitudes can usefully be involved
Agree	Active involvement of the patient in connection with goal setting regarding health-risk behavior change
Assist	Joint development of plan for health-risk behavior change
Arrange follow-up	Planning of the next steps at the GP or other (e.g. the municipality)

Group 3 – Participants engaging in health-risk behavior, and thus eligible for the offer of a targeted intervention at the municipality.

Group 4 – Participants with a healthy lifestyle and no need for further intervention.

Stratification to group 1

EPR data was collected via certified EPR-suppliers. We used International Classification of Primary Care-2 codes (ICPC-2) registered by the GP and/or Anatomical Therapeutic Chemical Classification (ATC) codes for prescribed medicine within the past 2 years, together with the indication for prescribing the medicine, to identify Group 1 participants (see Table 2).

Given the pre-existing diagnosis and/or treatment, Group 1 was excluded from the subsequent risk estimation and stratification into Group 2, 3, and 4.

Stratification to group 2

Next, participants at risk of lifestyle-related disease were identified using three validated risk scores: the Chronic Obstructive Pulmonary Disease Population Screener (COPD-PS), the Danish Diabetes Risk model, and a modified Heartscore BMI score [30–32]. The COPD-PS uses an algorithm accounting for age, lifetime use of cigarettes, and smoking-related symptoms to identify at-risk patients who may benefit from a spirometry to test for COPD (Table 3) [31]. The Danish Diabetes Risk score is based on an algorithm that incorporates age, sex, BMI, known hypertension, leisure activity level, and family history of diabetes (Table 4) [30]. The modified Heartscore BMI score accounts for age, sex, body mass index (BMI), and smoking status (Table 5) [32].

Consistent with the criteria of the four distinct stratification groups defined above, participants were categorized into Group 2 when one or more of the risk assessment algorithms indicated high likelihood of developing lifestyle-related disease (see Tables 3, 4 and 5).

Stratification to group 3 and 4

Finally, participants engaging in health-risk behavior with one or more risk factors were categorized in Group 3 (Group 3). Health-risk behavior was defined by the presence of at least one of the following behaviors: smoking tobacco on a daily basis, consuming more than 14/21 (male/female) standard units of alcohol per week, sustaining an unhealthy diet (diet score ≤ 4 on a 12-point score drawn from the Swedish National Guidelines on Disease Prevention) [4], maintaining a BMI $\geq$ 35, and/or engaging in a generally sedentary lifestyle. Lastly, participants with no lifestyle-related disease or risk thereof were stratified into Group 4.

Digital support system

All users had access to a digital support system in the form of a web page with a common database and specific user interfaces for the GP, the municipality health professionals, and the patient. No apps were developed. The system design drew inspiration from the work by Krist and colleagues' research on preventive EPRs, and was further inspired by the results of a Delphi process carried out to identify factors for optimal development of health-related websites [34–36]. Due to challenges in terms of interoperability between the eight suppliers of EPR systems used by GPs, and at least three suppliers of electronic care records (ECR) in the municipalities, it was not feasible to develop a support system that completely integrated the EPR and ECR systems. Instead, the digital support system was developed as a parallel system with an additional functionality facilitating the transfer of information (e.g. relating to lifestyle and/or

Table 2 Criteria for identification of participants with a pre-existing diagnosis and/or in current treatment for a lifestyle-related disease

Diagnosis	Diagnostic code(s) (ICPC-2)		ATC therapeutic code(s) for prescribed medicine and indicative texts for the prescription[a]
Hypertension	K86, K87	or	C0 *BT*, *bt*, *Bt*, *ypert*, *ldot*, *LODTR*, *lotr*, *lodptr*, *blodtryk* *bl. trykket*, *lodrtr*[b]
Hyperlipidemia	T93	or	C10 *kolesterol*
COPD	R95	or	R03AC18 (indacaterol), R03AC19 (Olodaterol), R03AL03 (vilanterol), R03AL04 (Indacaterol+Glycopyrroniumbromide), R03AL05 (Formoterol+Aclidiniumbromide) R03BB04 (tiotropium bromide), R03BB05 (Aclidiniumbromide), R03BB06 (Glycopyrroniumbromide) *obstruktiv*, *KOL*
T2DM	T90	or	A10(diabetes medicine) *sukkersyge*, *diabetes*
CVD	K74, K76[c]		

[a]The indicative text is in Danish and has not been translated as some indicative texts are only parts of the entire word and as such not translatable

[b]The reason for the large number of indicative text is misspellings by the GP when indicating the purpose of the prescription

[c]Diagnostic codes for ischemic heart diseases are transferred to the GP's EPR system when the patients are discharged from the hospital following an angina or a stroke. ATC codes for prescribed medicine will not provide further information

Table 3 Algorithm used for risk assessment of COPD

Characteristic		Score
During the past 4 weeks, how much of the time did you feel short of breath during every day activities? (e.g. Strolling, light gardening, cleaning, shopping etc.)	None of the time	0
	A little of the time	0
	Some of the time	1
	Most of the time	2
	All of the time	2
Do you ever cough up any "stuff," such as mucus or phlegm?	No, never	0
	Only when I have a cold, pneumonia or sore throat	0
	Yes a few days a month	1
	Yes most days a week	1
	Yes every day	2
Please select the answer that best describes you in the past 12 months. I do less than I used to because of my breathing problems.	Strongly disagree	0
	Disagree	0
	Unsure	0
	Agree	1
	Strongly agree	2
Have you smoked at least 100 cigarettes in your ENTIRE LIFE?	Yes	2
	No	0
Age	35–49 years	0
	50–59 years	1
	60–69 years	2
	+ 70 years	2

Cut off value: ≥5

prevention plans) to the EPR and ECR systems using Electronic Data Interchange (EDIfact) messages [22]. The patient controlled access to personal health information on the system, such that the GP and municipal health professional were only able to access this information with the explicit consent of the patient.

The digital support system was developed iteratively in collaboration with the users during the before mentioned workshops with municipality health professionals and GPs and in the form of usability tests with patients. The user interface for the patient was responsive and compatible with most devices, including mobile phones, tablets, laptops and stationary computers. Due to technical constraints in the secure log-in provided by NemID, the user interface for health professionals was only developed for laptops and stationary computers. In order to make the user interface for the patient as intuitive and user-friendly as possible, the digital support system made extensive use of simple visualizations, icons, and short information videos (Fig. 1). The primary text-based messages were kept short and concise with the provided possibility of accessing secondary in-depth information, retrieved from the Danish Health Portal, sundhed.dk [37].

Beyond facilitating the intervention, the digital support system also enabled data collection for research purposes. A number of questionnaires were sent from the digital support system to the participants at specific time-points, including immediately after consent, after receiving the personal health profile, following the health dialogue at the GP, and at the end of the implementation period. Questionnaire reminders were sent by e-mail with a link to the digital support system. The GPs and municipal health professionals received audits in the form of short questionnaires immediately after each consultation as well as before and after the study period (GPs only).

Personal health profile

Based on results of the stratification process, each patient received a personal health profile on the digital support system. The purpose of the health profile was to encourage patients to change their health-risk behavior and follow the tailored advice provided by the system. Patients who were at increased risk of developing a lifestyle-related disease (Group 2) were advised to consult their GP for further examination and advice. Similarly, patients engaging in health-risk behavior (Group 3) were offered lifestyle counseling, or lifestyle courses from the municipality health services.

Table 4 Algorithm used for risk assessment of T2DM

Characteristic	Score
Sex	
Male	1
Female	0
Age	
40–44 years	0
45–49 years	1
50–54 years	2
55–59 years	3
60–69 years	4
BMI	
25–30 kg/m^2	1
> 30 kg/m^2	2
Known hypertension	
Yes	2
No	0
Primary recreational activity level during the past year:	
Participating in sports competitions or hard exercise several times a week	0
Active with sports at least three times a week or regularly perform heavy house or garden work	0
Strolling, cycling or other light exercise at least 4 h a week (including Sunday walks, light gardening and cycling/walking to work)	1
Reading, watching television or other sedentary jobs	1
Family history of diabetes (Family includes grandparents, parents, sibling and children):	
No family member with diabetes before the age of 70	0
One family member with diabetes before the age of 70	1
More than one family member with diabetes before the age of 70	2
Having had diabetes including gestational diabetes	
Yes	2
No	0

Cut off value: ≥5

By definition, Group 4 patients lead a relatively healthy life with no need for health-risk behavior change. Group 1 patients were advised to continue their treatment and use the information provided to change health-risk behavior.

The personal health profile included individualized information on current health-risk behavior and risk of disease. The information was tailored based on the questionnaire, the information from the EPR, and the risk scores on COPD, T2DM, and CVD. It also included general health information and information about preventive health services concerning smoking, diet, exercise, and alcohol consumption. This information was provided by the municipality, the Region of Southern Denmark, or national health services, and targeted the individual (e.g. via links to apps and webpages) based on his/her specific health-risk behavior.

The targeted intervention

The intervention at the GP

The intervention at the general practice level consisted of a focused clinical examination and a subsequent health dialogue and was offered to patients who were at increased risk of developing a lifestyle-related disease (Group 2). Group 2 patients accepted the offer of the intervention by scheduling an appointment at the GP (either by phone or the GP's webpage). Whether the patient participated in the intervention or not was thus determined by their motivation and capabilities as well as the extent to which the content of the personal health profile motivated the patient to take action. The intervention was applied within the framework of the 5As model (see Table 1) [28]. The content of the focused clinical examination was based on the patient's health profile, and might include measurements of blood glucose (HbA1c) and cholesterol levels, as well as

Table 5 Algorithms used for risk assessment of CVD

Age	BMI	Daily smoker
Female		
> 50 years	> 40 kg/m^2	+
> 55 years	> 40 kg/m^2	–
> 58 years	35–40 kg/m^2	+
Male		
> 49 years	> 40 kg/m^2	+
> 55 years	> 40 kg/m^2	–
> 50 years	35–40 kg/m^2	+
> 55 years	35–40 kg/m^2	–
> 52 years	30–35 kg/m^2	+
> 56 years	25–30 kg/m^2	+

height, weight, blood pressure, and lung function measurements and Electrocardiogram (ECG). Results from the examinations were registered in the digital support system where both the patient and the GP could access them at any time. After the focused clinical examination all patients were given the opportunity to prepare for the subsequent health dialogue by answering a questionnaire inspired by three systematic reviews on the determinants of behavior change [38–40]. These included questions about motivation, resources, former experiences with behavior change,

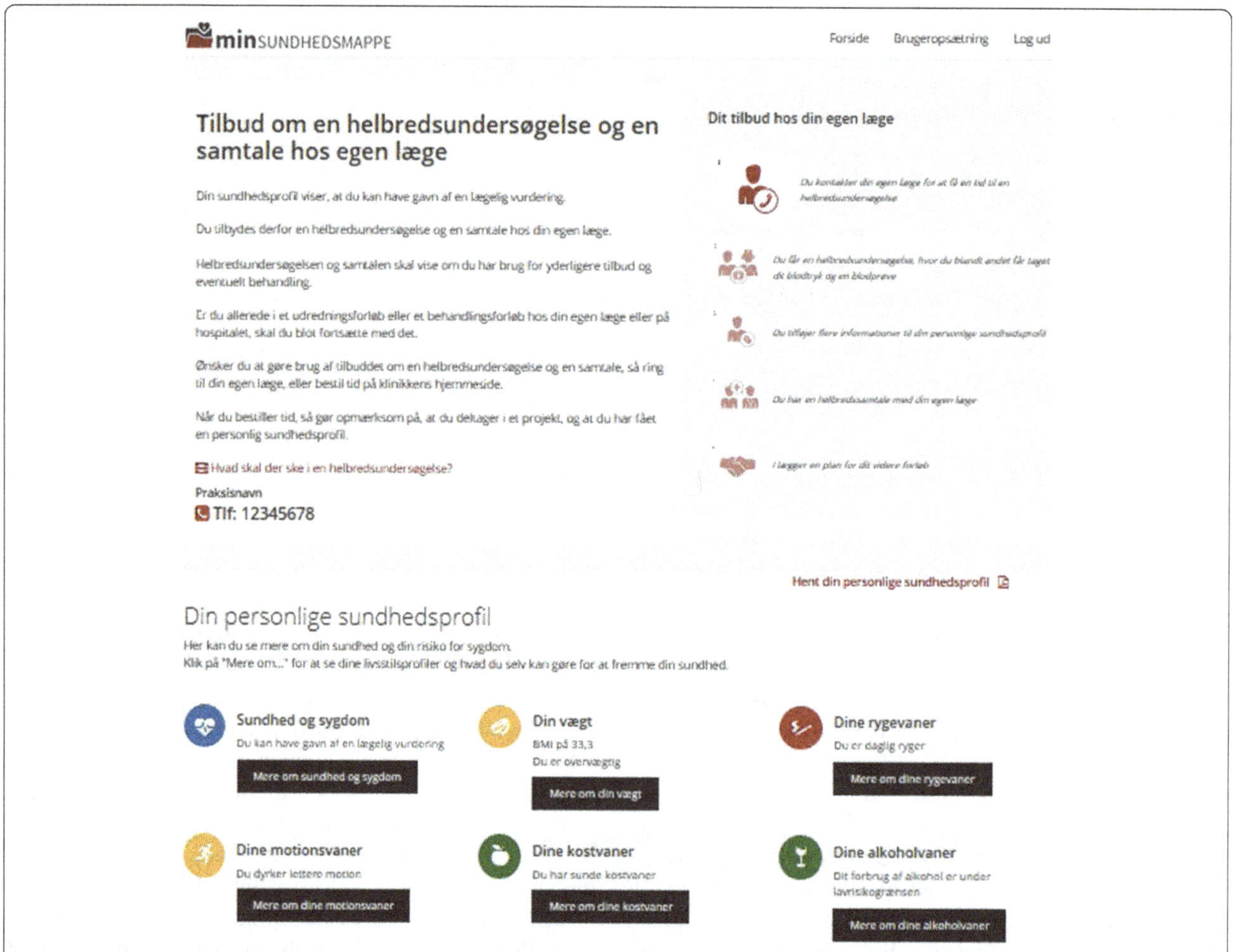

Fig. 1 Screen dump from digital support system (in Danish)

social network, mental health (WHO-5 for stress and Major Depression Inventory (MDI) for depression) [41, 42], and a scheme to qualitatively self-report on facilitators and barriers to behavior change (a so-called balance-sheet). The questionnaire results were shared with the GP on the digital support system. Based on the health dialogue, the GP and the patient developed a prevention plan that included a goal, a time frame, and identification of the appropriate means to fulfill the plan (e.g. reference to a smoking cessation course, or follow-up at the GP). The prevention plan was registered on the digital support system by the GP and was accessible to both the GP and the patient.

The intervention at the municipal level

The intervention at the municipal level was offered to patients exhibiting health-risk behavior (Group 3) and consisted of a short telephone consultation with a health professional – for example a nurse, a dietician, or a physiotherapist. A subsequent face-to-face health dialogue was offered to patients who were deemed to potentially benefit from more extensive support. Group 3 patients requested the intervention on the digital support system by filling in a short form and sending it by e-mail to the municipality. A municipal health professional would then call the patient within the following week. Similar to the GP intervention, the intervention at the municipal level was thus also determined by patient motivation and capabilities as well as the extent to which the content of the personal health profile motivated the patient to take action. Immediately after the intervention, a participation form was sent to the municipality. Patients could prepare for the upcoming call from a municipal health professional in the same way as Group 2 patients prepared for the health dialogue – that is, by answering a short questionnaire. Ultimately, a prevention plan, including concrete details on its execution, was developed based on the telephone consultation and the face-to-face health dialogue. The prevention plan was registered by the municipal health professional and presented on the user interfaces of both the municipality and the patient.

Sample size calculation

While aiming to test the acceptability, feasibility, and short-term effects of the pilot, we estimated a sample size for each GP that would allow the GP to familiarize him/herself with the intervention without unnecessary increases in workload during the intervention period. In agreement with the GP representative in the Region of Southern Denmark, we set a target of four health checks for each GP. From the feasibility study, we estimated that 60% would consent to the study, and that 75% of these participants would receive a personal digital health profile [22]. Also based on the feasibility study, we estimated that 12% of the study population would be recommended to consult their GP (Group 2). From results obtained in similar Dutch studies, we finally estimated that 35% of the these patients (Group 2) would eventually consult the GP [43]. Given these figures, we calculated that a total sample of approximately 200 patients from each GP would be required to reach the target of four completed health checks per GP.

Data collection and analysis

Evaluation outcomes

Evaluation of the study will be carried out using quantitative as well as qualitative research methods (Table 6). All outcome measures are based on validated instruments and aim to provide results pertaining to intervention acceptability, feasibility, and short-term effects. In addition, outcomes related to other associated topics will be included. The specific instruments used will be described in detail in later publications.

Qualitative data

Qualitative data will be derived from interviews (individual and focus groups comprising GPs, practice staff members, municipality staff members, patients from group 2 and 3, stakeholders, project leaders and researchers) and participant observations (during the health dialogues at the GP). The estimated number of participants is shown in Table 6.

Quantitative data

Quantitative data will be derived from questionnaires as well as Danish National registers (see section below). Table 7 shows the content of the questionnaires applied while a diagram, attached as Additional file 1, shows a flow of the entire intervention and the timing of the questionnaires during the intervention.

Register based data

Data from the Danish national registers concerning demographic information, prescriptions, and health care usage of the target population ($n = 9.400$) will be obtained from Statistics Denmark (https://www.dst.dk/da) [44]. Information from the different registers will be linked by the patients' Danish Personal Identification Number.

Socio-demographic variables

Information on socio-demography encompassed educational level, occupation, income, cohabitation status, ethnicity, and residency.

Education is defined as the highest formal educational attainment obtained on the first of October in each calendar year.

Occupation is defined as the occupational status on the first of November in each calendar year.

Table 6 Outcomes

Outcome	Data input
Change in proportion of patients at increased risk of lifestyle related disease from baseline to the 12 weeks follow up	Questionnaire at baseline (Q2) and end of study period (Q6 and Q7). Risk of lifestyle related disease is based on the algorithms previously described in the methods section and in Tables 3, 4 and 5
Determinants of participation and non-participation	Questionnaire at baseline (Q2). Participants and non-participants will be compared with regard to socio-demographic characteristics, morbidity and contextual characteristics
Evaluation of the digital support system with focus on design, usability and effect of the decision support system	Focus group interviews before study start comprising 6 GPs, 6 practice staff members, 6 municipality staff members, 6–8 patients and representatives from 6 to 8 stakeholder organizations, respectively
	Qualitative interviews with 8–10 patients before and after the health dialogue at the GP, and qualitative interviews with 6–8 GPs after health dialogues, focusing on the experienced usefulness of the digital support system
	Questionnaire to all participating patients immediately after signing the consent form (Q1) and after receiving the health profile (Q3 and Q4) and to all participating GPs and municipality staff members following each study related patient encounter (Q8-Q13)
Process evaluation focusing on the intervention in general practice and the municipality	Participant observation of 10–15 health dialogues in different general practices, followed by qualitative interviews with the participating patients, GPs and practice staff
	Focus group interviews with 6–8 municipality staff members involved in the study and interviews with 10–15 patients who have attended a health dialogue in the municipality
	Questionnaire to all participating GPs, practice staff members and municipality staff members following each study related patient encounter (Q8-Q13)
Process evaluation focusing on the organizational basis of the pilot implementation	Interviews with stakeholders involved in the planning, implementation and evaluation of the study; GPs, practice staff members, municipality staff members, patients, project leaders, researchers
Process evaluation focusing on the common training course for enrolled GPs, practice staff and health professionals from the municipalities	Interviews with GPs and municipal health professionals and questionnaire at the end of the course
GP and patients preferences with regard to the content of the health dialogue, and change in preferences during the study period	Questionnaire using discrete choice modelling (Q4, Q7, Q8, Q11)
Patients' perceptions of relational empathy following the health dialogue at the GP	Questionnaire including The Consultation And Relational Empathy (CARE) measure following each behavior counseling session in general practice (Q5)
Quality of Life Subscale on the Hip injury and Osteoarthritis Outcome Score (HOOS)/Knee Injury and Osteoarthritis Outcome Score (KOOS)	Questionnaire at baseline (Q2). Participants replying "yes" to any of the osteoarthritis related questions on hip/knee pain, GP care seeking or surgery at baseline will receive additional questions on knee/hip related quality of life and mechanical alignment of the leg and foot [55]
Patient enablement following the health dialogue at the GP	Questionnaire with Patient Enablement Instrument (PEI) (Q5)
Patient reported 1. Meaning-Making and Health, 2. Spiritual Wellbeing, 3. Religious belief and practices	Questionnaire items are sampled from the validated questionnaire SoMe (Sources of Meaning) and European Value Study (EVS) (Q6 and Q7)
GP reported 1. Perceived importance of communication on existential and spiritual issues, 2. Self-efficacy and barriers in communication on existential and spiritual issues, 3. Personal belief	Questionnaire items sampled from the validated Self-efficacy questionnaire, European Value Study (EVS) and two items developed for this study evaluation (Q6 and Q7)
Patient reported self-efficacy and change in self-efficacy during the study period as a result of participation	Questionnaire incl. The General Self-Efficacy Scale (Q3, Q4, Q6 and Q7)
Patient reported mental well-being and change in mental well-being during the study period as a result of participation	Questionnaire incl. The Warwick-Edinburgh Mental Well-being Scale (WEMWBS) (Q3, Q4, Q6 and Q7)

Table 7 The study questionnaires: Target groups and questionnaire items

Target group	Questionnaire	Items
Patients	Q1	Attitudes towards prevention, Risk-taking attitudes, Time preferences, Mental well-being, Self-efficacy, Evaluation of invitation and consent form
	Q2	Height, Weight, Self-perceived health status, Family history of lifestyle-related diseases, Known hypertension, COPD related symptoms, Osteoarthritis related risk factors, Smoking status, Leisure activity level, Alcohol consumption, Eating habits
	Q3	Evaluation of the personal health profile
	Q4	Evaluation of the personal health profile, Preferences with regard to the content of the health dialogue
	Q5	Patient Enablement Instrument, The Care Measurement
	Q6	Height, Weight, Self-perceived health status, Family history of lifestyle-related diseases, Known hypertension, COPD related symptoms, Osteoarthritis related risk factors, Smoking status, Leisure activity level, Alcohol consumption, Eating habits, Attitudes towards prevention, Mental well-being, Self-efficacy, Study participation, Study evaluation, Meaning-Making and Health, Spiritual Wellbeing, Religious belief and practices, Risk-taking attitudes, Time preferences
	Q7	Height, Weight, Self-perceived health status, Family history of lifestyle-related diseases, Known hypertension, COPD related symptoms, Osteoarthritis related risk factors, Smoking status, Leisure activity level, Alcohol consumption, Eating habits, Attitudes towards prevention, Mental well-being, Self-efficacy, Study participation, Study evaluation, Meaning-Making and Health, Spiritual Wellbeing, Religious belief and practices, Risk-taking attitudes, Time preferences, Preferences with regard to the content of the health dialogue
GPs	Q8	Attitudes towards prevention, Experiences with prevention, Preferences with regard to the content of the health dialogue, GPs health-risk behavior
	Q9	Content of the clinical examination, Staff and time consumption
	Q10	Evaluation of the quality of the stratification, Use and evaluation of the digital support system, The patients motivation and resources, The plan for the patient, Time consumption
	Q11	Attitudes towards prevention, Experiences with prevention, Preferences with regard to the content of the health dialogue
Municipality health professionals	Q12	Evaluation of the quality of the stratification, Use and evaluation of the digital support system, The patients motivation and resources, The plan for the patients, Time consumption
	Q13	Evaluation of the quality of the stratification, Use and evaluation of the digital support system, The patients motivation and resources, The plan for the patient, Time consumption

OECD-adjusted income level is defined as the individual's/family's disposable income, adjusted for family size and categorized in relative terms (low/middle/high income) [45].

Cohabitation status is defined as cohabitating or living alone.

Ethnicity is based on country of origin and descendance.

Morbidity

Information on health/disease status (hypertension, hypercholesterolemia, type-2 diabetes, cardio-vascular disease) is defined in terms of ICD-10 diagnosis codes and medical usage. The 'National Patient Registry' will provide information on ICD-10 diagnostic codes. The 'Register of Medicinal Product Statistics' provide information on medical usage [46, 47].

Contextual variables

Contextual variables include information on study site and neighborhood social deprivation. Neighborhood social deprivation will be derived on a census district level and is principally defined in terms of the following three variables: educational attainment, employment status (employed/social welfare), and income (mean family disposable income). Educational, employment, and income deprivation thus specifically refer to the proportion of citizens within each census district who has access to basic education (up to high school), who is unemployed (e.g. students, unemployed workers), and who belongs to the lowest income quartile, respectively. Each variable is ranked, grouped in quartiles, and given a value between 0 and 3 (3 = high deprivation). This results in an aggregated ranking system ranging from 0 (low deprivation) to 9 (high deprivation). The aggregated rank is then grouped in quartiles. A neighborhood social deprivation score will be calculated for all census districts in Denmark in order to obtain local deprivation scores that mirror the relative social deprivation of the individual census district [48].

Discussion

This pilot study will provide a solid empirical base from which to plan and implement a full-scale randomized study with the central aim of determining the efficacy of a preventive health intervention. The intervention was designed to systematically identify persons at risk of developing lifestyle-related disease or who engage in health-risk behavior, and provide targeted and coherent preventive services to these individuals.

Strengths and limitations

Much effort has been made to define the specific nature and objective of pilot and/or feasibility studies. In a scoping review of optimization strategies for complex interventions prior to randomized trials, Levati asserts the notion that different frameworks for intervention development, such as intervention mapping and the MRC framework for complex intervention, call for different approaches to pilot and feasibility studies [49]. As a common feature when developing complex randomized trials, the authors suggest "that the acceptability of the intervention to those directly involved in the delivery and receipt of the final intervention, together with the anticipated effect of the intervention, are important elements to take into account as early as possible in the pre-trial stage." [49].

Eldridge et al. used a Delphi survey to arrive at distinct definitions of feasibility and pilot studies [1]. They suggest that "feasibility study" is an overarching term with "pilot study" representing a subset of feasibility studies. Generally, feasibility studies ask whether something can be done, should we proceed with it, and if so, how? Pilot studies ask the same questions, but with a specific design feature of a larger study, conducted on a smaller scale. According to the authors, pilot studies can be separated in two distinct types: non-randomized and randomized. Non-randomized pilot studies do not include a control group and are usually external to the subsequent randomized controlled trial (RCT), that is, the participants are not included in the effect analysis of the RCT. Randomized pilot studies, on the other hand, randomize participants to an intervention or control group and can be internal to the subsequent RCT. Bowen et al. complement the work of Eldridge et al. and propose eight foci (design features) of feasibility studies: Acceptability, demand, implementation, practicality, adaptation, integration, expansion, and limited efficacy [50].

According to Eldridge et al., the study presented in this paper is a non-randomized pilot study. We chose a non-randomized design in order to examine the specific design features of a stepped wedge cluster randomized design for the full-scale randomized study. A stepped-wedge design is a type of cluster randomized design that meets the specific ethical and logistical demands of a delayed intervention performed in routine care where all participants will be offered the intervention [51]. The pilot resembles one cluster in a stepped wedge cluster randomized study, and will thus allow us to ascertain whether the intervention can be delivered during a three-month period, or if longer time is required to avoid carry-over effects [51]. In the event that more time is necessary to deliver the intervention, it will be difficult, if not impossible, to accurately determine the optimal duration of a cluster. This will likewise complicate the stepped wedge design. One way to compensate for incomplete knowledge on the optimal timeframe for the intervention may be to include a "wash out" period after every cluster allowing for any delay or lag in implementation before the next cluster is commenced [52]. The length of the "wash out" period can be estimated from the results of the pilot study.

We have randomly sampled 200 patients from each GP in order to have a source population that is representative of the target population. We have chosen to target people born between 1957 and 1986 to assess the risk of lifestyle-related disease and health-risk behavior at an age interval where changes in lifestyle will provide significant health effects and be cost-effective. To this end, we have chosen to assess variation in the proportion of patients at increased risk of lifestyle-related disease between baseline and the 12-week follow up as our primary health-related outcome. Further, given the fact that complex interventions, such as the one described here, usually have concurrent endpoints [23], we also collect data on a variety of other variables – both questionnaire- and register-based – related to both lifestyle and disease. We have yet to determine which of these endpoints to include in the full-scale randomized study.

We have planned the intervention in collaboration with the stakeholders, patients, and service providers in order to run a pilot study that is both acceptable and relevant for all user groups. We use quantitative as well as qualitative research methods to assess the acceptability, demand, implementation, and practicality of the pilot, from the viewpoint of both users and service-providers. In addition to evaluating the intervention, we assess the organizational challenges of planning and implementing IT-supported pilot studies [53]. At the same time we test different methods of data collection, including electronic collection of data from the digital support system and participant observations at the GP clinics. We also test various types of questionnaires, including ones that involve simple items with binary outcomes as well as others in more complex discrete choice format. The pilot will hence enable us to assess whether the intervention can be executed, and whether the organizational approach taken, fit the purpose. We will further be able to make an informed decision about how we can collect data during the full-scale study in the most efficient and cost-effective way that is also acceptable to both users and service-providers.

From pilot to full-scale randomized study

Another issue raised by Levati et al. and Eldridge et al. concerns pinpointing the appropriate time to move from piloting to full-scale RCT. That is, should we proceed with the project, and if so, how? [1, 49]. Proceeding from pilot to a full-scale randomized study is probably the most under-researched part of the implementation of complex interventions. Bugge et al. suggest a three step process to establish the best possible foundation on which to make a decision to advance a full-scale randomized study [54]. First, any problems should be categorized into three distinct types: Issues that are likely to complicate the full-scale study, issues that are likely to complicate both trial and real-world situations, and issues that are likely to complicate real-world situations only. Next, potential solutions should be identified for the expected issues, ideally with lay participation. Finally, the best of these solutions should be selected to determine the best way to proceed. With this strategy in mind, we will do a thorough assessment of the problems encountered in the pilot before advancing the full-scale study. We will thus identify solutions in collaboration with the service providers (GPs and municipal health professionals) who participated in the pilot study, as well as with those who took part in the design of the intervention. We will also seek patient-feedback on the technical and communicative properties of the digital support system before defining its final specifications. The final assessment is presented to the steering committee that will take the decision on the way forward.

Abbreviations

ATC: Anatomical Therapeutic Chemical Classification; BMI: Body mass index; COPD: Chronic Obstructive Pulmonary Disease; COPD-PS: Chronic Obstructive Pulmonary Disease Population Screener; CVD: Cardio vascular disease; EDIfact: Electronic Data Interchange messages; EPR: Electronic patient record; GP: General practitioner; ICD-10: International classification of diseases; ICPC-2: International classification of primary care; RCT: Randomized controlled trial; T2DM: Type 2 diabetes mellitus

Acknowledgements

Thanks to all the patients, GPs and municipal health professionals who provided valuable input to the development of the intervention. Also thanks to the steering committee members whose contribution to the realisation of the study was significant.

Funding

The project has received funding from the Region of Southern Denmark for secretarial support, participatory processes, digital support system and remuneration of the participating GPs; The joint Quality and educational committee (KEU) of the Region of Southern Denmark and the The Organization of general practitioners in Denmark for funding of research work-packages; And The Ministry of Health for testing and evaluation of the digital support system. The funders of the project have no role in the analysis, or interpretation of the data, writing of research papers, or the decision to submit a paper for publication.

Authors' contributions

All authors participate in the design and evaluation of the study. LBL, TT, JLT, AH and JS wrote the study proposal. NCH, TSM, LBP, PVP, EAH, LBL, TT and EMR supplied the study with research protocols and conduct the research. LBL, TT and ALS conduct the study and coordinate the evaluation. The manuscript for the study protocol was edited and revised by all authors. All authors read and approved the final manuscript.

Ethics approval and consent to participate

The study adheres to the SPIRIT guidelines and has been approved by the Danish Data Protection Agency (J.nr 2015-57-0008) and registered at Clinical Trial Gov (Unique Protocol ID: TOFpilot2016). According to Danish regulations (Act on Research Ethics Review of Health Research Projects (section 14,2)) this study does not need approval from a health research ethics committee as no research on human tissue or other biological material is performed. The study complies with the Helsinki declaration with informed consent to study participation and to disclosure of data from the GPs EPR obtained from all participants before enrolment. Participants were asked to read the information and electronically sign the consent form that was supplemented with short videos of the principal investigator and a GP describing the purpose of the study and the intervention. Before linking project data and national registers from Statistics Denmark participants will be pseudomized. Data management and data analysis of quantitative data will be performed on secure servers at Statistics Denmark.

Consent for publication

Not applicable.

Competing interests

The authors declare that they have no competing interests.

Author details

[1]Department of Public Health, Research Unit of General Practice, University of Southern Denmark, Odense, Denmark. [2]Department of Clinical Sciences, Center for Primary Health Care Research, Lund University, Lund, Sweden. [3]Department of Informatics, University of Oslo, Oslo, Norway. [4]Department of Business and Economics, COHERE, University of Southern Denmark, Odense, Denmark. [5]Department of Sports Science and Clinical Biomechanics, Research Unit for Musculoskeletal Function and Physiotherapy, University of Southern Denmark, Odense, Denmark. [6]National Institute of Public Health, University of Southern Denmark, Copenhagen, Denmark.

References

1. Eldridge SM, Lancaster GA, Campbell MJ, Thabane L, Hopewell S, Coleman CL, et al. Defining Feasibility and Pilot Studies in Preparation for Randomised Controlled Trials: Development of a Conceptual Framework. PLoS ONE. 2016;11(3). Available from: http://www.ncbi.nlm.nih.gov/pmc/articles/PMC4792418/. [cited 2016 Nov 10].
2. WHO. Global Status on Noncommunicable diseases. Geneva: WHO; 2010.
3. Juel K, Sørensen J, Brønnum-Hansen H. Supplement: risk factors and public health in Denmark. Scand J Public Health. 2008;36(1 suppl):1–227.
4. WHO TRS 916. Diet, Nutrition, and the Prevention of Chronic Diseases. 2003.
5. Glümer C, Hilding-Nørkjær H, Jensen H, Jørgensen T, Andreasen A, Ladelund S. Sundhedsprofil for region og kommuner 2008. Region Hovedstaden: Glostrup; 2008.
6. Shaw JE, Sicree RA, Zimmet PZ. Global estimates of the prevalence of diabetes for 2010 and 2030. Diabetes Res Clin Pract. 2010;87(1):4–14.
7. Yusuf S, Reddy S, Ounpuu S, Anand S. Global burden of cardiovascular diseases: part I: general considerations, the epidemiologic transition, risk factors, and impact of urbanization. Circulation. 2001;104(22):2746–53.

8. NCD Risk Factor Collaboration (NCD-RisC). Trends in adult body-mass index in 200 countries from 1975 to 2014: a pooled analysis of 1698 population-based measurement studies with 19·2 million participants. Lancet 2016; 387(10026):1377–1396.
9. Beaglehole R, Bonita R, Horton R, Adams C, Alleyne G, Asaria P, et al. Priority actions for the non-communicable disease crisis. Lancet. 2011;377(9775):1438–47.
10. The Role of General Practitioners in Preventing disease and promoting health in the Nordic countries [Internet]. Nordic Federation of General Practice; 2013. Available from: http://www.nfgp.org/files/8/policypaper_preventing_2.pdf. [cited 2016 Nov 6]
11. Si S, Moss JR, Sullivan TR, Newton SS, Stocks NP. Effectiveness of general practice-based health checks: a systematic review and meta-analysis. Br J Gen Pract. 2014;64(618):e47–53.
12. den Engelsen C, Koekkoek PS, Godefrooij MB, Spigt MG, Rutten GE. Screening for increased cardiometabolic risk in primary care: a systematic review. Br J Gen Pract. 2014;64(627):e616–26.
13. Jørgensen T, Jacobsen RK, Toft U, Aadahl M, Glümer C, Pisinger C. Effect of screening and lifestyle counselling on incidence of ischaemic heart disease in general population: Inter99 randomised trial. BMJ. 2014;348:g3617.
14. Krogsbøll LT, Jørgensen KJ, Grønhøj Larsen C, Gøtzsche PC. General health checks in adults for reducing morbidity and mortality from disease: Cochrane systematic review and meta-analysis. BMJ. 2012;345:e7191.
15. Dyakova M, Shantikumar S, Colquitt JL, Drew CM, Sime M, MacIver J, et al. Systematic versus opportunistic risk assessment for the primary prevention of cardiovascular disease. Cochrane Database Syst Rev. 2016;1:CD010411.
16. Badenbroek IF, Stol DM, Nielen MM, Hollander M, Kraaijenhagen RA, de Wit GA, et al. Design of the INTEGRATE study: effectiveness and cost-effectiveness of a cardiometabolic risk assessment and treatment program integrated in primary care. BMC Fam Pract. 2014;15:90.
17. Marshall T, Caley M, Hemming K, Gill P, Gale N, Jolly K. Mixed methods evaluation of targeted case finding for cardiovascular disease prevention using a stepped wedged cluster RCT. BMC Public Health. 2012;12:908.
18. Andersen JH, Thorsen T, Kousgaard MB. Samarbejde mellem kommuner og almen praksis om henvisning til kommunale sundhedstilbud for patienter med kroniske sygdomme [Internet]. København: Forskningsenheden for almen praksis; 2014. Available from: http://patientuddannelse.info/media/95449/samarbejde_mellem_almen_praksis_og_kommuner.pdf. [cited 2016 Oct 20]
19. Helbech hansen B. Omfanget af henvisninger fra alment praktiserende læger til kommunale sundheds- og forebyggelsestilbud [Internet]. København: Kommunernes Landsforening; 2015. Available from: http://www.kl.dk/ImageVaultFiles/id_74921/cf_202/Henvisninger_fra_almen_praktiserende_l-ger_til_kom.PDF. [cited 2016 Oct 20]
20. Porterfield DS, Hinnant LW, Kane H, Horne J, McAleer K, Roussel A. Linkages between clinical practices and community organizations for prevention: a literature review and environmental scan. Am J Public Health. 2012 Jun; 102(Suppl 3):S375–82.
21. Krist AH, Shenson D, Woolf SH, Bradley C, Liaw WR, Rothemich SF, et al. Clinical and community delivery Systems for Preventive Care. Am J Prev Med. 2013 Oct 1;45(4):508–16.
22. Bruun Larsen L, Soendergaard J, Halling A, Thilsing T, Thomsen JL. A novel approach to population-based risk stratification, comprising individualized lifestyle intervention in Danish general practice to prevent chronic diseases: Results from a feasibility study. Health Informatics J. 2017;23(4):249–59. https://doi-org.proxy1-bib.sdu.dk/10.1177/1460458216664514.
23. Craig P, Dieppe P, Macintyre S, Michie S, Nazareth I, Petticrew M. Developing and evaluating complex interventions: the new Medical Research Council guidance. BMJ. 2008;337. Available from: http://www.ncbi.nlm.nih.gov/pmc/articles/PMC2769032/. [cited 2014 Jan 16].
24. Pedersen KM, Andersen JS, Søndergaard J. General practice and primary health Care in Denmark. J Am Board Fam Med. 2012;25(Suppl 1):S34–8.
25. Pedersen KM, Søndergaard J. Det samarbejdende hospital: Almen praksis og kommuner. In: Fremtidens Hospital. København: Munksgaard; 2014. p. 115–26.
26. e-boks webpage. URL:http://www.e-boks.dk/default.aspx. Accessed: 2016 Oct 19. (Archived by WebCite® at http://www.webcitation.org/6lN8fheQf).
27. NemID webpage. The Danish Agence for Digitisation. URL:https://www.nemid.nu/dk-en/. Accessed: 2016 Oct 19. (Archived by WebCite® at http://www.webcitation.org/6lN81XyxY).
28. Whitlock E. Evaluating primary care behavioral counseling interventions an evidence-based approach. Am J Prev Med. 2002 May;22(4):267–84.
29. Den motiverende samtale [Internet]. Dansk selskab for almen medicin; 1999. Available from: http://www.dsam.dk/files/9/den_motiverende_samtale_1999.pdf. [cited 2014 Nov 16].
30. Christensen JO, Sandbaek A, Lauritzen T, Borch-Johnsen K. Population-based stepwise screening for unrecognised type 2 diabetes is ineffective in general practice despite reliable algorithms. Diabetologia. 2004;47(9):1566–73.
31. Martinez FJ, Raczek AE, Seifer FD, Conoscenti CS, Curtice TG, D'Eletto T, et al. Development and initial validation of a self-scored COPD population screener questionnaire (COPD-PS). COPD. 2008;5(2):85–95.
32. European Society of Cardiology. Heartscore webpage. URL: http://www.heartscore.org/en_GB/. Accessed: 2016 Oct 19. (Archived by WebCite® at http://www.webcitation.org/6lN9ncXMD).
33. Svenska Socialstyrelsen. Sjukdomsförebyggande metoder. Vetenskabeligt underlag för nationella riktlinjer. Svenska Socialstyrelsen; 2011.
34. Schneider F, van Osch L, de Vries H. Identifying factors for optimal development of health-related websites: a Delphi study among experts and potential future users. J Med Internet Res. 2012;14(1):e18.
35. Krist AH, Woolf SH. A vision for patient-centered health information systems. JAMA. 2011;305(3):300–1.
36. Krist AH, Beasley JW, Crosson JC, Kibbe DC, Klinkman MS, Lehmann CU, et al. Electronic health record functionality needed to better support primary care. J Am Med Inform Assoc. 2014;21(5):764–71.
37. sundhed.dk webpage. URL: https://www.sundhed.dk/. Accessed: 2016 Oct 19. (Archived by WebCite® at http://www.webcitation.org/710tT6aOg).
38. Murray J, Craigs CL, Hill KM, Honey S, House A. A systematic review of patient reported factors associated with uptake and completion of cardiovascular lifestyle behaviour change. BMC Cardiovasc Disord. 2012;12:120.
39. Murray J, Honey S, Hill K, Craigs C, House A. Individual influences on lifestyle change to reduce vascular risk: a qualitative literature review. Br J Gen Pract J R Coll Gen Pract. 2012;62(599):e403–10.
40. Murray J, Fenton G, Honey S, Bara AC, Hill KM, House A. A qualitative synthesis of factors influencing maintenance of lifestyle behaviour change in individuals with high cardiovascular risk. BMC Cardiovasc Disord. 2013;13:48.
41. Olsen LR, Jensen DV, Noerholm V, Martiny K, Bech P. The internal and external validity of the major depression inventory in measuring severity of depressive states. Psychol Med. 2003;33(2):351–6.
42. Topp CW, Østergaard SD, Søndergaard S, Bech P. The WHO-5 well-being index: a systematic review of the literature. Psychother Psychosom. 2015; 84(3):167–76.
43. Van der Meer V, Nielen MM, Drenthen AJ, Van Vliet M, Assendelft WJ, Schellevis FG. Cardiometabolic prevention consultation in the Netherlands: screening uptake and detection of cardiometabolic risk factors and diseases - a pilot study. BMC Fam Pract. 2013;14:29.
44. Thygesen LC, Daasnes C, Thaulow I, Brønnum-Hansen H. Introduction to Danish (nationwide) registers on health and social issues: structure, access, legislation, and archiving. Scand J Public Health. 2011;39(7 suppl):12–6.
45. What are the equivalence scales [Internet]. OECD Project on Income Distribution and Poverty. Available from: http://www.oecd.org/els/soc/OECD-Note-EquivalenceScales.pdf. [cited 2016 Mar 23].
46. Schmidt M, Schmidt SAJ, Sandegaard JL, Ehrenstein V, Pedersen L, Sørensen HT. The Danish National Patient Registry: a review of content, data quality, and research potential. Clin Epidemiol. 2015;7:449–90.
47. Pottegård A, Schmidt SAJ, Wallach-Kildemoes H, Sørensen HT, Hallas J, Schmidt M. Data resource profile: the Danish National Prescription Registry. Int J Epidemiol. 2017;46(3):798–798f. https://doi.org/10.1093/ije/dyw213.
48. Bender AM, Kawachi I, Jørgensen T, Pisinger C. Neighborhood deprivation is strongly associated with participation in a population-based health check. PLoS One. 2015;10(6):e0129819.
49. Levati S, Campbell P, Frost R, Dougall N, Wells M, Donaldson C, et al. Optimisation of complex health interventions prior to a randomised controlled trial: a scoping review of strategies used. Pilot Feasibility Stud. 2016;2:17.
50. Bowen DJ, Kreuter M, Spring B, Cofta-Woerpel L, Linnan L, Weiner D, et al. How we design feasibility studies. Am J Prev Med. 2009;36(5):452–7.
51. Hargreaves JR, Copas AJ, Beard E, Osrin D, Lewis JJ, Davey C, et al. Five questions to consider before conducting a stepped wedge trial. Trials. 2015; 16:350.
52. Copas AJ, Lewis JJ, Thompson JA, Davey C, Baio G, Hargreaves JR. Designing a stepped wedge trial: three main designs, carry-over effects and randomisation approaches. Trials. 2015;16:352.

Implementing telemonitoring in primary care: learning from a large qualitative dataset gathered during a series of studies

Janet Hanley[1*], Hilary Pinnock[2], Mary Paterson[3] and Brian McKinstry[3]

Abstract

Background: Telemonitoring for long term conditions such as hypertension and diabetes has not been widely adopted despite evidence of efficacy in trials and policy support. The Telescot programme comprised a series of seven trials and observational studies of telemonitoring for long term conditions in primary care, all with an explanatory qualitative component which had been analysed and published separately. There were changes to the models of care within and between studies and combining datasets would provide a longitudinal view of the evolution of primary care based telemonitoring services that was not available in the individual studies, as well as allowing comparison across the different conditions monitored. We aimed to explore what drove changes to the way telemonitoring was implemented, compare experience of telemonitoring across the range of long term conditions, and identify what issues, in the experience of the participants, need to be considered in implementing new telemonitoring systems.

Method: Synthesis and thematic reanalysis of transcribed qualitative interview and focus group data from the Telescot programme adopting an interpretive description approach. All transcribed and coded text was re-read and data relating to the experience of the telemonitoring services, perceptions of future use and strategies for implementation were recoded into one consistent system. This was analysed thematically.

Results: The combined dataset contained transcribed qualitative interview and focus group data from 181 patients and 109 professionals. Four major themes were identified, using data, empowering patients, adjusting the model of care and system design.

Conclusion: Telemonitoring was valued by patients who found it empowering and convenient. This, combined with initial professional concern that increased surveillance may create dependency led to the development of a more patient led service. However, despite a number of initial concerns being addressed as the service evolved, primary care professionals identified a number of barriers to widespread routine adoption of telemonitoring, many of which could be addressed by improved system design.

Keywords: Qualitative research, E-health, Primary care, Telemonitoring, Diabetes, Chronic Obstructive Pulmonary Disease (COPD), Hypertension

* Correspondence: j.hanley@napier.ac.uk
[1]School of Health and Social Care, Edinburgh Napier University, Sighthill Campus, Sighthill Court, Edinburgh EH11 4BN, UK
Full list of author information is available at the end of the article

Background

Home telemonitoring in long term conditions has been defined as *"an automated process for the transmission of data on a patient's health status from home to the respective health care setting."* [1]. The potential for telemonitoring to improve the management of long term conditions such as hypertension, diabetes, heart failure and chronic obstructive pulmonary disease (COPD) by enabling more frequent measurement of key parameters without the need to visit healthcare premises seems logical. However so far, despite strategy documents advocating its use [2, 3] and numerous pilot studies, this form of telemonitoring has not been widely adopted [4]. Randomised controlled trials (RCTs) have had mixed outcomes [5], although the positive effect of blood pressure (BP) telemonitoring is now firmly established [5–7]. In contrast to the low uptake of telemonitoring by healthcare services, there is public demand for increased monitoring in long term conditions with a profusion of apps available for recording home measured health data. The experience of those taking part in telemonitoring trials (both patients and professionals) could provide valuable guidance in developing effective telemonitoring services which would be widely adopted. This paper reports an analysis of combined qualitative data from the Telescot series of seven primary care based telemonitoring studies [8–14] carried out between 2009 and 2014 mainly in Scotland.

Table 1 summarises the trials and observational studies in hypertension, COPD, heart failure and type 2 diabetes in the programme, all of which were analysed and published as separate entities [8–17]. All studies had a qualitative component [8–14]. Because it was a series of studies rather than one large implementation of telemonitoring, the models of care were flexible and their evolution was observed both within and between studies. The combined dataset therefore provides a longitudinal view of the evolution of primary care based telemonitoring services that was not available in the individual studies, as well as allowing comparison across the different conditions monitored. The consistent aspect of the telemonitoring services were that home monitored data were shared with the healthcare practitioner. The main evolving aspect of the services was increasing patient responsibility for acting on the home monitored data and reducing professional responsibility from constant surveillance of the data to periodic review unless contacted by the patient.

The evolution of services is important. A number of intermediate level theoretical frameworks have been used to understand the dynamics and process of introducing new technologies into healthcare with the most frequently used being normalisation process theory with its important concept of 'fit' of the new technologies [18] and the diffusion of innovations [19]. Both these models highlight that ongoing use is unlikely if there is insufficient flexibility to enable new systems and care models to be adapted to meet the needs and expectations of the both patient and healthcare professional users (which in themselves will evolve as they become familiar with the technologies).

The experience of participants in trials and pilot studies can identify and illuminate the complexities and unexpected consequences surrounding home telemonitoring and guide decision making about future implementation. We therefore synthesised and re-analysed the qualitative data from all these studies with the aim of exploring what drove the changes in the way telemonitoring was implemented, comparing experience of telemonitoring across

Table 1 The Telescot studies

	Telemonitoring Study	Design	Number in RCT	Primary Outcome	Patients interviewed	Healthcare providers interviewed
1.	COPD telemonitoring pilot [8]	Observational and qualitative study (27 participants). Monitoring symptoms, O2 saturation and FEV1)			20	25
2.	BP Telemonitoring trial (HITS) [9, 15]	RCT of BP telemonitoring with nested qualitative study	401	Systolic BP significantly lower in intervention group	25	20
3.	BP after stroke pilot trial [10]	Pilot trial of BP telemonitoring plus qualitative study	55		16 (plus 23 in 3 focus groups)	4
4.	COPD Trial [12, 16]	RCT of COPD telemonitoring with qualitative evaluation	256	No difference in days to first hospital admission	38	31
5.	Heart Failure [11]	Qualitative study			18	5
6.	Diabetes trial [13, 17]	RCT of blood glucose and BP telemonitoring with qualitative evaluation	321	HbA1c and systolic BP significantly lower in intervention group	23	10
7.	COPD "light touch" [14]	Observational and qualitative study (51 participants)			20	14 (8 in focus group)

the range of long term conditions, and identifying what issues, in the experience of the participants, need to be considered in implementing new telemonitoring systems.

Methods

Context

Details of seven qualitative studies within the Telescot programme are shown in Table 1.

All the studies had been approved via the UK national research ethics service (references 12/EM/0359, 11/S1102/23, 10/S1102/160, 08/S1101/34, 08/S1101/38, 08/S1101/60) and participants gave specific written consent to the qualitative component [8–14]. This combined and comparative reanalysis of the qualitative data was carried out by the core research team for all these studies with no external transfer of data and was within the scope of the initial ethical approvals. The qualitative studies were all embedded in trials or observational studies gathering quantitative usage and outcome data except study 5 (heart failure) which was purely qualitative. In studies 1–6 telemonitoring was based on a surveillance model where the patient took their readings at agreed intervals and these were regularly reviewed by professionals (daily for COPD and heart failure, weekly- fortnightly for hypertension and type 2 diabetes). The professionals interpreted the data and contacted the patient if there were any concerns. In study1 (COPD pilot study) a call centre acted as an intermediary between the patient and their primary care practice and reviewing readings daily and contacting both the patient and practice according to a protocol if they breached any limits. (In this study healthcare professionals also initially had an associated advisory treatment protocol linked to the patient monitored parameters but this was dropped within a few weeks due to concerns that it would lead to overtreatment). In all other studies, the patients' own doctor, nurse or therapist reviewed patient readings (only on request in study 7). The telemonitoring systems varied. The system used in the first two COPD (studies 1 and 4) and the heart failure studies (Study 5) as well as transmitting readings provided the patient with PC based educational material but no on-going record of their readings. In the hypertension and type 2 diabetes studies (studies 2,3 &6) readings were transmitted via Bluetooth/ mobile phone and patients had access to a web portal where they could view a record of their readings. The system also provided simple automated feedback via SMS text or email, but did not provide any educational material. In the final COPD study (Study 7) a much more patient-led approach was adopted and the professionals did not review the patients' data unless the patient contacted them via a hotline and asked for advice. Due to technical issues patients initially kept a paper record of their readings which some opted to continue when the SMS based system became available. The professional interface for all systems required logging on to a separate system where readings submitted by all their patients could be reviewed.

Qualitative approach

An interpretive description approach was adopted for qualitative studies throughout the programme [20]. This adopts a constructivist approach to knowledge using rigorous methods employed in more traditional approaches to qualitative research, but acknowledges that the purpose of the researcher is to gain insight which will be of use in a clinical context.

Data collection

Qualitative data were gathered by JU, PF and SL (one male and one female social science researchers, one female nurse researcher, all educated to masters or doctoral level and previously unknown to the interviewee), through audio recorded semi structured face to face or telephone interviews and focus groups with patients, healthcare professionals and other stakeholders involved in the studies between 2009 and 2014. These were transcribed verbatim. Patients had been sampled purposively from participants in the associated trial or observational study to gain a maximum variation sample based on age, sex and location and all signed an additional consent for the qualitative study. In all cases the purpose of the interviews was stated as being to elicit the individuals' experiences and opinions about telemonitoring and interviewees were aware that the interviewer was not involved in either providing the service or collecting quantitative outcome data. Full details about recruitment can be found in relevant papers [8–14]. Each qualitative dataset had been inductively coded by the relevant researcher using constant comparison to ensure consistency, with review by the full research team, and where possible by participants, to ensure viewpoints have been accurately represented. However, there had been no attempt to match coding frames across the different studies.

These data were anonymised and combined to form the dataset for this analysis. Four interviews with nurses involved in study 3 that had not previously been analysed were added to the dataset.

Data synthesis and analysis

All transcribed and coded text was re-read and data relating to the experience of the telemonitoring services, perceptions of future use and strategies for implementation were recoded into one consistent system. Data relating to trial management issues or specific obsolete hardware were excluded. However data relating to software and hardware design which may be relevant to future systems were included. The initial re-reading and development of provisional codes was done on paper. Subsequently the recoded data were extracted from electronic (word) versions of the documents into tables. Steps to ensure this was a rigorous process included constant comparison and search for negative cases. The recoding was done by JH, and the recoding was reviewed and discussed by BM, HP and MP. Base codes were then grouped into sub themes and themes, again reviewed by the whole research team.

Data saturation, defined as no new themes or ideas arising in consecutive interviews when the research team were satisfied that a wide range of individuals had been interviewed, had been used to guide sampling in each of the studies (subject to minimum numbers agreed with funders). In this reanalysis of data the researcher re-read all the transcribed data but stopped adding data extracts to the coding frame when numbers became very large, having ensured that a wide range of individuals and all studies were represented.

Having identified the main themes and sub-themes emerging from this large recoded dataset, we mapped the data to Rogers [19] description of the characteristics of an innovation which are likely to lead to its adoption. The purpose of this additional step in the analysis was to illuminate both the aspects of telemonitoring which are likely to drive its adoption (including those which evolved through the series of studies) and those which require attention if they are not to become barriers to future adoption of telemonitoring.

Results

The characteristics of the participants are summarised in Table 2.

The thematic analysis led to four main themes: Data use, empowering patients, adjusting the model of care and system design. These themes and their subthemes are shown in Table 3 and presented below.

Theme 1. Data use

Telemonitoring provides patients and professionals with regular measurements of a range of symptom and physiological parameters. This generates a large volume of data and potential insights into the patient's condition which had not previously been available. However, this series of studies demonstrated variation in the way these measurements were used. Regular home monitored blood pressure (BP) readings were useful to both patients and professionals who considered that they provided a more reliable assessment than BP measured occasionally in the surgery. Importantly they provided a trusted basis for treatment change which previously may have been delayed because of concerns about the representativeness of surgery based measurement.

> *[prior to telemonitoring] ... We're all guilty of it...'we'll just see how it goes, you know, maybe watch it. I'll check it again tomorrow' and they probably maybe sit on it a bit longer* (Practice Nurse 9, BP trial)

In contrast, blood glucose data were often not used in the management of type 2 diabetes by the professionals, who used HbA1c measured at surgery-based routine reviews as a basis for care, although there was general agreement that home monitored blood glucose data could be useful when medication changes were being considered or had been initiated. Blood glucose data was seen to be of greater use to the patients in guiding their day-to-day self-management of the condition. Regular data sharing had a motivating effect on patients in relation to diet and medication adherence, as they were aware that at some point the readings may be reviewed.

> *But knowing that everything's going to be looked at on a regular basis by somebody else, it's actually, it's not bad to have a policeman somewhere ....* (Patient 6, Diabetes trial)

Table 2 Characteristics of participants in the qualitative studies

Study	Patients		Professionals (number)			
	Mean age of patients	Proportion of male patients	Doctors (all general practitioners (GPs) except where stated)	Nurses	Therapists	Managers and Administrators
COPD pilot [8]	68	59%	4	6	3	12
BP trial [9]	61	60%	9	11		
BP after stroke pilot trial [10]	66	75%		4		
COPD Trial [11]	68	47%	3 GPs, 1 respiratory specialist	9	6	12
Heart Failure [12]	75	61%	1	4		
Diabetes trial [13]	60	65%	4	6		
COPD "light touch" [14]	67	50%		3	5	6

Table 3 Themes and sub themes

Theme	Associated sub themes
Using data	BP data • Measurement more trusted than surgery measurement • Patients and professionals confident to use as a basis for treatment change Blood sugar data • Not used by all professionals, some waited for HbA1c • Useful when treatment change contemplated • Sharing data motivated patients – diet and medication COPD data (O_2 saturation, symptoms, FEV_1) • Not discriminatory for severe exacerbation/ lots of false alarms • Complex, need to know the patient – can change fast • Overtreatment • Other symptoms Patients use of data • Previously not told their readings. • Understanding their normal • Reduced dependency on readings • Data providing motivation • Sharing data motivated patients • Not willing to keep manual record of self monitoring
Empowering patients	• Empowering patients o Use shared readings to actively negotiate care o Self management and reassurance • Confidence - patients/ families o Reassurance o Guardian angel/ access to care • Potential negative effects o Anxiety o Concern about dependency • Valuing convenience
Adjusting the model of care	• Scaling up • Workloads: o Fitting telemonitoring into practice workflows o Increasing or decreasing workloads • Communication channels with patient and within the team • Letting go • 'How does this affect my role?'
System design	• Hardware • Reliability • Professional interface • Easy access via patient records • Easy two way communication • Feedback and decision support

The motivating effect was also seen to some extent with blood pressure readings.

> *When I was taking the blood pressure I couldn't bear looking at 140, 150 over 110 and I wanted to just be able to see better readings in a way. So over the summer as well, starting to get more walking exercise, that kind of thing.... I didn't want beta blockers because they had various side effects ...so it did spur me on to look for alternative...* (Patient 2, BP trial)

The purpose of telemonitoring in COPD was to spot signs of impending exacerbations and intervene early. In practice the data were difficult to interpret and staff reported many false positives. Daily monitoring by a professional was not thought to be useful in preventing hospital admission as healthcare staff were not convinced enough was known for clear signals in the data to be recognised.

> *this patient's peak flow's up or down, all this... oxygen saturation might have dropped or increased a little bit, but we are not quite sure what that... means in the clinical context with all the other conditions.* (GP 11, COPD trial)

There was also concern amongst professionals that acting on the additional data provided by telemonitoring could lead to overtreatment. This was mainly seen in COPD although there was also an example relating to blood pressure management.

> *You can't just continually prescribe antibiotics for these people. .... But then if you're scoring 9 - and some of these people can go down SO quickly...* (Practice Nurse 1, COPD pilot study)

> *He was quite surprised when I said "We're aiming for a target here of 130/80." Because his blood pressure readings have been 148/86, which really for most people they would look at that at 92 years old and think that's quite acceptable* (Practice nurse 5, BP following stroke)

Although healthcare staff did not find COPD data particularly useful, patients used their data, particularly oxygen saturation, to guide day-to-day management of their health. Although they found it difficult to tell if changes in their respiratory symptoms were leading to acute exacerbation, the steady oxygen saturation readings and absence of non respiratory symptoms they associated with the onset of an exacerbation (such as sore legs) gave them confidence to go about their normal activities.

> *Sometimes I wouldnae (would not) go out for six or eight weeks. Now I know and I take my reading, I can go out any day I want. I have my confidence back and that is what it's done for me* (Patient 10, light touch telemonitoring)

2. Empowering patients

Overall, generating and recording the telemonitoring data empowered patients. They now had information about their health which previously had been in the domain of the healthcare providers and frequently had not previously been shared with them. They felt more able to participate actively in consultations and manage their own health.

It's certainly given me more meaningful data to speak to the doctor rather than, "Well, I think my BP has probably gone up." (Patient 6, BP trial)

He's more aware of his symptoms. He understands when he should be seeking help, so he's not just tending to phone up every time that he gets a cough or a bit more breathless because, unless he's got all the symptoms, that's when he would contact us. So it's helped him to manage his own condition better (Nurse 17, COPD trial)

Most patients found the ability to take their own readings reassuring, particularly when they were normal and, as noted above, for some it increased their confidence. Another source of confidence, particularly for those with COPD, was that the telemonitoring data enabled them to negotiate prompt access to care. The convenience of taking readings at home, particularly blood pressure readings, was also highly valued.

For me personally just taking it in the house, rather than go up there and sit with the coughs and splutters (patient 1, BP following stroke study)

Some patients felt empowered to take a more proactive approach to their health care based on their readings and made appointments rather than waiting for professionals to contact them, if necessary circumventing the supporting advice services. For example, if patients felt they needed a new prescription and thought the nurse or therapist who managed their telemonitoring data could not prescribe, they would go directly to a GP. On occasions, this disrupted the usual workflows and communication channels within the practice, and illustrated the need for telemonitoring data to be easily available with the medical records.

... so I'm not even going to bother with her [member of respiratory team], ... I'll just use the wee oxygen monitor and just use it every day,... if it goes below two for two or three days, then I know to go along to the doctor. (Patient 7, COPD light touch study)

However, although many patients described taking a proactive approach to their long term condition, occasional review of the data by a healthcare professional was appreciated, particularly when blood pressure or blood glucose readings were in the normal range but could be better.

And then I was getting higher readings, and I thought... I thought, 'Oh well somebody's monitoring it. If there's something dangerous, somebody's going to tell me.' I hope! (Patient 28, diabetes trial)

All patients taking part in these studies were eligible because their condition was sub-optimally controlled, but as control improved they tended to reduce the frequency of their readings. This was particularly noticeable in the 'light touch' COPD telemonitoring where people tended to monitor until they recognised their usual pattern of measurements and then stopped until they felt something was wrong.

Although most patients were empowered and reassured by telemonitoring, a very small number were made anxious by it. Of all the patients interviewed, only one reported increased anxiety, but several professionals commented on this possibility. Across all the early studies, professionals were concerned that the surveillance model of care, in which professionals reviewed and interpreted the submitted data, would lead to anxious patients becoming dependent.

...they like it because they're getting somebody that's looking at their symptoms every day of the week... And that's why we need to be careful over this group of patients who are already quite anxious anyway, I think we're making a dependency (Therapist 8, COPD trial)

The model of care used in the final study (study 7) where the monitoring data provided by COPD patients was only viewed if the patients were concerned and contacted the helpline addressed the concerns about dependency.

Theme 3. Adjusting the model of care

This theme was generated largely by the professionals and service providers interviewed. Many professionals were happy to contribute to research by participating in the trials where only a small proportion of their patients were using telemonitoring but would not have been willing to implement the systems widely until their intertwined concerns about both the care model underpinning telemonitoring and design of telemonitoring systems were addressed. Associated with these were concerns about workloads, workflows and role.

I think at the moment it is totally appropriate for us as practitioners to do [tele-monitoring], but again I think it's because the numbers are manageable. I wonder how it would be if we had 60 or 70 or 80 patients with telehealth ... (nurse 13, COPD trial)

The care model employed in the COPD pilot study which used a call centre to review telemonitoring data was changed in subsequent trials to one where the GP practice or specialist respiratory service was responsible for daily monitoring. Generally this was preferred by many practitioners who felt that it was important to know the patient, although not all thought this essential.

I would probably think it's better done within the practice ... I know you have the team that they can contact, but rather than taking it outwith the practice, I think they're probably more comfortable with the practice itself and the people that they know here. (Practice nurse 9, diabetes trial)

However, as noted above, there was concern that the surveillance model of telemonitoring employed in studies 1–6 could create dependency and professionals taking part in the early trials expressed a preference for a model which shifted responsibility to the patient to a greater extent.

... if your weight goes up, you get these symptoms, you must phone, you have to take responsibility for your health and in one way you're taking that responsibility away from them cause all they've to do is to slap a machine on every day... and not necessarily think about it so much...(Nurse 2, heart failure study)

I think, patients are more and more, you know, will be self-managing,... (Practice nurse 2, diabetes trial)

Professionals were also concerned about workloads. Both patients and professionals thought that in the longer term telemonitoring would reduce the number of visits required but during the trials professionals experienced increased workloads for a number of reasons (except in study 7 where use of the hotline was lower than expected). Professionals, mainly practice nurses, had to find regular time to log into systems to monitor the data across the patient group with the unprocessed stream of raw data taking some time to interpret. This did not fit with their normal workflows where reports relating to individual patients arrived mainly through a single electronic transfer system and could be added to the electronic medical record after review. Some professionals tried to fit logging on to the telemonitoring systems into their normal workload between patients; others put a specific time aside. However these studies took place during a well documented time of increasing pressure on primary care in the UK and finding time to log in and review telemonitoring data became more difficult.

I think we weren't as busy with [previous study] and that's why it didn't feel quite as intense but this time we just haven't had... we have catch up slots and admin time and we're squeezing people into that time, so all of time is just being eaten up by appointments at the minute. (Practice nurse 5 BP following stroke trial)

However, they also found that with experience, and forced by the pressure of work, they were able to reduce the level of supervision and contact with patients without adverse effects.

I was a lot more involved with the patients [in previous study], I seemed to communicate more with patients than I did this time. (Practice nurse 1 BP following stroke trial)

Although there were concerns about the additional workload generated by telemonitoring there was also recognition that there were some elements of personal practice which professionals needed to let go for telemonitoring to make an efficient contribution to care. This included stopping the reliance on clinic measurements and using the patients' self-measurements. For example, in all three studies involving BP monitoring incidents were reported where patients had high self-monitored BP, but treatment decisions had been made on a single measurement taken when they visited the surgery.

...So they're coming in to see the doctor, the doctor takes their BP, one forty five ninety; 'oh, that's fine, what are you worried about?' ... And then you go and you look at it the next week and you think; they've seen the doctor and yet their BP's still really high (Practice Nurse 11 BP study)

On a practical level, this problem was potentially caused by the patients' readings not being available from within the electronic medical record (see data on system design below).

A small number of professionals were concerned that although telemonitoring could potentially reduce primary care workloads it may change individuals' roles in a way they would not like.

It is not my type of medicine I have to say. I don't monitor patients remotely by means of electronic equipment. I would rather actually see a patient, discuss them on telephone, to make a clinical decision about seeing them, assessing, examining them, knowing their history. (GP11, COPD trial)

Reducing the level of face to face contact with the patients was a concern for professionals, but this concern was not universally shared by patients, some of whom experienced the non face to face contact as additional and efficient input.

Theme 4. System design

Contacting patients by phone in relation to their telemonitoring data was found to be very time consuming and the need for agreement about who (professional or patient) should initiate contact if readings were abnormal was raised. Both patients and professionals commented that the telemonitoring systems lacked the ability to send ad hoc messages so there was no easy way of letting patients know that a professional had reviewed and was happy with their data leading to some patients wondering if anyone was looking at their records.

> *I've heard from [healthcare professional's name], a couple of times he has phoned... The first time in response to you having pressed the opposite answer to every morning's answer just to see what would happen. I thought, you know, I'm doing this and I don't know if anybody is looking at it...* (Patient 11, Heart Failure study)

By the final study (study 7) the issues relating to contact had largely been resolved by making patients responsible for initiating contact if they were concerned about their readings and the provision of a telephone hotline.

Another aspect of system design which caused concern was the inability to access the telemonitoring data via the electronic the medical records without a separate log in, which complicated consultations. Unreliable systems, inadequate maintenance of peripherals, poorly designed professional interfaces which were time consuming to navigate, and lack of intelligent decision support also caused frustration.

> *there was a problem with the system. So again that was a time consuming thing that I had to chase up....* (Practice nurse 5, BP following stroke trial)

Although professionals thought that systems could be better designed to fit with their own workflows rather than them adjusting their workflows to the system, some also found that they needed to reconsider how information flowed within the practice to use the patient generated data efficiently and coherently.

Mapping the data to the characteristics of an innovation likely to influence its adoption

The data relating to the experience of patients and professionals in trials of telemonitoring were mapped to Rogers [19] list of characteristics of an innovation likely to influence its adoption (see Table 4). This provided a useful framework for summarising the aspects of telemonitoring which would be likely to encourage its adoption, and those which, based on the experience in these trials, would need careful consideration in any future implementation.

Discussion

This analysis explored the experience of patients and professionals in trials of telemonitoring in the management of a range of long term conditions in primary care in the UK, mainly in Scotland. The additional value of the combined dataset is that provides a longitudinal focus on telemonitoring services which were evolving from trial to trial based on experience in the previous trial.

The experience of implementing telemonitoring for long term conditions challenged the simple model in which the patient takes measurements and shares them telemetrically with the professional who then adjusts treatment based on the readings. Not all data could be used in this way, particularly in COPD where no strong and reliable signal of the early stages of an exacerbation could be identified. However, generating their own measurements empowered patients who used them in managing their health and accessing appropriate healthcare, although they also valued occasional routine review of their data by primary healthcare professionals. Additionally professionals were wary of the initial surveillance model of care which they thought would increase dependency on health services and the evolution of the services was towards a more patient led approach.

Both patients and professionals found it more efficient for telemonitoring to be situated in existing primary care services. However, professionals found that system design limited their ability to integrate telemonitoring into normal primary care workflows and there were concerns from a small number of healthcare professionals that a reduction in face to face contact with the patient would negatively impact on their role. Mapping the experiences of both patients and professionals against the characteristics influencing the adoptability of a technology from the diffusion of innovations model [19] suggest that from the patients' viewpoint adoption of telemonitoring is highly feasible. Challenges relating to the usability of systems by primary care professionals need to be considered if there is to be widespread adoption of telemonitoring in primary care in the UK.

Strengths and limitations

The strengths of this study are that it is based on a large dataset and the themes emerged strongly. The analysis of the combined dataset showed that, apart from a few very condition-specific issues, there was substantial commonality in the experience of telemonitoring across the different conditions and different technologies used. Indeed the technology used to enable the telemonitoring service appeared to be of secondary importance to the redesign of the care model. Although qualitative data is situated in context and not generalisable, the dataset incorporates wide experience of using telemonitoring in long term conditions and the learning is likely to be transferable. However, the studies

Table 4 Mapping to the characteristics of an innovation likely to affect its adoption

Characteristic of the innovation (from Rogers (1995) The diffusion of innovations) [19]	Positive findings from this study	Negative findings from this study
Relative advantage (the perceived efficiencies gained by the innovation relative to current tools or procedures)	• Convenience • Empowerment • Confidence • Motivation • Better measurements • Could potentially reduce workloads	• Anxiety/dependence in small numbers of patients • Professional concerns about creating dependency • Concern about workloads
Complexity/ difficulty to learn	• Most patients found telemonitoring easy	• Professional interfaces complex • No clear signals for professionals in COPD data • Lack of intelligent decision support
Compatibility with the pre-existing system	• Preference for adoption within current system which influenced later implementations	• Lack of fit of professional system interfaces with workflows within practices • Concern about roles
Trialability or testability	• High –particularly for patients	
Potential for reinvention (using the tool for initially unintended purposes)	• Patients used data to manage day to day activity	
Observed effects	• Higher workloads – reduced with learning and external drivers such as pressure on the system. • Patients using data to support self management. • Increased responsibility for the patient in study 7 was acceptable	• Limitations and extra work created by system design • Empowered patients bypassing nurses or therapists, particularly with regard to prescribing

were limited to primary care in the UK (mainly Scotland) and may not reflect responses to telemonitoring in other health care systems. A further limitation is that the interviewees were participating in trials so their exposure to telemonitoring was relatively short term. The semi structured interview guides were designed separately for each study and although similar were not fully consistent across the studies. A strength is that despite this, the themes reported emerged strongly across the studies.

Interpretation in the light of published literature

No comparable qualitative studies based on this level of telemonitoring experience across an evolving telehealth service have been found. The European Union *Renewing Health* project [21] which involved over 7000 patients across Europe gathered qualitative data from patients, and reported a similarly positive response from them. Evaluation of this project was guided by the model for assessment of telemedicine (MAST) framework [22] which does not include healthcare professionals' responses, although one recommendation of the Renewing Health project was that the healthcare professionals viewpoint should be included in MAST. Our findings support this, suggesting that it is the professional experiences of systems which are currently likely to prevent them from being widely adopted. The UK based Whole Systems Demonstrator project included a qualitative study amongst healthcare professionals [23] which reported findings broadly consistent with those reported here, apart from their finding of a much more negative response from GPs. This may have been because in some areas the nurse-led telemonitoring service was separate from the GP practices. The wider literature suggests that grafting a new technology in pilot form to an existing management system seldom produces time savings in the short run [24] and in general needs it to be a good 'fit' with current systems before it is normalised [18]. Greenhalgh [25] warns that forcing professionals to drop their existing routines and adopt new, seemingly more efficient, ones may inadvertently create inefficiency, which was what was reported by the professionals in this study. However, subsequent research within the Telescot programme has suggested that by working with the healthcare professionals it would be possible to develop telemonitoring systems which could be integrated seamlessly within current primary care systems and working practices [26].

Conclusion

This synthesis of the qualitative findings of a series of telehealth studies found that telemonitoring was generally valued by patients with a range of long term conditions who found it to be both empowering and convenient. This, combined with professional concern that the surveillance model of telemonitoring may create dependency led to the development of a more patient led service. In contrast, despite a number of initial concerns being addressed as the service evolved, primary care professionals identified a number of barriers to widespread routine adoption of telemonitoring. In particular professional facing aspects of the systems tested did not fit with General Practice workflows and all were perceived to be excessively time consuming. If the potential benefits of telemonitoring are to be achieved on a widespread basis, system designers and system evaluation must address the needs of both patients and practitioners.

Abbreviations

BP: Blood pressure; COPD: Chronic obstructive pulmonary disease; RCT: Randomised controlled trial

Acknowledgements

The design and implementation of the initial studies was the responsibility of the Telescot grantholders who, in addition to BM, JH and HP, were Sarah Wild, John McKnight, Paul Padfield, William McNee, Aziz Sheikh, Claudia Pagliari, Jim Forrest and Steff Lewis, with support from Lucy McCloughan and MP. The interview data were gathered and initially coded by Jenny Ure, Peter Fairbrother and Siew Hwa Lee.

Funding

Funding for the initial studies was provided by BUPA Foundation, Chief Scientist Office, Scottish Centre for Telhealth and Telecare, NHS Lothian and Edinburgh and Lothian Health Foundation. The views expressed in this paper are those of the authors and not necessarily those of the funders.

Authors' contributions

JH analysed the combined dataset and led the drafting this paper. HP, BM and MP contributed to the detailed coding checks. All authors commented on drafts and contributed to revisions. All authors read and approved the final manuscript.

Consent for publication

Not applicable

Competing interests

JH is an associate editor for BMC Family Practice. No other competing interests.

Author details

[1]School of Health and Social Care, Edinburgh Napier University, Sighthill Campus, Sighthill Court, Edinburgh EH11 4BN, UK. [2]Allergy and Respiratory Research Group, Usher Institute of Population Health Sciences and Informatics, University of Edinburgh, Teviot Place, Edinburgh EH8 9AG, UK. [3]E-Health Research Group, Usher Institute of Population Health Sciences and Informatics, University of Edinburgh, Nine Edinburgh BioQuarter, Edinburgh EH16 4UX, UK.

References

1. Paré G, Jaana M, Sicotte C. Systematic review of home telemonitoring for chronic diseases: the evidence base. J Am Med Inform Assoc. 2007;14(3):269–77.
2. NHS Scotland: eHealth Strategy 2014–2017. http://www.gov.scot/Publications/2015/03/5705/downloads Accessed 11 Jul 2017.
3. European Commission Information Society. European countries on their journey towards national eHealth infrastructures: Final European progress report 2011. http://www.ehealth-strategies.eu/report/eHealth_Strategies_Final_Report_Web.pdf Accessed 11 Jul 2017.
4. Zanaboni P, Wootton R. Adoption of telemedicine: from pilot stage to routine delivery. BMC Med Inform Decis Mak. 2012;12:1. https://doi.org/10.1186/1472-6947-12-1.
5. Hanlon P, Daines L, Campbell C, McKinstry B, Weller D, Pinnock H. Telehealth interventions to support self-Management of Long-Term Conditions: a systematic Metareview of diabetes, heart failure, asthma, chronic obstructive pulmonary disease and cancer. J Med Internet Res. 2017;19(5):e172.
6. Agarwal R, Bills JE, Hecht TJ, Light RP. Role of home blood pressure monitoring in overcoming therapeutic inertia and improving hypertension control. A systematic review and meta-analysis. Hypertension. 2011;57:29–38.
7. Omboni S. Clinical usefulness and cost effectiveness of home BP telemonitoring: meta-analysis of randomized controlled studies. J Hypertens. 2013;31(3):455–67.
8. Ure J, Hanley J, Pinnock H, Pagliari C, Kidd G, Sheikh A, et al. Piloting telemonitoring in COPD: a qualitative exploration of issues in design and implementation for research and service development. Prim Care Respir J. 2012;21(1):57–64. https://doi.org/10.4104/pcrj.2011.00065
9. Hanley J, Ure J, Pagliari C, Sheikh A, McKinstry B. Experiences of patients and professionals participating in the HITS home blood pressure telemonitoring trial: a qualitative study. BMJ Open. 2013;3:e002671. https://doi.org/10.1136/bmjopen-2013-002671.
10. Hanley J, Fairbrother P, Krishan A, McCloughan L, Padfield P, Paterson M, et al. Mixed methods feasibility study for a trial of blood pressure telemonitoring for people who have had stroke/transient ischaemic attack. (TIA). Trials. 2015;16:117. https://doi.org/10.1186/s13063-015-0628-y.
11. Fairbrother P, Ure J, Hanley J, McCloughan L, Denvir M, Sheikh A, et al. Telemonitoring for chronic heart failure: the views of patients and healthcare professionals – a qualitative study. J Clin Nurs. 2014;23:132–44. https://doi.org/10.1111/jocn.12137.
12. Fairbrother P, Pinnock H, Hanley J, McCloughan L, Sheikh A, Pagliari C, et al. Exploring telemonitoring and self-management by patients with chronic obstructive pulmonary disease: a qualitative study embedded in a randomized controlled trial. Patient Educ Couns. 2013;93(3):403–10.
13. Hanley J, Fairbrother P, McCloughan L, Pagliari C, Paterson M, Pinnock H, et al. Qualitative study of telemonitoring of blood glucose and blood pressure in type 2 diabetes. BMJ Open. 2015;5:e008896. https://doi.org/10.1136/bmjopen-2015-008896.
14. MacNab M, Lee SH, McCloughan L, Hanley J, McKinstry B, Pinnock H. Oximetry-supported self-management for chronic obstructive pulmonary disease: mixed method feasibility pilot project. BMC Health Serv Res. 2015;15:485. https://doi.org/10.1186/s12913-015-1135-2.
15. McKinstry B, Hanley J, Wild S, Pagliari C, Paterson M, Lewis S, et al. Telemonitoring based service redesign for the management of uncontrolled hypertension: multicentre randomised controlled trial. BMJ. 2013;346:f3030. https://doi.org/10.1136/bmj.f3030.
16. Pinnock H, Hanley J, McCloughan L, Todd A, Krishan A, Lewis S, et al. Effectiveness of telemonitoring integrated into existing clinical services on hospital admission for exacerbation of chronic obstructive pulmonary disease: researcher blind, multicentre, randomised controlled trial. BMJ. 2013;347:f6070. https://doi.org/10.1136/bmj.f6070.
17. Wild SH, Hanley J, Lewis SC, McKnight JA, McCloughan LB, Padfield P, et al. Supported Telemonitoring and Glycaemic control in people with type 2 diabetes: the Telescot diabetes pragmatic multicenter randomized controlled trial. PLoS Med. 2016;13(07):e1002098. https://doi.org/10.1371/journal.pmed.1002098.
18. May C, Finch TL, Cornford J, Exley C, Gately C, Kirk S, et al. Integrating telecare for chronic disease management in the community: what needs to be done? BMC Health Serv Res. 2011;11:131. https://doi.org/10.1186/1472-6963-11-131.
19. Rogers EM. Diffusion of innovations. 5th ed. New York: Simon and Schuster; 2003.
20. Thorne S. Interpretive Description. New York: Routledge; 2008.
21. Renewing Health Deliverable D1.12 Final report 2014. http://www.renewinghealth.eu/documents/28946/1008625/D1.12+v1.5+Renewing+Health+Final+Project+Report+-+Public.pdf / Accessed 11 Jul 2017.
22. Kidholm K, Ekeland AG, Jensen LK, Rasmussen J, Pedersen CD, Bowes A, et al. A model for the assessment of telemedicine applications: MAST. Int J Technol Assess Health Care. 2012;28(1):44–51.
23. MacNeill V, Sanders C, Fitzpatrick R, Hendy J, Barlow J, Knapp M, et al. Experiences of front line professionals in the delivery of telehealth: a qualitative study. Br J Gen Pract. 2014;64(624):e401–7. https://doi.org/10.
24. Leonard KJ. Critical factors to healthcare's adoption of new technology: a guide to increasing the likelihood of successful implementation. Electron Healthc. 2004;2:72–81.
25. Greenhalgh P. Role of routines in collaborative work in healthcare organisations. BMJ. 2008;337:a2448.
26. Davidson E, Simpson CR, Demiris G, Sheikh A, McKinstry B. Integrating telehealth care-generated data with the family practice electronic medical record: qualitative exploration of the views of primary care staff. Interact J Med Res. 2013;2(2):e29. https://doi.org/10.2196/ijmr.2820.

Development of an evidence-based brief 'talking' intervention for non-responders to bowel screening for use in primary care: stakeholder interviews

Debbie Cavers[1*], Natalia Calanzani[1], Sheina Orbell[2], Gabriele Vojt[3], Robert J. C. Steele[4], Linda Brownlee[5], Steve Smith[6], Julietta Patnick[7], David Weller[1] and Christine Campbell[1]

Abstract

Background: Bowel cancer is the third most common cause of cancer death worldwide. Bowel screening has been shown to reduce mortality and primary care interventions have been successful in increasing uptake of screening. Using evidence-based theory to inform the development of such interventions has been shown to increase their effectiveness. This study aimed to develop and refine a brief evidence-based intervention for eligible individuals whom have not responded to their last bowel screening invitation (non-responders), for opportunistic use by primary care providers during routine consultations.

Methods: The development of a brief intervention involving a conversation between primary care providers and non-responders was informed by a multi-faceted model comprising: research team workshop and meetings to draw on expertise; evidence from the literature regarding barriers to bowel screening and effective strategies to promote informed participation; relevant psychological theory, and intervention development and behaviour change guidance. Qualitative telephone interviews with 1) bowel screening stakeholders and 2) patient non-responders explored views regarding the acceptability of the intervention to help refine its content and process.

Results: The intervention provides a theory and evidence-based tool designed to be incorporated within current primary care practice. Bowel screening stakeholders were supportive of the intervention and recognised the importance of the role of primary care. Interviews highlighted the importance of brevity and simplicity to incorporate the intervention into routine clinical care. Non-responders similarly found the intervention acceptable, valuing a holistic approach to their care. Moreover, they expected their primary care provider to encourage participation.

Conclusions: A theory-based brief conversation for use in a primary care consultation was acceptable to bowel screening stakeholders and potential recipients, reflecting a health promoting primary care ethos. Findings indicate that it is appropriate to test the intervention in primary care in a feasibility study.

Keywords: Cancer, Primary care, Behaviour change, Bowel screening, Intervention

* Correspondence: debbie.cavers@ed.ac.uk
[1]The Usher Institute of Population Health Sciences and Informatics, Medical School, University of Edinburgh, Doorway 1, Teviot Place, Edinburgh EH8 9AG, UK
Full list of author information is available at the end of the article

Background

Bowel cancer is an important public health issue; it is the third most common cancer and the fourth most common cause of cancer death worldwide [1]. Screening has been shown to reduce bowel cancer mortality, but high levels of participation are required [2]. In Europe, national screening programmes are still being implemented across all EU member states following European Council recommendations for consistency in coverage and the type of test used [3]. In the UK, a rolled-out national programme in all constituent countries has been delivered centrally via regional hubs since 2010, where a guaiac-based Faecal Occult Blood test (FOBt) is sent by post to eligible patients (those aged 60–74 years; 50–74 in Scotland) every two years [4]. Overall participation is currently 57.5% (45.1% vs 66.5% for the most deprived and least deprived groups respectively) [5].

Policy initiatives in the UK have focused on the prevention and early detection of cancer (including screening and early diagnosis) in order to reduce overall mortality [6, 7]. Although bowel screening kits are sent straight from the regional hubs, and therefore primary care has no direct involvement in the delivery of bowel screening, there is increasing recognition that primary care is well placed to mediate between bowel screening programmes and the public [8]. As such, general practices are provided with a regular list of non-responders and, in Scotland, have been financially incentivised to increase bowel screening participation among their patients [9]. In this context, a number of bowel screening interventions have been trialed [10]. Interventions shown to be successful in increasing uptake include those using patient reminder letters [11] and General Practitioner (GP) endorsements of patient invitation letters [12]. Brief interventions have been effective in relation to alcohol consumption and smoking cessation in primary care [13, 14], but less is known about their use in relation to the topic of bowel screening.

We aimed to develop and refine a theory-driven brief 'talking' intervention for opportunistic use in primary care consultations with non-responders to bowel screening. The use of robust theories enhances intervention implementation and evaluation, helping to determine why an intervention was (or was not) effective [15] – indeed, theory-driven interventions have been tested widely in the field of screening, including strategies to increase bowel screening uptake [16, 17]. In this paper we describe the process of developing the brief intervention and a preliminary evaluation of its content and acceptability using qualitative interviews with bowel screening stakeholders and bowel screening non-responders.

Methods

Developing the Brief Intervention

The development process to design a theory-driven conversation between a primary care provider (PCP) and their eligible patient (a non-responder to their last bowel screening invitation) is illustrated by the flowchart (Fig. 1). Initially, relevant motivational and behavioural targets were identified based on our previous work on bowel screening interventions [18]. Existing evidence on factors associated with screening participation and effective strategies to improve participation was incorporated [10, 19]. The intervention drew on a variety of theoretical frameworks and relevant guidance. The second stage involved a workshop to develop supporting materials and identify implementation challenges. This included the identification of barriers or 'bottlenecks' when implementing each stage of the intervention such as the primary care provider having too many issues to deal with, the patient not being receptive to the intervention or the patient requesting a new kit but not ultimately completing it (Additional file 1: Intervention bottlenecks). Feedback on the draft materials was then requested from the Scottish Bowel Screening Centre (SBSC) and used to finalise them.

Theoretical underpinnings

In developing our intervention we sought to draw on psychological theories commonly utilised in screening studies that target the active components of behaviour change. This approach allows an understanding of the barriers and incentives to changing behaviour; it can guide analysis, and it offers a consistent and transparent implementation framework that is generalisable across populations and health care settings [15]. The theoretical underpinnings include tenets from the implementation literature, motivational interviewing, the Health Behaviour Framework, and implementation intentions as well as guidance on complex interventions, behaviour change and informed choice that have been effective in previous work [20]. Further details on the included theory can be found in Additional file 2: Theoretical underpinnings.

Consultation interviews

As part of the development and refinement process, one -to -one semi-structured telephone interviews were conducted with UK bowel screening stakeholders with a systems-level perspective of the screening landscape, and with potential intervention recipients (non-responders) to ensure a patient-centred approach. Interviews assessed the acceptability, and potential challenges of the intervention content and process before testing its feasibility in a primary care setting. Feedback therefore reflected the views of both those involved in delivering the intervention at the interface between public health and primary care, and those who would be eligible to receive it.

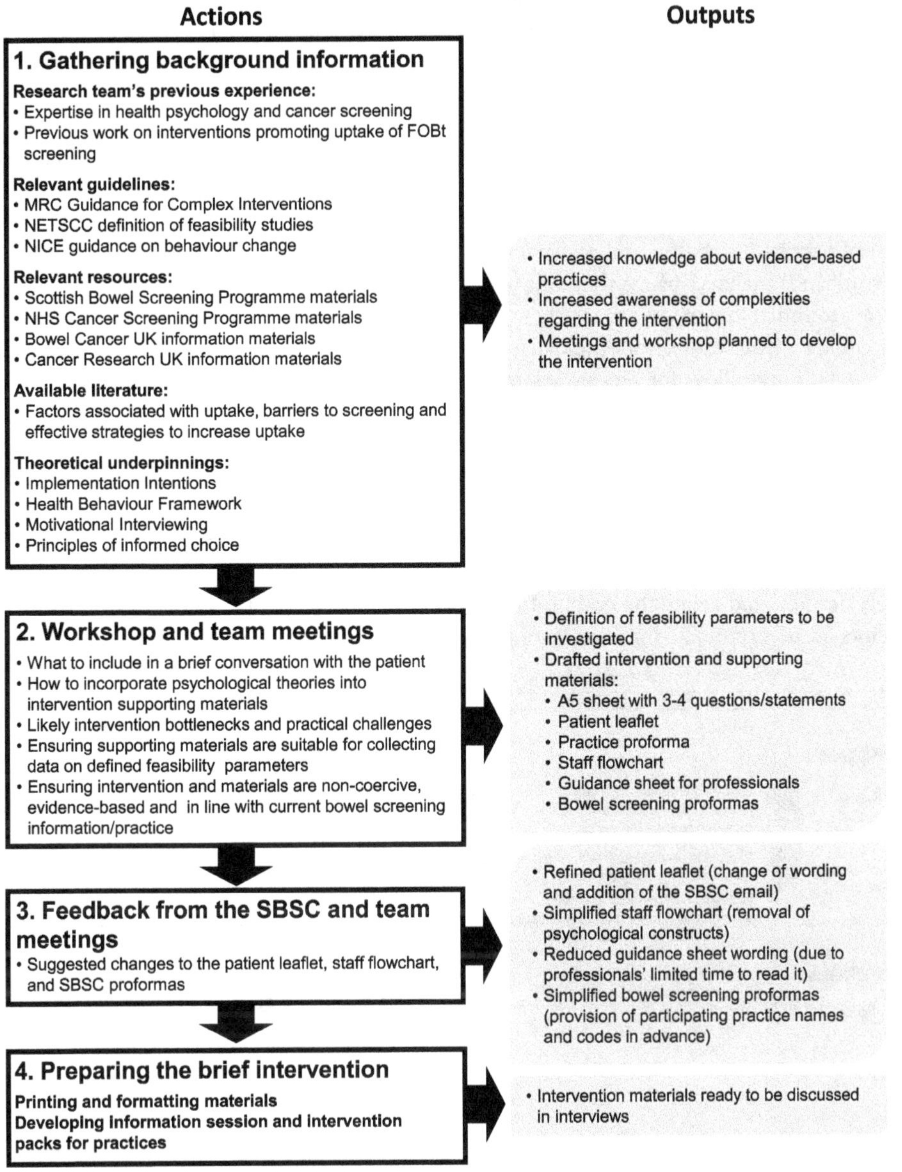

Fig. 1 Developing the bowel screening brief intervention

Recruitment and Sampling

Stakeholder interviews

Bowel screening stakeholders were identified from around the UK and sampled to include senior staff within the national screening programmes in England, Northern Ireland and Wales, health board coordinators in Scotland, a lead cancer GP and a practice manager; representing a range of professional roles and geographical locations with varying screening uptake rates. Intervention supporting materials were shared with this group of interviewees.

Non-responder interviews

Non-responders were recruited via two bowel screening centres: the Scottish Bowel Screening Centre in Dundee (Scotland) and the Midlands and North West Bowel Screening Hub in Rugby (England). Potential participants were identified from records of non-responders to the most recent round of bowel screening invitations. Letters of invitation to interview, an information sheet detailing the study, and a response card with FREEPOST envelope were delivered to 500 non-responders by the NHS screening centre managers on behalf of the research team. Potential respondents were purposively selected based on age, gender, socio-economic status, geographical location (six Scottish health boards: NHS Lothian, NHS Tayside, NHS Lanarkshire, NHS Argyll and Clyde, NHS Shetland and NHS Orkney, and one large English region: The Midlands and North West), and number of times the kits were not returned, to represent a range of views and experiences. A total of 33 reply cards (6.6%) were returned to the research team, of which 24 were eligible for interview (the remaining nine turned out to be responders or were being followed up with regular colonoscopies). Individuals were offered a £15 high street shopping voucher.

Analysis

All interviews were transcribed verbatim and anonymised. Transcripts were read and analysed using thematic analysis informed by a grounded theory approach [21, 22]. Open, line by line coding of the transcripts took place to stay close to the raw data and allow for any issues to be identified beyond those assumed significant by the researcher (DC). All were read and a proportion coded by three researchers. This was followed by focused and axial coding to formulate a structured set of codes rooted in and explained by the data. Constant comparison within and across transcripts took place as part of the coding process to iteratively develop and refine the coding framework. The transcripts were examined for contrasting or deviant cases and these were interpreted in the context of the data and through discussion within the research team.

Results

The Intervention

Our developmental process resulted in a 'talking' intervention, which comprised a brief guided conversation between a PCP and a patient non-responder attending a routine primary care consultation. The conversation was supported by a number of materials to inform and guide it (Fig. 2). These comprised 3–4 suggested questions the PCP could use to introduce the topic of non-response to a bowel screening invitation, a patient leaflet with an included implementation intention plan and details of how to request a new screening kit, a flowchart, and a guidance sheet for PCPs. Intervention proformas were also developed to be completed by 1) primary care staff after each intervention, and 2) SBSC staff after each kit request and summarising all kit requests.

In addition, a planned package of support was developed to help practices implement and sustain the intervention,

Intervention materials	Aim(s)	Adopted principles	Full description
1. Information for practice staff			
Guidance sheet • A4 coloured and laminated • Given to primary care staff	To provide practice staff with relevant information regarding the research study	Not applicable (N/A)	Described supporting materials, intervention steps and timelines, study rationale and who (and how to) contact the research team
Staff flowchart • A4 coloured and laminated • Given to primary care staff	To provide practice staff with relevant information regarding the study To describe barriers to screening, corresponding psychological concepts and evidence-based approaches	Health Behaviour Framework Motivational interviewing	Evidence-based barriers categorised into 7 response categories Original version had health psychology concepts alongside screening barriers; removed from final version to ease reading
2. Implementation in consultation			
3-4 questions/statements • A5 coloured and laminated	To guide discussion & address concerns	Non-directive Non-coercion Informed choice Implementation Intentions theory	Issue of non-participation raised using a non-directive statement Patients' concerns explored and discussed; informed choice ensured Patient offered the opportunity to request a new kit (i.e. via leaflet) If there was time, the patient and health professional would work together to develop an implementation plan
Patient leaflet and envelope • A5 coloured, perforated so slip could be posted • Given to patients who accepted the intervention • FREEPOST envelope addressed to the Scottish Bowel Screening Centre (SBSC)	To provide information with individual relevance To address beliefs associated with low uptake To allow for the patient's implementation plan To offer the opportunity to request a new kit	Health Behaviour Framework Non-coercion Informed choice Implementation Intentions theory	Based on the research team's expertise, evidence from the literature and official bowel screening leaflets Design reflects leaflets from the Scottish Bowel Screening Programme and Bowel Cancer UK for credibility and relevance By email (address provided), post or telephone (free phone number provided) - email added after consulting the SBSC
3. Data capture			
Practice Proforma • Green A4 with perforations (3 proformas in each sheet) • Given to primary care staff	To collect intervention data so the feasibility outcomes could be assessed	N/A	Requesting: Intervention date, staff name/role, duration of intervention, patient age/gender, reasons for consultation, whether the intervention was accepted, the leaflet was given and completed in practice and additional comments. Designed to be completed in approximately 2 minutes
Bowel screening proformas • A4 sheet with three proformas to be used daily • A4 sheet to be completed at the end of study • Given to SBSC staff	To collect individual data on bowel screening requests To summarise total number of requests and returned kits	N/A	Daily proforma for phone and email requests: date of request, practice name/code, type of request (phone/email) and comments End of study proforma for information on all requests: practice name/code, total requests, total requests by post/email/phone and number of returned kits Practice names/codes to be added for practices included in the study so SBSC staff did not have to check for these

Fig. 2 Intervention supporting materials

including: a briefing session to provide background information on the intervention and its theoretical and evidential underpinnings; support to set up the intervention according to practice needs; and regular appropriate practice contact.

Stakeholder interviews

Eight individuals were identified and invited to interview via email and telephone: two declined but suggested others who would be suitable. Seven semi-structured qualitative interviews were carried out by telephone and lasted approximately 30 min (see Table 1) (Additional file 3). Stakeholders are not named and details of their precise role are not included to protect confidentiality.

Bowel screening stakeholders were involved in a number of local initiatives, sometimes linked to national campaigns, to increase uptake of bowel screening in their local area. Initiatives included working with general practices, public information campaigns, workshops to increase awareness among health professionals and work visits.

Themes identified in these interviews are: *the role of primary care, feedback on the intervention,* and *potential obstacles.*

The Role of Primary Care

Bowel screening stakeholders recognised the significant role for primary care in promoting bowel screening uptake; PCPs provided a trusted source of information, support and encouragement for patients,

> "I think the big involvement of general practice has probably contributed quite a lot to that increase in uptake [...] where you've got the GPs engaged and they are talking to patients opportunistically." (Bowel screening stakeholder 1)

Stakeholders also mentioned the importance of multi-disciplinary working in the primary care context and the necessity to make sure PCPs had up to-date knowledge of bowel screening and bowel cancer to pass on to their patients. Targeting interventions for specific groups was also reported as important. Interviewees recognised that there would be variability between practices and it would be important to adapt to their existing practices and working style.

Table 1 Characteristics of bowel screening experts[a]

Pseudonym	Sex	Region
Bowel Screening Expert 1	Female	Lanarkshire, Scotland
Bowel Screening Expert 2	Female	Belfast, Northern Ireland
Bowel Screening Expert 3	Female	Rhondda Cynon Taf, Wales
Bowel Screening Expert 4	Female	Shetland, Scotland
Bowel Screening Expert 5	Male	Forth Valley, Scotland
Bowel Screening Expert 6	Female	Tayside, Scotland
Bowel Screening Expert 7	Female	Lothian, Scotland

[a]All participants occupied a senior position in their specific areas (Bowel Screening leads, Cancer leads, GP leads or practice managers)

Feedback on the Intervention

Bowel screening stakeholders were supportive of the intervention and its objectives: to promote a clear and coherent bowel screening message, raise awareness and normalise its practice, and discuss screening as part of a proactive approach to people's own health,

> "I thought actually it was a really good idea. I think it's really important that there's a consistent message from the professionals going out. [...] I thought it was really straightforward and should be very effective." (Bowel screening stakeholder 3)

A face-to-face approach was also considered more personal and thus more likely to meaningfully connect with individuals and feel relevant to them,

> "Having that targeted and it might not be very much that's needed on a personal level to, for somebody to decide they will go and do it." (Bowel screening stakeholder 4).

The intervention was considered workable in a primary care setting and the wording was acceptable and non-coercive,

> "I think they're (the questions) good because they're open questions they're not direct...and they're allowing the person to respond in a number of different ways; you're not pushing down on one particular response."(Bowel screening stakeholder 5)

Stakeholders also suggested particular opportunities for delivering the intervention, such as chronic disease or flu clinics, and stressed the importance of utilising the whole primary care team.

Potential Obstacles

Potential challenges related to the time and resource-constrained primary care environment, the risk of overwhelming PCPs with too much paperwork and being too prescriptive, thus belittling their wealth of experience in patient communication and care.

The main reservation and anticipated obstacle was lack of time and competing priorities for health promotion,

> "I think the GP will be stretched in their ten minutes they have or less [...] to actually sort out their

immediate problem [...] They've also to look at other things like smoking, weight management, all these other things that they're being bombarded with in terms of health messages; it's how do they prioritise? Which of these things do they pick?" (Bowel screening stakeholder 2)

Reservations were voiced about the time it would take to address implementation intentions; although it was viewed as a helpful 'stem', participants indicated that the use of materials may vary across different PCPs. Additionally, stakeholders cautioned that it would be difficult to measure the impact of the intervention in the context of other ongoing efforts to increase screening participation.

Non-responder Interviews

Twenty-four telephone interviews were conducted exploring experiences of being invited to take part in bowel screening, reported reasons for not completing the test, and responses to the proposed brief intervention scenario as described above, including the opportunity to request a new bowel screening kit (Additional file 4). Non-responders did not see the supporting materials for the intervention as these had not yet been piloted in primary care and thus shown to be acceptable. The intervention scenario was described to them in detail. Participants in five interviews were subsequently deemed ineligible due to ongoing bowel investigations, leaving 19 interviews in the final analysis (9 female, 10 male) (Table 2). Data on age were not obtained due to confidentiality issues. All interviewees were within the eligible age groups for screening (50–74 in Scotland and 60–74 in England), with two years added to the maximum age to include non-participants who were last invited at the age of 74 (invitations happen every two years).

Interviews lasted approximately 30 min and participants have been given pseudonyms to protect their identity. Core themes were common to almost all of the interviews.

Themes identified from non-responder interviews are: *screening and the wider health care environment, expected role of the PCP* and *responses to the proposed intervention.*

Screening and the Wider Health Care Environment

Participants demonstrated some knowledge of bowel cancer symptoms and screening, although they reported the need for further awareness-raising and, for the most part, more open discussion of bowel screening to remove stigma. At odds with their actual screening behaviour, interviewees

Table 2 Characteristics of interviewed non-responders

Pseudonym	Sex	Region	Country	SIMD/IMD decile[a]	Regular GP attendance
Sarah	female	Greater Glasgow & Clyde	Scotland	10[b]	No
Bill	male	Lothian	Scotland	8	No
Andrew	male	Lothian	Scotland	8	No
Fred	male	Lothian	Scotland	not available	No
Maureen	female	Lothian	Scotland	6	No
Elsie	female	Lothian	Scotland	9	No
Joyce	female	Lanarkshire	Scotland	3	Yes, regular bloods
Sandra	female	Lanarkshire	Scotland	4	No
William	male	Lothian	Scotland	3	Yes
Angela	female	Lothian	Scotland	7	No
Flora	female	Lanarkshire	Scotland	2	No
Gregor	male	Lanarkshire	Scotland	9	Yes
Gavin	male	Greater Glasgow & Clyde	Scotland	10	Yes
Gillian	female	Tayside	Scotland	5	No
Alan	male	Midlands and North West	England	not available	Unknown
Clark	male	Midlands and North West	England	not available	"Used to"
Catherine	female	Midlands and North West	England	1	Yes
Dean	male	Midlands and North West	England	7	Yes
Graham	male	Midlands and North West	England	7	No

[a]SIMD, Scottish Index of Multiple Deprivation; IMD, Index of Multiple Deprivation. SIMD (http://www.gov.scot/Topics/Statistics/SIMD/SIMDPostcodeLookup/ScotlandPostcodeLookup) and IMD (http://imd-by-postcode.opendatacommunities.org/ found using postcode search. SIMD refers to the year 2012, while the IMD refers to 2015. Recent or very old postcodes did not retrieve SIMD details in three cases (hence the missing data). Deciles were used instead of quintiles as the latter were not available for England

[b]1 = most deprived; 10-least deprived

were largely supportive of screening (as well as engaging in discussion on the topic during their consultation), believing it to be important and effective in diagnosing bowel cancer at an earlier stage,

> *"Well I think it's positive, I'm pretty much in favour of health screening although I am aware of some of the arguments against it but no I think that sort of early identification of problems has got to be a good thing."*
>
> *(Andrew, Lothian)*

Interviewees also viewed bowel screening as part of a holistic approach to their care and demonstrated appreciation of their wider health needs being taken into consideration,

> *"I went in about something and he raised a couple of other things, [...] right how much alcohol do you drink, things like that. And that felt good. It felt like, you know, you're there about your health but somebody is thinking about it in a slightly wider, more holistic sense."*
>
> *(Angela, Lothian)*

Participants reported variable contact with primary care, with a mix of those consulting regularly for long term conditions to those who visited their GP 'once in a blue moon'. However, participants suggested that the endorsement of their trusted GP would add credibility to the information they were being communicated,

> *"It would be a good idea because that then strikes home on the medical side, it reinforces that it's a health issue. I go to the doctors pretty regularly for blood tests and cholesterol tests and if he was saying to me have I done it, well maybe I should be doing it or even offered me the kit to do it then it would maybe reinforce it."*
>
> *(Gregor, Lanarkshire)*

Expected Role of the PCP

With the exception of two participants who reported damaged relationships, interviewees valued their PCP being involved and there was an expectation that they would consider their overall health and wellbeing,

> *"I think the more joined up, coordination in the NHS the better. So I don't see that as an issue, I see that as almost part of wellbeing."*
>
> *(Graham, Midlands and North West)*

Many participants reported that they would welcome a proactive and fairly hard line approach from their PCP in promoting bowel screening,

> *"It should be encouraged a lot more by the GPs encouraging them."*
>
> *(Bill, Lothian)*

> *"You know, more in your face kind of thing."*
>
> *(Joyce, Lanarkshire)*

Participants also reported that making a personal commitment to their PCP meant they were more likely to perform a particular behaviour,

> *"If I made that promise to the GP, yeah, I'll do it, you're more likely to send it back to whoever it is."*
>
> *(Fred, Lothian)*

Responses to the Proposed Intervention

When asked to consider how they would hypothetically respond to the proposed intervention, participants were broadly supportive of it and felt that it would fit well with their expected care.

Participants noted the primary care consultation as a good opportunity to engage with people about bowel screening, suggesting it was a good chance to 'seize the moment' despite being there for another reason,

> *"Actually I'm type two diabetic so I'm there seeing the practice nurse as well so questions like that wouldn't bother me."*
>
> *(Gavin, Greater Glasgow & Clyde)*

Participants were in favour of the proposed approach and language used,

> *"It never is intrusive when it comes to your health, but most GPs know...they deal with the public all the time. [...] I think it's non-threatening what you've said."*
>
> *(Catherine, Midlands and North West)*

They emphasised the need for sensitivity and an avoidance of attributing blame,

"I think you've got to be aware of how you approach a person over anything as delicate as that, that's down to a doctor's demeanour."

(Clark, Midlands and North West)

Participants reported that receiving a leaflet would be good to reinforce the message but a few cautioned against the use of unnecessary words or paperwork, and were unsure whether they would use the implementation intentions.

Overall, interviewees conveyed that the intervention was a good opportunistic approach and went further to suggest handing out kits directly through general practice or using other technology such as text messaging to engage with non-responders.

Discussion

Summary

Theoretical concepts of behaviour change, together with the evidence base on bowel screening and complex interventions, were used to develop a brief intervention for opportunistic use in engaging with bowel screening non-responders in primary care. This approach was validated through consultation with stakeholders and bowel screening non-responders.

The professional stakeholders were supportive of the approach and considered it an effective tool to contribute to an increased role for primary care to support participation in bowel screening. They predicted that the intervention acceptance would be variable and adaptations would be made to suit each practice. The planned intervention, including discussions with practices on how to implement it, were therefore modified slightly to allow for greater flexibility when delivering it in practice.

Bowel screening non-responders were similarly supportive of the proposed intervention and indicated that they expected and appreciated a broader view of their health. Interviewees were happy to have the topic of screening raised while visiting their GP for another reason, suggesting the intervention is acceptable for use in a number of different consultation scenarios. Interviewees favoured a proactive approach to promoting their participation in bowel screening. Figure 3 summarises the main recommendations for developing the intervention that were subsequently incorporated into the finished product.

Strengths and limitations

This was a small scale study focusing on providing a theoretical and evidence-based platform for developing an intervention and obtaining feedback on its acceptability.

Non-responder interviewees were a self-selecting group; they indicated support for the screening programme and it is possible those strongly opposed to screening may have not responded to the invitation to participate.

Screening expert interviewees were chosen to access the views of those working at the interface between public health, screening and primary care. One GP was included at this stage. However, further PCP views were obtained when testing the implementation of the intervention in general practice; these are reported separately [23].

There was a low response rate for non-responder interviews so that some perspectives were likely not included. However, key common issues arose in this hard to reach group. This is a sensitive topic area and these recruitment difficulties are encountered in similar studies [24].

Advantages of our development process

Using a theory and evidence-based approach informed the development of a brief intervention to influence bowel screening uptake. Adopting a multi-stage development method allowed the identification of potential bottlenecks when implementing the intervention and provided scope to make changes, such as adding an email address as a way to request a new test kit. Furthermore, discussion of the proposed intervention during interviews provided a forum for consideration of the real world applicability of the intervention.

Comparing patient and provider views

Both stakeholders and non-responders reported similar views that informed the ethos of the intervention: their belief in bowel screening, the need for further promotion to raise awareness of screening, and the role of PCPs in

Bowel screening experts

- Minimise paperwork; consider electronic versions of all documents
- Minimise the length of time the intervention takes
- Be aware of the busy and pressurised environment PCPs are working in

Patient interviews

- The intervention is acceptable for use in a range of primary care consultations
- People appreciated having their holistic health needs considered
- Sensitivity of language - be careful to avoid an accusatory tone and respect patient privacy

Fig. 3 Consultation interviews – main recommendations

adopting a holistic view of patient care; within a model of primary care reflecting a health promoting approach.

Although non-responders' positive view of bowel screening was seemingly at odds with their behaviour, reported barriers to bowel screening are rarely related to a negative view of screening per se; more so to practical barriers or relative priority [19, 25]. This finding also reflects the evidence for the gap between intention and behaviour [26], with scope for these barriers to be explored between the PCP and the patient during the intervention. Participant reported barriers to bowel screening participation reflect those found elsewhere in the literature, including barriers such as practical issues with completing the test; embarrassment, privacy and competency concerns; fear, and busy lives mediating the intention to complete the test. These barriers are reported in more detail separately [23].

Non-responders in this study referred to PCPs adopting a proactive or even hard line approach to encouraging bowel screening participation. This raises the question of how people use information to make informed decisions and the extent to which it actually mediates their behaviours, an issue addressed elsewhere in the literature [27]. The finding also reinforces the evidence for the weight placed on an NHS recommendation to participate in screening in addition to full disclosure of information [28, 29].

Conclusion

Developing and refining a complex intervention based on relevant evidence and theory provides a robust product and increases confidence in its implementation and suitability for evaluation in feasibility study. Feedback from potential users of the intervention provides further insights to its real world applicability and inform feasibility testing that predicates its effective delivery in practice [23].

Abbreviations

FOBt: Faecal occult blood test; GP: General Practitioner; NHS: National Health Service; PCP: Primary Care Provider; SBSC: Scottish Bowel Screening Centre; UK: United Kingdom

Acknowledgements

With thanks to all those interviewed for this study.

Funding

The study was funded by Cancer Research UK's NAEDI 2 initiative, grant number: C12357/A13965. The funding body approved the design of the study but were not involved in the data collection, analysis and interpretation of the data or the drafting of this manuscript.

Authors' contributions

DC, NC, SO, GV, JP, SS, RS, LB, DW and CC contributed to the design of the study and the intervention. GV, DC, NC, CC, SO and DW consulted on the relevant theory applicable to the intervention and attended the workshop described in the methods section. DC carried out the qualitative interviews and analysis (NC and CC read and analysed a proportion of the transcripts and SO, GV, JP, SS, RS, LB, and DW gave comments and critical feedback). DC and NC drafted the manuscript and SO, GV, JP, SS, RS, LB, DW and CC gave comments and critical feedback on it. All authors have read and approved the final version of this manuscript for publication.

Consent for publication

Not applicable.

Competing interests

The authors have no competing interests to declare.

Author details

[1]The Usher Institute of Population Health Sciences and Informatics, Medical School, University of Edinburgh, Doorway 1, Teviot Place, Edinburgh EH8 9AG, UK. [2]Department of Psychology, University of Essex, Wivenhoe Park, Colchester CO4 3SQ, UK. [3]Department of Psychology, Social Work and Health Sciences, Glasgow Caledonian University, 70 Cowcaddens Road, Glasgow, UK. [4]Division of Cancer Research, Ninewells Hospital and Medical School, Mailbox 4, Level 6, Dundee DD1 9SY, UK. [5]Scottish Bowel Screening Centre, Kings Cross Hospital, Clepington Road, Dundee DD3 8EA, UK. [6]NHS Bowel Cancer Screening Midlands and North West Programme Hub, St. Cross Hospital, Barby Road, Rugby CV22 5PX, UK. [7]Cancer Epidemiology Unit, Oxford University, Richard Doll Building, Roosevelt Drive, Oxford OX3 7LF, UK.

References

1. World Cancer Research Fund and American Institute for Cancer Research. Food, nutrition, physical activity, and the prevention of Cancer: a global perspective. Washington, DC: American institute for Cancer Res; 2007.
2. Weller DP, Patnick J, McIntosh HM, Dietrich AJ. Uptake in cancer screening programmes. Lancet Oncol. 2009;10(7):693–9.
3. Altobelli E, Lattanzi A, Paduano R, Varassi G, di Orio F. Colorectal cancer prevention in Europe: burden of disease and status of screening programs. Prev Med. 2014;62:132–41.
4. Bowel Cancer Screening [https://www.bowelcanceruk.org.uk/about-bowel-cancer/screening/]. Accessed 7 Jan 2017.
5. Scottish Bowel Screening Programme. Key Performance Indicators Report: May 2015 data submission. Invitations between 1st November 2012 and 31st October 2014.
6. Be Clear on Cancer [http://www.cancerresearchuk.org/health-professional/early-diagnosis-activities/be-clear-on-cancer]. Accessed 7 Jan 2017.
7. Detect Cancer Early [http://www.gov.scot/Topics/Health/Services/Cancer/Detect-Cancer-Early]. Accessed 7 Jan 2017.
8. Rubin G, Berendsen A, Crawford SM, Dommett R, Earle C, Emery J, Fahey T, Grassi L, Grunfeld E, Gupta S, et al. The expanding role of primary care in cancer control. Lancet Oncol. 2015;16(12):1231–72.
9. The Scottish Government. Detect Cancer Early - Bowel Screening Initiative. In: Health and Social Care Integration Directorate Primary Care Division; 2013.
10. Hewitson P, Ward AM, Heneghan C, Halloran SP, Mant D. Primary care endorsement letter and a patient leaflet to improve participation in colorectal cancer screening: results of a factorial randomised trial. Br J Cancer. 2011;105(4):475–80.
11. Wardle J, von Wagner C, Kralj-Hans I, Halloran SP, Smith SG, McGregor LM, Vart G, Howe R, Snowball J, Handley G et al: Effects of evidence-based strategies to reduce the socioeconomic gradient of uptake in the English NHS bowel Cancer screening Programme (ASCEND): four cluster-randomised controlled trials. Lancet 2015, 387(10020):751–759.
12. Raine R, Duffy SW, Wardle J, Solmi F, Morris S, Howe R, Kralj-Hans I, Snowball J, Counsell N, Moss S, et al. Impact of general practice endorsement on the social gradient in uptake in bowel cancer screening. Br J Cancer. 2016;114(3):321–6.

13. Kaner EF, Beyer F, Dickinson HO, Pienaar E, Campbell F, Schlesinger C, Heather N, Saunders J, Burnand B: Effectiveness of brief alcohol interventions in primary care populations. The Cochrane Database Syst Rev 2007(2):Cd004148.
14. Bauld L, Bell K, McCullough L, Richardson L, Greaves L. The effectiveness of NHS smoking cessation services: a systematic review. J Public Health. 2010;32(1):71–82.
15. Michie S, Fixsen D, Grimshaw JM, Eccles MP. Specifying and reporting complex behaviour change interventions: the need for a scientific method. Implementation science : IS. 2009;4:40.
16. Greiner KA, Daley CM, Epp A, James A, Yeh H-W, Geana M, Born W, Engelman KK, Shellhorn J, Hester CM, et al. Implementation intentions and colorectal screening: a randomized trial in safety-net clinics. Am J Prev Med. 2014;47(6):703–14.
17. O'Carroll RE, Steele RJ, Libby G, Brownlee L, Chambers JA. Anticipated regret to increase uptake of colorectal cancer screening in Scotland (ARTICS): study protocol for a randomised controlled trial. BMC Public Health. 2013;13(1):1–8.
18. Campbell C, Techer L, Crawford F, Orbell S, Szczepura A, Gumber A, Steele R, Weller D. Primary care based strategies to increase uptake of colorectal cancer screening. USA: Report to the National Cancer Institute; 2009.
19. Palmer CK, Thomas MC, von Wagner C, Raine R. Reasons for non-uptake and subsequent participation in the NHS bowel Cancer screening Programme: a qualitative study. Br J Cancer. 2014;110(7):1705–11.
20. Sheeran P, Orbell S. Using implementation intentions to increase attendance for cervical cancer screening. Health Psychol. 2000;19(3):283–9.
21. Charmaz K: Constructing grounded theory: a practical guide through qualitative analysis, 2nd edn. London: SAGE; 2013.
22. Glaser B, Strauss A. The discovery of grounded theory: strategies for qualitative research. Chicago: Aldine publishing Group; 1967.
23. Calanzani N, Cavers D, Vojt G, Orbell S, Steele RJC, Brownlee L, Smith S, Patnick J, D W CC. Is an opportunistic primary care-based intervention for non-responders to bowel screening feasible and acceptable? A mixed methods feasibility study in Scotland. BMJ Open. 2017;7(10):e016307.
24. Jepson RG, Hewison J, Thompson A, Weller D. Patient perspectives on information and choice in cancer screening: a qualitative study in the UK. Soc Sci Med. 2007;65(5):890–9.
25. Javanparast S, Ward PR, Carter SM, Wilson CJ. Barriers to and facilitators of colorectal cancer screening in different population subgroups in Adelaide, South Australia. Med J Aust. 2012;196(8):521–3.
26. Power E, Van Jaarsveld CH, McCaffery K, Miles A, Atkin W, Wardle J. Understanding intentions and action in colorectal cancer screening. Ann Behav Med. 2008;35(3):285–94.
27. Smith SK, Kearney P, Trevena L, Barratt A, Nutbeam D, McCaffery KJ. Informed choice in bowel cancer screening: a qualitative study to explore how adults with lower education use decision aids. Health Expect. 2014;17(4):511–22.
28. Woodrow C, Watson E, Rozmovits L, Parker R, Austoker J. Public perceptions of communicating information about bowel cancer screening. Health Expect. 2008;11(1):16–25.
29. Waller J, Macedo A, von Wagner C, Simon AE, Jones C, Hammersley V, Weller D, Wardle J, Campbell C. Communication about colorectal cancer screening in Britain: public preferences for an expert recommendation. Br J Cancer. 2012;107(12):1938–43.

Development and validation of a Malawian version of the primary care assessment tool

Luckson Dullie[1,2,3*], Eivind Meland[1], Øystein Hetlevik[1], Thomas Mildestvedt[1] and Sturla Gjesdal[1]

Abstract

Background: Malawi does not have validated tools for assessing primary care performance from patients' experience. The aim of this study was to develop a Malawian version of Primary Care Assessment Tool (PCAT-Mw) and to evaluate its reliability and validity in the assessment of the core primary care dimensions from adult patients' perspective in Malawi.

Methods: A team of experts assessed the South African version of the primary care assessment tool (ZA-PCAT) for face and content validity. The adapted questionnaire underwent forward and backward translation and a pilot study. The tool was then used in an interviewer administered cross-sectional survey in Neno district, Malawi, to test validity and reliability. Exploratory factor analysis was performed on a random half of the sample to evaluate internal consistency, reliability and construct validity of items and scales. The identified constructs were then tested with confirmatory factor analysis. Likert scale assumption testing and descriptive statistics were done on the final factor structure. The PCAT-Mw was further tested for intra-rater and inter-rater reliability.

Results: From the responses of 631 patients, a 29-item PCAT-Mw was constructed comprising seven multi-item scales, representing five primary care dimensions (first contact, continuity, comprehensiveness, coordination and community orientation). All the seven scales achieved good internal consistency, item-total correlations and construct validity. Cronbach's alpha coefficient ranged from 0.66 to 0.91. A satisfactory goodness of fit model was achieved (GFI = 0.90, CFI = 0.91, RMSEA = 0.05, PCLOSE = 0.65). The full range of possible scores was observed for all scales. Scaling assumptions tests were achieved for all except the two comprehensiveness scales. Intra-class correlation coefficient (ICC) was 0.90 ($n = 44$, 95% CI 0.81–0.94, $p < 0.001$) for intra-rater reliability and 0.84 ($n = 42$, 95% CI 0.71–0.96, $p < 0.001$) for inter-rater reliability.

Conclusions: Comprehensive metric analyses supported the reliability and validity of PCAT-Mw in assessing the core concepts of primary care from adult patients' experience. This tool could be used for health service research in primary care in Malawi.

Keywords: Primary care, Primary care assessment tool, Patient centeredness, Patient experience, Primary care quality measurement

Background

Evidence from both developed and developing countries indicates that well established primary care is the backbone of effective, efficient and equitable health care delivery systems [1–7]. Investing more in primary health care interventions is likely to accelerate progress towards achieving the sustainable development goal of universal health coverage [8]. A growing focus is also emerging to investigate primary care performance and organization in different settings using data from patients' assessment of service delivery [9–12].

Malawi is a signatory to global declarations on primary health care and has a health sector strategic plan "that is inspired by the primary health care approach" [13]. Malawi's health system is faced with the most severe shortage of healthcare personnel in sub-Saharan Africa with only two (2) physicians and 34 nurse/midwives per 100,000 inhabitants [14]. Mid-level health care workers

* Correspondence: ldullie@pih.org; Luckson.Dullie@student.uib.no
[1]Department of Global Public Health and Primary Care, University of Bergen, Bergen, Norway
[2]Partners In Health, Neno, Malawi
Full list of author information is available at the end of the article

such as clinical officers and medical assistants form the bulk of the work force as providers of primary care [15]. Most health indicators, while slowly improving, remain poor. Access, equity and financial risk protection are still major challenges [14–16].

There are three levels of health care in Malawi. Primary care consists of dispensaries and health centers which target a coverage radius of 8 km. Secondary level care is provided in district hospitals while tertiary care is delivered in three regional and two mental hospitals. There is an essential health package of services since 2004 that is offered in all public facilities as well as those belonging to the faith based organizations. Patients enter the system at first level and are referred higher up depending on the need [13].

To augment this primary health care structure, Malawi's sole medical school has since 2015 started a specialist family medicine training program to train family physicians who will lead district health systems towards primary health care implementation. This approach is already showing evidence of positive impact on health systems elsewhere in sub-Saharan Africa [17, 18]. Earlier similar findings have come from developed and mid-level emerging countries like China and Brazil [19].

The Ministry of Health in Malawi has established a memorandum of understanding with the non-governmental organization Partners In Health to use the rural district of Neno in the South-west part of the country as a model of primary care delivery. As a result, novel models of primary care interventions are being implemented in the district to reflect program integration of programmatic interventions, [20] community orientation [21] and financial risk protection [22].

As an integral part of these primary care reforms, there is need for assessment of primary care performance in order to describe, compare and follow-up services from patients' perspectives. Several instruments have been developed in order to make this assessment structured and standardized way in different settings [23–27]. Some instruments assess many aspects of primary care services (or key dimensions) whereas others only target specific dimensions, like accessibility or continuity of care [28].

Within primary health care research, the US Primary Care Assessment Tool (PCAT) has been widely adapted and used in patient surveys in many countries including South Africa [29–34]. Based on the 1994 American Institute of Medicine's definition of primary care [35], the PCAT aims at a global assessment of primary care organizations and their achievements around the core dimensions of accessibility, comprehensiveness, coordination and continuity, and accountability. In addition, it also assesses derivative dimensions of family orientation, community orientation, and cultural competence.

The aim of this study was therefore to develop a reliable and valid instrument that could be used to assess primary care performance from adult patients' perspective of the Malawian health system in order to facilitate future evaluation of heath care services and to compare performance and development over time. The Specific objectives were to adapt the South African PCAT (ZA-PCAT) to the Malawian health system and culture, and to analyze its feasibility, reliability and validity.

Methods

Instrument

The ZA-PCAT questionnaire is similar to the original American PCAT. Through 114 items, it measures eight domains of primary care: first contact (access and utilization), on-going care, coordination (patient care and information systems), comprehensiveness (services available and services provided), family orientation, community orientation, cultural competence and primary care team. Each item is answered on a 4-point Likert-type scale (1 = definitely not; 2 = probably not; 3 = probably; 4 = definitely) with an additional possibility to respond "not sure". The questionnaire includes 26 additional questions to determine the user's primary care facility/person and socio-demographic data. The ZA-PCAT was chosen for the study because of proximity and similarity of health systems to the study setting. Adapted versions of the PCAT have been used to measure primary care organization and performance, and to assess performance of primary care in different settings [9–11].

Face and content validity

The cross cultural validation from ZA-PCAT to PCAT-Mw is illustrated in Fig. 1.

Face and content validity of the questionnaire were assessed through a modified Delphi [36] and nominal group technique process [37] using a panel of 9 experts that included 2 primary care providers, 2 primary care managers, 2 primary care policy makers, 2 Family Medicine academics and 1 patient representative. The ZA-PCAT was sent to the 9 experts by e-mail. To assess content validity, each expert was asked to rate each dimension and item for relevance to the Malawi health system on Likert scale: 5 – highly relevant, 4 – relevant, 3 – not decided, 2 – not relevant, 1- highly irrelevant. Additionally, experts were asked if items were appropriately phrased and if there were additional dimensions or items to be added. Criteria for retention was at least 7 experts scoring 4 and above while exclusion was when at least 7 experts scored 2 or 1. Dimension and items with any other score results, additional dimensions and items proposed and suggested rephrasing of items were brought for the nominal group technique session using the same group of experts convened by three of the investigators. During this session, suggested new phrasing and items were discussed and experts were asked to reassess those items that had not

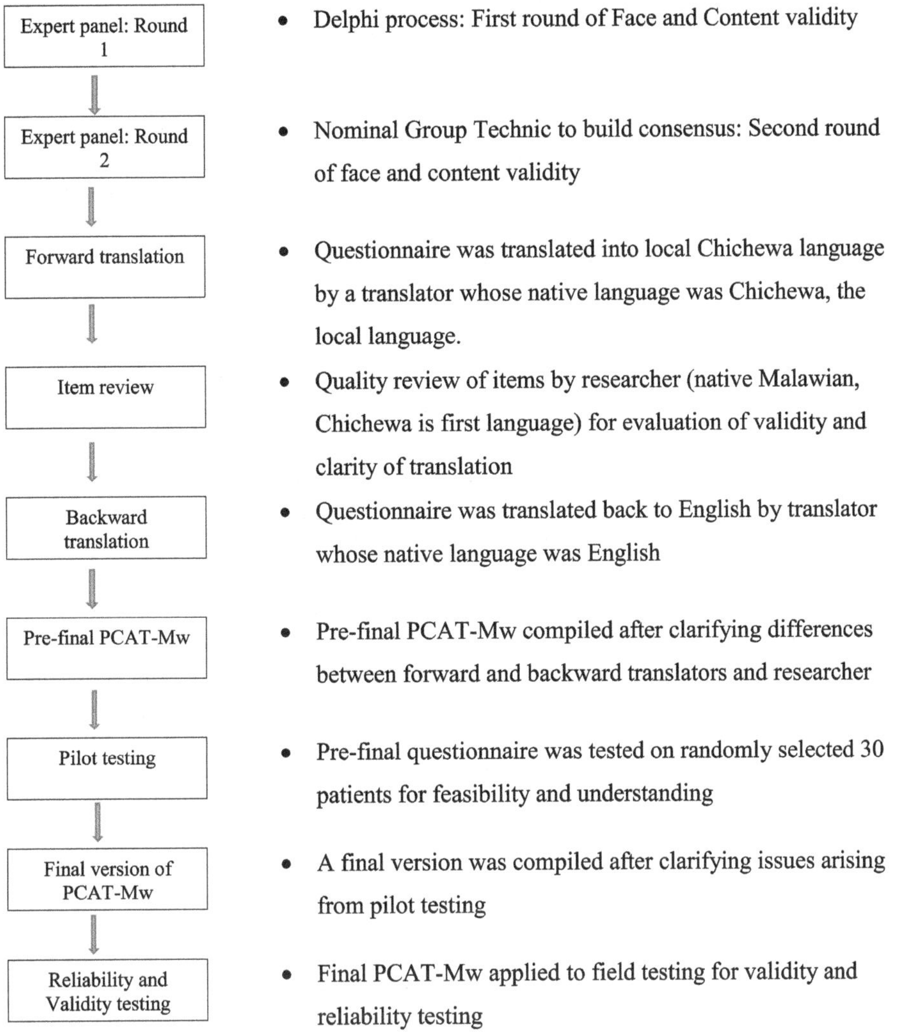

Fig. 1 Process of cross cultural validation from ZA-PCAT to PCAT-Mw before metric analysis

achieved adequate consensus during the first round. Criteria for inclusion or exclusion were as described above.

For face validity, we used the definition "the degree to which a measurement instrument looks as though it is an adequate reflection of the construct to be measured" [38] and thus asked each expert to indicate whether or not the questionnaire was generally adequate to be used in the Malawian context. Results were collated to form the questionnaire that was to be translated.

Translation and cultural adaptation

Forward translation was done by a translator whose native language was Chichewa, the most widely spoken national language (used by about 65% of the population) which was to be used in the study. A review was done by the principal investigator, a native Malawian with Chichewa as first language for clarity of the translation. A backward translation was then done by a translator whose native language was English. Any differences were sorted out through a reconciliation discussion between the translators and the principal investigator.

Feasibility and understanding of the questionnaire- pilot testing

Six interviewers with prior experience in patient interviews were trained in the PCAT interviews. The interviewers administered the questionnaire to 30 randomly selected patients at Neno district hospital out-patient clinic. In addition to responding to the items, patients were also asked for comprehensibility of the questions, the overall relevance of the items to the Malawi setting and for suggestions for any changes to the wording. The pilot study also assessed how long the questionnaire took to complete and the feasibility of carrying interviews in the out-patient clinic. From this phase a version was obtained which was used for the survey.

Data collection, setting and study population

A cross sectional study was carried out in August – September, 2016 in Neno, a rural district in South-West of Malawi with a population of 150,000 people, two hospitals and 11 health centers. Out-patient clinics in the two hospitals and 8 health centers were selected based on high patient volumes. Study participants were at least 18 years of age, must have been using the facility for at least six months and must have visited the facility for at least 3 times. Patients that were acutely ill, frail looking or with severe mental health disorders were excluded in order to allow for the immediate medical attention that they needed. Sample size was calculated based on similar studies using at least 5:1 subject to item ratio [30–34]. Sample size of 600 was targeted. From this it was calculated that each interviewer needed to administer seven questionnaires per day. The sampling frame was the 40–50 patients waiting to be seen on each working day. These patients were asked for permission to participate in the interview with a full explanation of the research purpose and were told that the survey would not influence their consultation. The sampling interval was calculated by dividing the number of available waiting patients by seven. The random starting point was identified using a smart phone random number generator.

Statistical analysis

Data were entered into and analyzed using the IBM SPSS Statistics 24.0.0 (2016) package. For consistency with methods used in PCAT studies in other countries, a mid-scale value of 2.5 was assigned to "not sure" answers while the mean item score was used for missing data [26, 29–31].

First, each item responses were inspected for floor or ceiling effect and a correlation analysis was run to ensure sufficient correlation between the items.

Secondly, the data file was split randomly into 50% subsets to allow for exploratory factor analysis with sample 1 and confirmatory factor analysis with sample 2.

Prior to exploratory factor analysis of sample 1, the overall Kaiser-Meyer-Olkin (KMO) statistic and Bartlett's test for sphericity were calculated to evaluate whether the sample was large enough to perform a satisfactory factor analysis. The KMO statistic is a measure of the shared variance in the items to justify factor analysis. On a range of 0 to 1, the desirable result is closer to 1 and the minimum recommended value is 0.6 [39]. Bartlett's test is a chi squared test whose null hypothesis states that there are no relationships between the items. A significant test confirms that linear combinations exist between the items and that the matrix is suitable for factor analysis [40]. Factor extraction was done through principal axis factoring and varimax rotation. Principal axis factoring was chosen because it allows for the exploration of underlying constructs, which cannot be measured directly, through items thought to be reflective measures of the construct especially where there are few items per component and low component loadings [41]. Theoretically, oblique rotation should be used in the case where factors were assumed to possess underlying correlations [41]. However, the varimax rotation rendered the matrix more reproducible and easier to interpret.

Determining scale structure and item reduction was based on multiple steps. First the scree plot, which is a graphical representation of the factors and their corresponding eigenvalues, was used. Factors above the bend or elbow cut-off point were retained. Additionally, items were retained when they attained factor loadings of at least 0.32, without cross loadings of the same significance and shared the same underlying meaning of construct and had inter-item correlation between 0.2 and 0.5.

Next, internal consistency was assessed by Cronbach's alpha and item-total correlation. For a scale to be considered sufficiently reliable, minimum Chronbach's alpha value of 0.5 is accepted as adequate. Within the scale, all the retained items were to exceed the minimum acceptable item-total correlation of 0.30 [39].

Likert scaling assumptions were tested by assessment of equal item convergence through the range of item-total correlation; domain score reliability through Cronbach's alpha; item-convergent validity through item-scale correlations (minimum 0.3); and item-discriminant validity using scaling success rate (correlation of each item with other items within the same scale being greater than with items from different scales).

Construct validity was analyzed throughout the measures of convergent validity and discriminant validity explained above. Further construct cross-validation was done through confirmatory factor analysis (CFA) using IBM Amos Graphics package 24.0.0 (2016) on sample 2 which was subjected to structural equation modeling. Maximum likelihood estimation was chosen with output of squared multiple correlations, maximization history, standardized estimates and index modification. The model's overall goodness of fit was assessed using a combination of indices: chi squared test, goodness of fit index (GFI), the root mean square error of approximation (RMSEA), and an incremental fit index, the comparative fit index (CFI). Some authors advocate for an insignificant chi squared test to show model fitness [42]. This is known to be unlikely possible especially when a large sample size is used [43]. The GFI was created as an alternative to the Chi squared test and calculates the proportion of variance that is accounted for by the estimated population covariance. The statistic ranges from 0 to 1 and a minimum cut off of 0.9 is recommended [44]. RMSEA estimates how well the model would fit the sample if optimal parameters were available and uses the chi squared statistics taking degrees of freedom into account. Most authors will accept values below 0.08 but recommend those under 0.06 to indicate a sufficient fit between the specified model and the data [45]. The CFI evaluates the difference between an independent model and a specified model without being affected by the sample size and values > 0.9 are acceptable [45].

Lastly, descriptive statistics were performed for the revised PCAT domains, including the mean, standard deviation, range, skewness and kurtosis. The results of the study were planned for both local and international dissemination through meetings with local authorities, scientific conference presentations and publication in an appropriate journal.

Further reliability tests

A subset of patients had second interviews after 4 weeks to assess consistency of the item scores through intra-rater and inter-rater reliability analysis. To do this 2 of the 10 facilities where data was collected were selected randomly. One was assigned for test –retest intra-rater reliability and patients from this facility were asked to return for a second interview by the same interviewer after 4 weeks. At the inter-rater facility, patients were asked to return after 4 weeks and were interviewed by a different interviewer from the one who did the first. Intra-class correlation coefficient (ICC) was calculated for the sum scores of the domain means of the responses of the participants with the two rounds of interviews to measure intra-rater and inter-rater reliability.

Table 1 Comparison of number of items and structure of ZA-PCAT and PCAT-Mw

Parts of the Questionnaire	ZA-PCAT	PCAT-Mw before metric analysis	Final PCAT-Mw
Core domains			
B - First contact: utilization	3	3	
C - First contact: access	19	18	3
D - Continuity of care	15	16 (plus 2 open question)	8
E - Coordination	10	9 (plus 7 open questions)	3
F - Coordination – Health information	3	4	
G - Comprehensiveness			
Services available	28	28	6
H - Comprehensiveness			
Services provided	15	14	6
Ancillary domains:			
I - Family orientation	3	3	
J - Community orientation	6	6	3
K - Cultural competence	5	5	
P - Primary care team	7		
About PC provider information	8	8	8
Socio-demographic data	18	18	18
Core domains (B-H)	93	92	26
All domains (B-P)	114	106	29
Total:	140	132 (plus 9 open questions)	47

Results

Face and content validity

The ZA PCAT was rated to be generally relevant to the Malawi health system. Table 1 compares the item and domain structures of the ZA PCAT and the initial version of the PCAT-Mw. The general structure and content was largely similar. The modified Delphi and nominal group technique process eliminated the domain "primary care team" and modified "coordination – Health information" because patients in Malawi use patient held health passports for their medical records. There was also substitution of services available and provided to fit context in Malawi.

Pilot study

During the pilot study, it was found that the questionnaire took approximately 45 min to complete. There were no substantial changes suggested by patients to the content of dimensions or items. All items and dimensions were thought to be relevant to the Malawi setting. Suggestions were however made to the local language translation to improve comprehensibility of items in the continuity dimension. A further suggestion concerned timing of interviews to fit better into normal flow of services as patients were waiting to be attended to.

Study participants

Out of 649 patients approached, 18 (2.8%) declined to participate in the study. These results are based on 631 completed questionnaires. Missing data accounted for approximately 1.9% of all data. Table 2 shows the socio-demographic characteristics of the 631 study participants of which 65.1% were female, 74.1% were under the age of 40 years and 2.7% were above 65 years. Education was generally low with 80.9% having only attended 8 years of primary school or less. We found that 41.7% of the patients were unemployed themselves while 52.5% came from homes where the household head was unemployed. Access to safe water and electricity were major challenges as only 21.9% of households had access to safe water while access to electricity was at 6.3%.

Of the total interviewees, 75.6% had been in contact with their health center for at least 3 years and 65.9%

Table 2 Sociodemographic characteristics of total study subjects ($N = 631$) and comparison of Sample 1 and 2

	Total sample ($N = 631$)	Sample 1($n = 323$)	Sample 2 ($n = 308$)	p value
Gender				
Male	220 (34.9)	110 (34.4)	110 (35.7)	0.37
Female	411 (65.1)	213 (65.6)	198 (64.3)	
Age (years)				
Up to 40	467 (74.1)	242 (74.9)	225 (73.4)	0.33
41–65	146 (23.2)	75 (23.2)	71 (22.9)	
> 65	18 (2.7)	6 (1.9)	12 (3.7)	
Education				
< 5 years of primary school	271(43.0)	132 (40.9)	139 (45.1)	0.14
6–8 years of primary school	239 (37.9)	128 (39.6)	111 (36.4)	
Attended secondary school	113 (17.9)	60 (18.6)	53 (17.2)	
Post-secondary education	8 (1.3)	3 (0.9)	5 (1.2)	0.36
Employment				
Full time	54 (8.6)	31 (9.6)	23 (7.5)	0.17
Part time	103 (16.3)	52 (16.1)	51 (16.6)	
Self-employed	211 (33.4)	101 (31.3)	110 (35.7)	
Unemployed	263 (41.7)	139 (43.0)	124 (40.2)	0.24
Piped water/protected well nearby within compound or nearby				
Yes	138 (21.9)	69 (21.1)	69 (22.4)	0.35
No	493 (78.1)	254 (78.9)	239 (77.6)	
Electricity in the home				
Yes	41 (6.3)	23 (7.1)	18 (5.8)	0.25
No	590 (93.7)	300 (92.9)	290 (94.2)	
Head of house employment status				
Employed	301 (47.5)	158 (48.9)	143 (46.4)	0.27
Unemployed	330 (52.5)	165 (51.1)	165 (53.6)	
Health status				
Good to Excellent	418 (66.2)	208 (64.4)	210 (68.2)	0.16
Poor to Fair	213 (33.8)	115 (35.6)	98 (31.8)	
Years in contact with HC				
Up to 2 years	154 (24.4)	82 (25.4)	72 (23.4)	0.28
3–4 years	69 (10.9)	30 (9.3)	39 (12.6)	
> 4 years	408 (64.7)	211 (65.3)	197 (64.0)	
Contact times with HC in past 2 years				
0–4 times	215 (34.1)	107 (33.1)	108 (35.1)	0.30
5–9 times	171 (27.1)	81 (25.1)	90 (29.2)	
> 10 times	245 (38.8)	135 (41.8)	110 (35.7)	0.06
Chronic condition				
Yes	254 (39.6)	139 (43.0)	115 (36.7)	0.06
No	377 (60.4)	184 (57.0)	193 (63.3)	

had visited their health center at least 5 times within two years. 39.6% reported having a chronic condition and 33.8% indicated poor to fair health.

Table 2 also shows that the socio-demographic characteristics of sample 1 and 2 had no statistical difference across all parameters.

Exploratory factor analysis (EFA)

Initially, the factorability of the 106 items was examined on the one half of the data set. Firstly, it was observed that all the items correlated at least 0.3 with at least one other item. Secondly, the Kaiser-Meyer-Olkin measure of sampling adequacy was calculated to be 0.72, above the commonly recommended value of 0.6 and Bartlett's test of sphericity was significant ($\chi 2$ (4278) = 10,951.7, $p < .01$). Finally, the communalities were above 0.3 for 101 items, further confirming that most items shared some common variance with others. Given these overall indicators, factor analysis was deemed to be suitable with all 106 items.

Construct validity

Results of the rotated matrix after principal axis factoring, varimax rotation and Kaiser normalization are found in Additional file 1. Seven common factors were extracted based on the initial exploratory factor analysis and were named first contact - access, continuity of care (communication), continuity of care (personal relationship), coordination, comprehensiveness (services available), comprehensiveness (services provided) and community orientation. Initial item reduction was based on the scree test and then retaining items with factor loadings of at least 0.32, items sharing the same underlying meaning of construct without cross loadings of the same significance and inter-item correlation between 0.2 and 0.5. As a result, from the preliminary number of items those retained were as follows: 3 of the 18 items in the first contact - access domain, 4 of the 7 items in the continuity of care (communication) domain, 4 of the 9 items in continuity of care (personal relationship) domain, 3 of the 13 items in the coordination domain, 6 of the 28 items in the comprehensiveness (services available) domain, 6 of the 19 items in the comprehensiveness (services provided) domain and 3 items from the community orientation domain.

As shown in Table 3, factor loadings ranged from 0.34 to 0.89. The coordination domains were analyzed separately to include only those patients that had experienced referral.

Internal consistency

The Cronbach's alpha coefficient results ranged from 0.66 (first contact) to 0.91 (coordination) for all revised multi-item scales. The item-total correlations ranged from 0.31 to 0.87, meeting the acceptable standard of > 0.30 (Table 3).

Likert scale assumptions

Tables 3 and 4 show the results of Likert scaling assumptions using the seven revised multi-item scales. All item-scale correlations were above the accepted minimum (0.30) with the majority being greater than 0.50. All scales demonstrated a relatively narrow range of item-scale correlations. Five of the seven scales showed 100% discriminant validity. The two comprehensiveness available and comprehensives provided had items that correlated higher in other scales but were retained because of other favorable metric properties.

Confirmatory factor analysis (CFA)

The structural equation model (SEM) for sample 2 is illustrated in Fig. 2. After allowing for some covariations between unique variables, this model produced a satisfactory goodness of fit to the model: chi squared test = 462.59, df = 270, CMIN/df = 1.71, $p = < 0.001$, GFI = 0.90, CFI = 0.91, RMSEA = 0.05, PCLOSE = 0.65.

Descriptive features of PCAT-mw

Table 5 presents estimates of central tendency, dispersion, and other features of the seven revised scales representing four core primary care principles and one derivative domain. The full range of possible scores was observed for all scales. Continuity (personal relationship) and the two comprehensiveness domains were positively skewed, indicating distributions with more negative ratings of primary care. The other four scales were negatively skewed indicating more positive ratings among patients.

Further reliability

Forty four out of 50 patients (88%) returned for a second interview at the intra –rater reliability chosen facility while

Table 3 Results of exploratory factor analysis[a] and internal consistency (n = 323) of PCAT-Mw

Scale	Number of retained items/original items	Factor loadings on the scale	Item-total correlation range	Cronbach's alpha
First contact- access	3/18	0.34–0.59	0.31–0.62	0.66
Continuity of care - communication	4/7	0.36–0.62	0.39–0.56	0.73
Continuity of care- personal relationship	4/9	0.47–0.70	0.53–0.63	0.78
Coordination	3/13	0.81–0.89	0.78–0.87	0.91
Comprehensiveness -services available	6/28	0.34–0.52	0.42–0.46	0.71
Comprehensiveness -services provided	6/14	0.50–0.68	0.43–0.59	0.80
Community orientation	3/6	0.41–0. 57	0.49–0.67	0.78
Total	29/95			0.82

[a]Principal axis factoring, varimax rotation

Table 4 Results of item convergent and discriminant validity testing ($n = 323$) of PCAT-Mw

Scale	Number of items	Item- scale correlation	Item- other scale correlation	Scaling success rate (%)
First contact - access	3	0.31–0.65	0.03–0.21	21/21 = 100%
Continuity of care - communication	4	0.46–0.72	0.01–0.41	28/28 = 100%
Continuity of care - personal relationship	4	0.34–0.70	0.10–0.33	28/28 = 100%
Coordination	3	0.69–0.81	0.02–0.41	21/21 = 100%
Comprehensiveness- services available	6	0.33–0.65	0.07–0.39	40/42 = 95%
Comprehensiveness- services provided	6	0.31–0.92	0.03–0.39	46/49 = 94%
Community orientation	3	0.36–0.52	0.05–0.38	21/21 = 100%

42 out of 50 patients (84%) returned for a second interview at the inter – rater chosen facility. A high level of reliability was found between the sum scores of the domain mean scores in both the intra-rater test re-test and the inter-rater reliability. The Intra-class Correlation Coefficient (ICC) for the intra-rater test re-test was 0.90 with a 95% confidence interval (CI) of 0.81–0.95 ($n = 44$, $p < 0.001$). The ICC for inter-rater reliability was 0.84, 95% CI 0.71–0.96 ($n = 42$, $p < 0.001$).

The final version of the adult PCAT-Mw questionnaire is attached as Additional file 2.

Discussion

This study developed a 29 item PCAT-Mw with seven scales as a tool for measuring the performance of primary care from adult patients' experience in the Malawian context. The items in the PCAT-Mw measure the four core dimensions of primary care: first contact - access, continuity of care, coordination and comprehensiveness of services as well as the derivative dimension of community orientation. The PCAT-Mw is significantly shorter making it time efficient in administration and will contribute to the evaluation of primary care performance in Malawi.

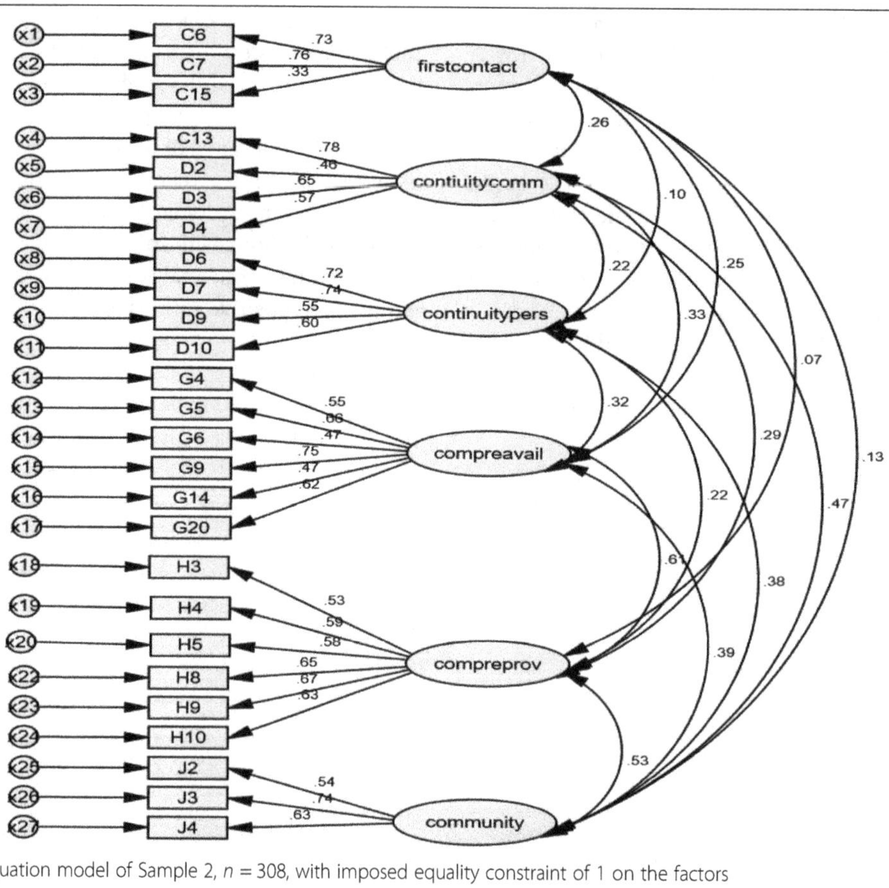

Fig. 2 Structural equation model of Sample 2, $n = 308$, with imposed equality constraint of 1 on the factors

Table 5 Descriptive features of PCAT-M

Scale	Number of items	Mean	Standard deviation	25th percentile	50th percentile	75th percentile	Range	Skewness	Kurtosis
First contact - access	3	8.48	2.44	7	9	10	3–12	−1.62	0.32
Continuity of care-communication	4	14.53	2.53	9	16	16	4–16	−.2.18	3.84
Continuity of care- personal relationship	4	9.26	4.26	4	7	16	4–16	0.99	−1.68
Coordination	3	9.64	3.43	8	12	12	3–12	−1.14	−0.54
Comprehensiveness – services available	6	14.5	5.01	7	12	23	6–24	0.38	−1.04
Comprehensiveness – services provided	6	22.25	5.86	15	28	28	7–28	1.09	−0.36
Community orientation	3	11.80	3.79	7	16	16	4–16	−0.65	1.36

Accepted methods of cross-cultural adaptation were carried out on the South African version. The resultant PCAT-Mw underwent standard metric analyses to assess reliability and validity. The high ICC observed for both intra-rater and inter-rater reliability could be due to the fact that the PCAT-Mw measures patients' experience rather than satisfaction with care and that the 4 weeks' interval was optimal for repeat measurements.

The dimension of coordination was not included in the structural equation model (SEM) because of limited data as only 16% of patients reported to have been referred to a higher level of care. However confirmatory factor analysis performed on the items under first contact - access, continuity of care, comprehensiveness of services and community orientation yielded results that indicated that the retained items sufficiently represented the conceptual multidimensional nature of primary care. Models of these core dimensions and the one derivative dimension of community orientation showed satisfactory statistical fit.

This also supports the idea that the creation of effective primary care systems is context dependent and that the strength of a country's primary care system is determined by the degree of development of a combination of core primary care dimensions in the context of its health care system [46, 47]. With regards to Likert scale assumptions, the two comprehensiveness scales had some items that correlated with other scales. However, the other five scales achieved 100% item-other scale discriminant validity, and the other Likert scaling assumptions, including item convergent validity, equal item-scale correlation, and score reliability, were satisfied, which suggests by and large the appropriateness of the usage of the Likert scales in this study which can be used without standardization.

PCAT-Mw is different in the factor structure from the original PCAT adult expanded version and ZA-PCAT on which adaptation was based. The original version consists of four core dimensions represented by six scales and three derivative domains while the South African version has an additional derivative domain "the primary care team". Nonetheless, the final PCAT-Mw scales are consistent with the theoretical four core principles of primary care. While the domain "primary care team" was eliminated at content validity stage, "family orientation" and "cultural competence" did not satisfy metric analysis requirements for retention similar to other studies [30–32].

There are a number of ways in which a reliable and valid tool such as the PCAT-Mw would be applied in health services research. This study shows that although primary care in Malawi is structured differently, it does conform to the accepted definition and reflects the multi-dimensionality as proposed by the Institute of Medicine [35]. The instrument can be used to assess the content and organization of primary care in Malawi in the regions where Chichewa is the main language. Another application is the use of the PCAT-Mw to set the standards of quality of primary care based on data on patients' experience of service delivery. In this regard, the PCAT-Mw can be used on its own as well as in combination with clinical outcome measures. Users of the PCAT-Mw should review the adequacy and relevance of the comprehensiveness domains to the context in which they are to be applied. Similarly, those items that showed lower item-total correlation may be considered to be used when more information on accessibility is desired.

The study had a number of potential limitations. First is that although an adequate sample size as confirmed by the Kaiser-Meyer-Olkin and Bartlett's test results, the study was carried out in one rural district, which may limit its generalizability to the national scale particularly in those regions where people largely speak another language other than Chichewa. This currently accounts for about 35% of the population. Cross cultural adaption will be needed when another language should be used. Another potential limitation on generalizability is the exclusion of acutely ill, frail and patients with severe mental illness. Further studies should consider different settings to include patients that initially presented with conditions that needed immediate attention to assess their experience of primary care. Second is the potential for recall bias inherent with this nature of studies. The intra-rater and inter-rater reliability tests and the one to one interviewing sought to ascertain minimal measurement error that would arise from it.

The PCAT-Mw is a new instrument in this setting. However, it is based on a standardized and widely used questionnaire and a full validation procedure was undertaken. Further, future application of the tool in more regions and populations could add to its validation on a wider scale. Future studies could also develop tools for providers, managers and children to provide a comprehensive assessment of primary care as was developed in the original set of tools and could combine this methodology and disease specific quality of care measurement.

Conclusion

This study indicates that the PCAT Mw is a reliable and valid tool to assess core concepts of primary care as seen from patients' perspective in Malawi. It can be used to establish baseline and to compare primary care performance from patients' perspectives over time. Further studies could focus on assessing responsiveness and developing tools for providers, managers and children and to compare measures of patients' experiences with disease specific outcomes in Malawi.

Abbreviations

CFA: Confirmatory Factor Analysis; CFI: Comparative Fit Index; CI: Confidence Interval; EFA: Exploratory Factor Analysis; GFI: Goodness of Fit Index; ICC: Intra-class correlation coefficient; PCAT - Mw: Primary Care Assessment Tool – Malawian version; PCAT: Primacy Care Assessment Tool; PCLOSE: *P* value of close fit; RMSEA: Root Mean Squared Error of Approximation; SEM: Structural Equation Model; ZA-PCAT: Primary Care Assessment Tool – South African version

Acknowledgements

The authors thank the participants in the survey and the expert panel for their enormous contribution towards this study. Special mention goes to Dr. Graham Bresick for providing insights in the initial processes of the study, Constance Kantema for her role in translation and data collection; Joe Lusaka and Beth Dunbar in the back translation process.

Funding

Funding for the study was provided by Partners In Health and The University of Bergen. The Principal Investigator and corresponding author is employed by Partners In Health and a PhD student at the University of Bergen.

Authors' contributions

LD conceived, designed and carried out the study, the data analysis and drafting of the paper. EM took part in the development of the study, the analysis, interpretation of data and critically revised the paper. SG took part in the development of the study, supported interpretation of the results and critically revised the paper. ØH, TM and SG supported interpretation of the results and critically revised the paper. All authors read and approved the final paper.

Competing interests

The authors declare that they have no competing interests.

Author details

[1]Department of Global Public Health and Primary Care, University of Bergen, Bergen, Norway. [2]Partners In Health, Neno, Malawi. [3]University of Malawi College of Medicine, Blantyre, Malawi.

References

1. Shi L. The relationship between primary care and life chances. J Health Care Poor Underserved. 1992;3(2):p321–35.
2. Starfield B. Primary care: is it essential? Lancet. 1994;344(8930):p1129–33.
3. Shi L. Primary care, specialty care, and life chances. Int J Health Serv. 1994; 24(3):p431–58.
4. Franks P, Fiscella K. Primary care physicians and specialists as personal physicians: health care expenditures and mortality experience. J Fam Pract. 1998;47(2):p105–9.
5. Farmer FL, Stokes C, Fiser R, Papini DP. Poverty, primary care and age-specific mortality. The Journal of Rural Health. Spring. 1991;7(2):153–69.
6. Shi L, Starfield B. Primary care, income inequality, and self-rated health in the United States: a mixed-level analysis. Int J Health Serv. 2000;30(3):p541–55.
7. Starfield B, Shi L, Macinko J. Contribution of primary care to health systems and health. Milbank Q. 2005;83(3):457–502.
8. WHO. World Health Report: Primary health care (now more than ever). World Health Organisation; 2008. http://www.who.int/whr/2008/en/. Accessed 25 May 2017.
9. Bresick G, Sayed A, le Grange C, et al. Western cape primary care assessment tool (PCAT) study: measuring primary care organization and performance in the western Cape Province, South Africa. Afr J Prm Health Care Fam Med. 2016;8(1):a1057. https://doi.org/10.4102/ phcfm.v8i1.1057.
10. Wei X, Li H, Yang N, et al. Comparing quality of public primary care between Hong Kong and shanghai using validated patient assessment tools. PLoS One. 10(3):e0121269. https://doi.org/10.1371/journal. pone.0121269.
11. Hu R, Liao Y, Du Z, et al. Types of health care facilities and the quality of primary care: a study of characteristics and experiences of Chinese patients in Guangdong Province, China. BMC Health Serv Res. 2016;16:335. Available on : doi. https://doi.org/10.1186/s12913-016-1604-2.
12. Browne K, Roseman D, Shaller D, et al. Analysis & commentary measuring patient experience as a strategy for improving primary care. Health Aff. 2010;29:921–5.
13. Malawi Government Ministry of Health. Health sector strategic plan II 2017–22. Lilongwe; 2017. Available on www.health.gov.mw/index.php/policies-strategies?download=47:hssp-ii-final (Accessed on 21 July, 2017)
14. WHO. Malawi factsheet of health statistics, 2016: WHO-AFRO; 2016. Available on http://aho.afro.who.int/profiles_information/images/d/d8/Malawi-Statistical_Factsheet.pdf. Accessed 25 May 2017.
15. Abiiro GA, Mbera GB, De Allegri M. Gaps in universal health coverage in Malawi: a qualitative study in rural communities. BMC Health Serv Res. 2014; 14:234. Available from http://www.biomedcentral.com/1472-6963/14/234 (Accessed on 20 Feb 2017)
16. Zere E, Moeti M, Kiringa J, et al. Equity in health and healthcare in Malawi: analysis of trends. BMC Public Health. 2007;7:78. Available from https:// bmcpublichealth.biomedcentral.com/articles/10.1186/1471-2458-7-7. Accessed 12 Feb 2017.
17. Swanepoel M, Mash B, Naledi T. Assessment of the impact of family physicians in the district health system of the western cape, South Africa. Afr J Prim Health Care Family Med. 2014;6(1):8. https://doi.org/10.4102/ phcfm.v6i1.695. pages. Art. 695
18. Mash R, Ogunbanjo G, Naidoo S, et al. The contribution of family physicians to district health services: a national position paper for South Africa. South Afr Fam Pract. 2015;57(3):p54–61. S
19. Kidd M. The contribution of family medicine to improving health systems: a guidebook from the world Organization of Family Doctors, Second Edition. p. 10–21.
20. Wroe EB, Kalanga N, Mailosi B, et al. Leveraging HIV platforms to work toward comprehensive primary care in rural Malawi: the integrated chronic care clinic, healthcare; 2015. https://doi.org/10.1016/j.hjdsi.2015.08.002i.
21. Dullie L, Wroe E B, Dunbar E et al Evaluating the impact of a community health worker program in Neno, Malawi (protocol). https://clinicaltrials.gov/ ct2/show/NCT03106727.
22. Watson SI, Wroe EB, Dunbar EL, et al. The impact of user fees on health services utilization and infectious disease diagnoses in Neno District, Malawi: a longitudinal, quasi-experimental study. BMC Health Serv Res. 2016;16:595. https://doi.org/10.1186/s12913-016-1856-x.

23. Flocke SA. Measuring attributes of primary care: development of a new instrument. J Fam Pract. 1997;45:64–74.
24. Safran DG, Kosinske M, Tarlov AR, et al. The primary care assessment survey: tests of data quality and measurement performance. Med Care. 1998;36:728–39.
25. Casady CE, Starfield B, Hurtado MP, et al. Measuring consumer experiences with primary care. Pediatrics. 2000;105:998–1003.
26. Shi L, Starfield B, Xu J. Validating the adult primary care assessment tool. J Fam Pract. 2001;50:161.
27. Mead N, Bower P, Roland M. The general practice assessment questionnaire (GPAQ) – development and psychometric characteristics. BMC Fam Pract [serial online]. 2008;9:13. http:// www.biomedcentral.com/1471-2296/9/13
28. Barker I, Steventon A, Deeny SR. Association between continuity of care in general practice and hospital admissions for ambulatory care sensitive conditions: cross sectional study of routinely collected, person level data. BMJ. 2017;356:j84. https://doi.org/10.1136/bmj.j84.
29. Pasarin MI, Berra S, Rajmil L, et al. An instrument to evaluate primary health care from the population perspective. Aten Primaria. 2007;39(8):395–401.
30. Pasarin MI, Berra S, Gonzalez A, et al. Evaluation of primary care: the "primary care assessment tools - facility version" for the Spanish health system. Gac Sanit. 2013;27(1):12–8. https://doi.org/10.1016/j.gaceta.2012.03.009.
31. Yang H, Shi L, Lebrun L, et al. Development of the Chinese primary care assessment tool: data quality and measurement properties. Int J Qual Health Care. 2013;25(1):92–105.
32. Lee JH, Choi YH, Sung NJ, et al. Development of the Korean primary care assessment tool—measuring user experience: tests of data quality and measurement performance. Int J Qual Health Care. 2009;21(2):103–11.
33. Aoki T, Inoue M, Nakayama T. Development and validation of the Japanese version of primary care assessment tool. Fam Pract. 2016;33(1):112–7. https://doi.org/10.1093/fampra/cmv087.
34. Bresick G, Sayed A, Le Grange C, et al. Adaptation and cross-cultural validation of the United States primary care assessment tool (expanded version) for use in South Africa. Afr J Prim Health Care Fam Med. 2015;7(1) https://doi.org/10.4102/phcfm.v7i1.783.
35. Institute of Medicine. Defining primary care: an interim report. Washington: National Academy Press; 1994.
36. Hsu C, Sandford BA. The Delphi technique: making sense of Consensus Practical Assessment Research & Evaluation. 2007;12(10) Available online: http://pareonline.net/getvn.asp?v=12&n=10
37. McMillan SS, King M, Tully MP. How to use the nominal group and Delphi techniques. Int J Clin Pharm. 2016;38:655–62. https://doi.org/10.1007/s11096-016-0257-x.
38. De Vet HCW, Terwee CB, Mokkink LB, et al. Measurement in Medicine. A Practical Guide. Cambridge CB2 8BS. United Kingdom: Cambridge University Press; 2011. p. 155.
39. Beavers AS, Lounsbury JW, Richards JK, et al. Practical considerations for using exploratory factor analysis in educational research. Pract Assess Res Eval. 2013;18(6) Available online: http://pareonline.net/getvn.asp?v=10&n=7
40. Bartlett MS. A note on multiplying factors for various chi square approximations. J R Stat Soc. 1954;16(Series B):296–8.
41. Osborne JW, Costello AB. Best practices in exploratory factor analysis: four recommendations for getting the best out of your analysis. Pan-Pacific Manag Rev. 2009;12(2):136–45.
42. McIntosh CN. Improving the evaluation of model fit in confirmatory factor analysis: A commentary on Gundy CM, Fayers PM, Groenvold M, Petersen MAa, Scott NW, Sprangers MAJ, Velikov G, Aaronson NK. Comparing higher-order models for the EORTC QLQ-C30. 2011; Quality of Life Research. 2012; 21(9):1619–21. https://doi.org/10.1007/s11136-011-0082-6.
43. Schumacker RE, Lomax RG. A beginner's guide to structural equation modelling (2nd Ed). Mahwah: Lawrence Erlbaurn Associates, Inc.; 2004.
44. Marsh HW, Balla JR, McDonald RP. Goodness of fit indexes in confirmatory factor analysis: the effect of sample size. Psychol Bull. 1998;103:391–410.
45. Hu L, Bentler PM. Cutoff criteria for fit indexes in covariance structure analysis: conventional criteria versus new alternatives. Struct Equ Model Multidiscip J. 1999;6:1. https://doi.org/10.1080/10705519909540118.
46. Kringos DS, Boerma WGW, Hutchinson A, et al. BMC Health Serv Res. 2010; 10:65. http://www.biomedcentral.com/1472-6963/10/65
47. Martin R. Measuring and improving patient experience in primary care. Prim Health Care Res Dev. 2012;13(2):103–5. https://doi.org/10.1017/S1463423612000084.

21

Medical overuse and quaternary prevention in primary care

Kathrin Alber*, Thomas Kuehlein, Angela Schedlbauer and Susann Schaffer

Abstract

Background: Medical overuse is a topic of growing interest in health care systems and especially in primary care. It comprises both over investigation and overtreatment. Quaternary prevention strategies aim at protecting patients from unnecessary or harmful medicine. The objective of this study was to gain a deeper understanding of relevant aspects of medical overuse in primary care from the perspective of German general practitioners (GPs). We focused on the scope, consequences and drivers of medical overuse and strategies to reduce it (=quaternary prevention).

Methods: We used the qualitative Grounded Theory approach. Theoretical sampling was carried out to recruit GPs in Bavaria, Germany. We accessed the field of research through GPs with academic affiliation, recommendations by interview partners and personal contacts. They differed in terms of primary care experience, gender, region, work experience abroad, academic affiliation, type of specialist training, practice organisation and position. Qualitative in-depth face-to-face interviews with a semi-structured interview guide were conducted (n = 13). The interviews were audiotaped and transcribed verbatim. Data analysis was carried out using open and axial coding.

Results: GPs defined medical overuse as unnecessary investigations and treatment that lack patient benefit or bear the potential to cause harm. They observed that medical overuse takes place in all three German reimbursement categories: statutory health insurance, private insurance and individual health services (direct payment). GPs criticised the poor acceptance of gate-keeping in German primary care. They referred to a low-threshold referral policy and direct patient access to outpatient secondary care, leading to specialist treatment without clear medical indication. The GPs described various direct drivers of medical overuse within their direct area of influence. They also emphasised indirect drivers related to system or societal processes. The proposed strategies for reducing medical overuse included a well-founded wait-and-see approach, medical education, a trustful doctor-patient relationship, the improvement of primary/health care structures and the involvement of patients and society.

Conclusions: GPs are frequently located at the starting point of the diagnostic and treatment process. They have the potential to play a vital role in quaternary prevention. This requires a debate going beyond the medical profession and involving society as a whole.

Keywords: Medical overuse, Over investigation, Overtreatment, Quaternary prevention

* Correspondence: kathrin.alber@web.de
Institute of General Practice, Friedrich-Alexander-University Erlangen-Nuernberg (FAU), Universitaetsstr. 29, 91054 Erlangen, Germany

Background

Medical overuse has become a problem of increasing importance to patients and health care systems. A variety of interrelated or even competing concepts of medical overuse exists and a consensus on a detailed terminology is not yet achieved [1]. Morgan et al. summarise definitions of medical overuse including overdiagnosis, diagnosis of abnormalities not related to disease, unnecessary medical evaluation, overtesting, overtreatment, wrong practice or unwanted care – processes which could be provider- or patient driven [2]. There is a growing awareness among clinicians and health care scientists, that medical overuse comprises unnecessary health care lacking benefit for patients [3] or putting them at risk of harm outweighing a potential benefit [4]. Moreover, unnecessary medicine adds to rising health care expenditures [5] and a misallocation of scarce resources [6]. Asymptomatic individuals are at risk of being labelled as patients, causing anxiety and affecting their quality of life [7].

Moreover, in secondary prevention, risk factors are increasingly treated as diseases [8]. There is a tendency to screen asymptomatic populations at low risk and to label pre-diseases as manifest diseases [1]. Serum cholesterol levels are a good example of threshold lowering by shifting the boundary between health and disease [9].

A growing number of research and health care campaigns show the worldwide importance of this topic. "Choosing wisely", an initiative founded in 2015 by the American Board of Internal Medicine, addresses unnecessary medical procedures via top five recommendation lists in cooperation with a growing number of specialty societies [10]. In primary care, the "quaternary prevention concept" [11] was introduced (see Fig. 1) in order to protect individuals from unnecessary investigations and treatment. Quaternary prevention is a "new term for an old concept: first, do not harm" [12]. It refers to actions "taken to identify [a] patient at risk of overmedicalisation [= in the sense of medical overuse, author's note], to protect him from new medical invasion, and to suggest to him interventions, which are ethically acceptable" [13].

The complex influencing factors of medical overuse and the possibilities to reduce it have to be interpreted in a system-specific context. The German health insurance system comprises several coverage schemes for out-patient and in-patient care: First, the statutory health insurance (about 86% of residents), financed by compulsory contributions as a percentage of income (up to an income ceiling) including employed persons and their non-earning dependents (free of charge). Second, private health insurance (about 11% of the population) for persons above the income threshold for compulsory insurance (opt out), self-employed persons and civil servants.[1] Patients have free access to primary care, out-patient secondary care and in-patient care (with referral), including diagnostics, treatment and preventive services. There is no mandatory enrolment in a specific primary care model. There has been an ongoing discussion on a compulsory gate-keeping function of GPs, but to date, this has not been implemented. Health care spending also includes out-of-pocket spending and co-payment (pharmaceuticals, aids, in-patient treatment). In out-patient care, so-called individual health services are offered. These extra services are not included in the statutory health insurance coverage and are reimbursed as direct payment (out-of-pocket) to the provider [14].

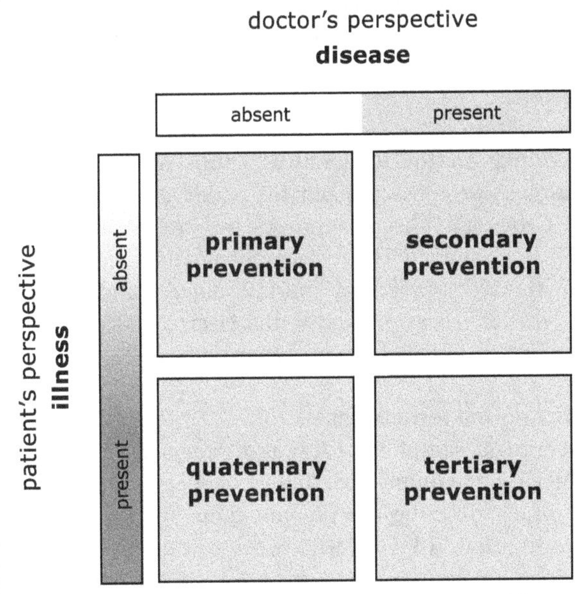

Fig. 1 The concept of quaternary prevention. Source: [11] Kuehlein T, Sghedoni D, Visentin G, Gérvas J, Jamoulle M. Quaternary prevention: a task of the general practitioner. PrimaryCare. 2010;10:350–4, and [12] Jamoulle M. Quaternary prevention, an answer of family doctors to overmedicalization. Int J Health Policy Manag. 2015;4:61–4

The primary care perspective plays an important role in tackling the challenge of unnecessary medicine. General practitioners (GPs) face an unselected patient population with a low prevalence of manifest disease. They are confronted with a higher level of uncertainty regarding the correct and final diagnosis [11]. Preventing patients from broad diagnostic testing for unspecific symptoms [15] is an essential task in this setting: Once a cascade of unnecessary medical interventions has been started, it might almost become impossible to stop it [16].

Although a broader research agenda on medical overuse has been suggested [2], there has been little focus on primary health care. This is why our study aims at a deeper understanding of the definitions of medical overuse, its scope, consequences and its drivers, as well as quaternary prevention strategies from the GPs' point of view.

We were especially interested in the aspects of medical overuse within the GPs' direct area of influence.

Methods

Study design

According to the explorative nature of our research question, we chose a qualitative study design and used the Grounded Theory approach by Strauss and Corbin [17]. In Grounded Theory, sampling, data collection and analysis are defined as an interrelated and iterative process [18]. Figure 2 shows the interrelated process of sampling, data collection and analysis.

Sampling and recruitment

Theoretical sampling [17] was performed in order to achieve a maximum variation of concepts and categories which describe the phenomenon of medical overuse. In total, 13 GPs who work within the German health care system were included in the study. The development of sampling criteria was a combined deductive and inductive process. We focused on a sampling based on relevant data to identify, substantiate, dismiss or broaden concepts and categories. Due to an initially easier access to the field of research, we first recruited GPs who had an affiliation to the Institute of General Practice, Friedrich-Alexander-University Erlangen-Nuernberg (FAU), taking the sampling criteria age/work experience into account. Through personal contacts and recommendations by interviewed GPs we found additional interview partners with similar or different opinions or behaviour related to the phenomenon of medical overuse. Throughout the course of the study, the sampling was done stepwise and empirically-driven as theoretical sensitivity increased [18]. Finally, GPs differed with regard to the following sampling criteria: years of primary care experience, gender, region (urban/rural), work experience abroad (in our study: none, UK, Ireland, Denmark, Guatemala), academic affiliation to an institute of general practice, type of specialist training, practice organisation and position (group/single practice, practice owner/employee). Sampling was continued until theoretical saturation [17] of information was achieved. Participants were approached face-to-face and via email. There were no drop outs. Prior to the interview, the involved GPs received a fact sheet including a description of the research goals, the interviewer, the research team and data protection.

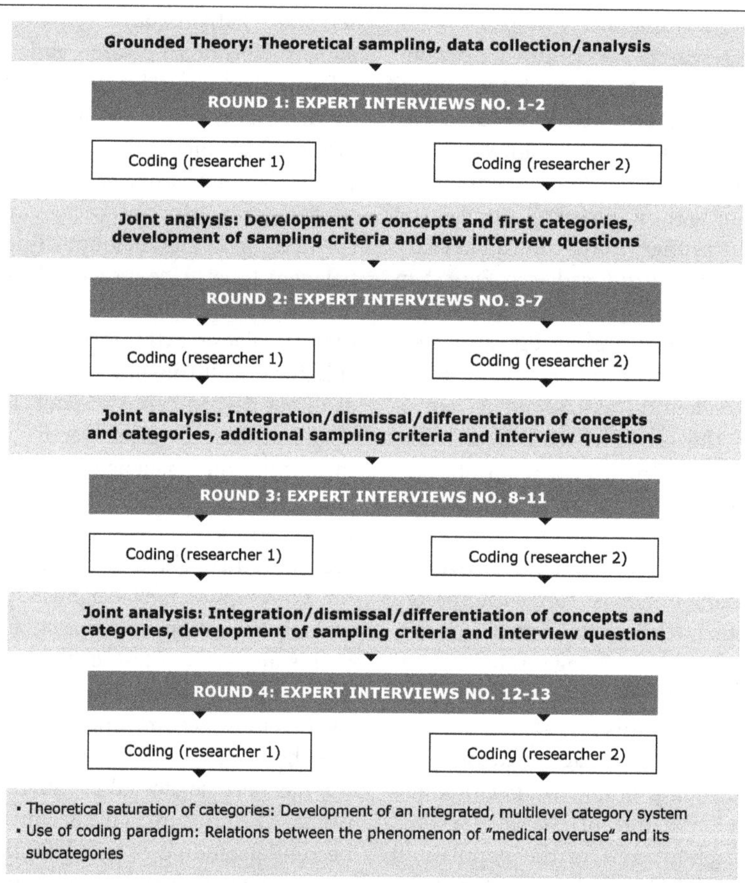

Fig. 2 Interrelated process of theoretical sampling, data collection and analysis

Data collection

For data collection, the method of in-depth expert interviews based on a semi-structured guide with mostly open-ended questions was chosen. The interview guide was pilot tested. At the beginning, we only had a few open interview questions, always depending on the interview partner's fluency. The guideline was extended and adjusted (more back-up questions and prompts) with growing insight into the research topic throughout the course of the inquiry [17]. Main interview topics (see Additional file 1) were a) relevance and definitions of medical overuse, b) examples of unnecessary investigations and treatment in own daily work routine and/or observed in other colleagues, c) drivers and consequences of medical overuse, d) strategies to prevent patients from medical overuse in general and/or applied by the interviewed GP (quaternary prevention). In order to reduce negative effects of social desirability, the interview questions started with the GPs' observations and opinions in general or also their perception of other GPs' work routines. In a second step, they were encouraged to reflect on their own potential contribution to medical overuse. All interviews were conducted by the same interviewer (KA), face-to-face at the GPs' workplace. They had an average duration of 64 min, were tape-recorded and transcribed verbatim in German. The translation process of the quotes used in this manuscript was supervised by one of the authors (AS) with long-standing work experience within the NHS primary care services and UK health care sciences.

Data analysis

Two independent researchers (KA and TK) coded the transcripts sequentially. After interview 2, 7, 11 and 13, the codes were compared with each other and either consolidated or further specified adding new interview questions (investigator triangulation). Analysis was supported using RQDA software [19]. We applied the following interrelated coding approaches:

First, open coding [17] lead to data-based concepts which were grouped in categories on a higher level. We examined our data for concepts, categories and its properties and dimensions. We used the method of constant comparison to substantiate those categories and to develop new interview questions. Flip-flop techniques (for example in terms of the rationale of medical overuse to be located between necessary economic survival and profit maximisation) were applied. A special focus lay on red flags (one GP held the belief that medical overuse only takes place in secondary care, not in primary care, for example). The extent to which we added new interview questions to differentiate and specify newly found properties and dimensions again was defined according to its importance to help explain the phenomenon of medical overuse.

Second, the coding paradigm used in axial coding helped to relate the data-based categories to subcategories (causal conditions, context and intervening conditions, strategies and consequences) to get a deeper understanding of the phenomenon of medical overuse. Due to the immense amount of categories we found, we were not able to give a full, comprehensive figure (based on the coding paradigm), but included figures and tables to the individual results paragraphs instead. Throughout the course of the analysis, the method of constant comparison [18] allowed to challenge existing concepts and relations between categories with new data. It helped to avoid bias in the combined inductive-deductive analytical process and improved the precision, consistency and congruence of emerging concepts and its relations [18].

We continued this iterative process until theoretical saturation [17] of information was achieved and answers kept repeating (see timeline in Additional file 2 as an example for this iterative process and theoretical saturation of information). Memo writing in terms of categories, properties, hypotheses and newly evolved interview questions was applied [18]. It led to an integrated and multi-level classification system of concepts and categories related to the phenomenon of medical overuse.

In order to conduct a full Grounded Theory study, selective coding and theory building as a third coding step could be applied. Strauss and Corbin [17, see axial coding chapter] explain that in case of thematic analysis or development of concepts, open and axial coding might be sufficient. As there has been little research background on the topic of medical overuse in German primary care, we think it would be too early to present a theory of this phenomenon yet. Our focus lay on a comprehensive description of its scope and context, relevant drivers, conditions, consequences and strategies to avoid it.

Results

1. Overview

1.1 Main results

The main results of our inquiry are related to GPs' definitions of medical overuse, its scope and consequences, including examples of over investigation and overtreatment and also the country-specific aspect of referrals to secondary out-patient care. We then focus on direct and indirect drivers of medical overuse (related to a direct or indirect area of influence from a GP's perspective), paying attention to vulnerable groups. Finally, various strategies for reducing medical overuse from the interviewed GPs' point of view are described.

1.2 Study population

Background information and demographics of the study population (see further information in the methods section) are shown in Fig. 3.

THEORETICAL SAMPLING

- n = 13
- In-depth expert interviews
- Semi-structured interview guide

GENDER	
Female	6
Male	7

POSITION	
Practice owner	6
Employed	7

REGION	
Rural	7
Urban	6

PRACTICE ORGANISATION	
Group practice	10
Single practice	3

WORK EXPERIENCE ABROAD	
Yes	4
No	9

ACADEMIC AFFILIATION	
Yes	8
No	5

TYPE OF SPECIALIST TRAINING	
General medicine	9
Internal and general medicine	2
Internal medicine	2

YEARS OF PRIMARY CARE EXPERIENCE	
≤ 10 years	4
11 to 30 years	5
≥ 30 years	4

Fig. 3 Study population

2. GPs' definitions of medical overuse

Although there was a broad variation in the GPs' perception of medical overuse, all had experienced it in their working environment. They generally defined medical overuse as unnecessary medicine that lacks benefit for patients or could even harm them in terms of morbidity, health-related quality of life or mortality. They distinguished between a number of negative consequences: First, they observed a spiral of diagnostic testing including short re-visit intervals without patient benefit or treatment consequences. Second, in their opinion, unnecessary testing increased the risk of finally irrelevant incidental findings, which nonetheless required further diagnostic workup. Third, they saw the risk of rising health care expenditures. Fourth, GPs were concerned that medical overuse promotes a misallocation of scarce resources that leads to undertreatment in other health care areas.

Quotation: "There is always the danger of harming my patient. For example with certain prevention examinations such as screening for mamma carcinoma which is up for discussion at the moment." (General Practitioner, A11).

Quotation: "People are suddenly confronted with diagnoses and diseases, where nobody knows, whether it is a disease or not. A debate which already started in screening. You pay a high price trying to examine everything and everyone." (General Practitioner, A06).

Quotation: "(...) through this approach (author's note: extended laboratory diagnostics) you sometimes find borderline values, which require subsequent explanations." (General Practitioner, A01).

Quotation: "Would it have consequences which change our further treatment? Or do we get results which do not change our actions? Then we must ask ourselves: do we need this test at all?" (General practitioner, A09).

Their definition was either acquired by evidence from study findings (in the sense of formal, published peer reviewed evidence) or, in a more subjective approach, by their individual expertise from personal work experience. Some of the interview partners emphasised the challenge of clear inclusion and exclusion criteria in the search for a sound definition of medical overuse and quaternary prevention strategies.

Quotation: "The reference base would be, as almost always in our profession: Does it make a difference? Sometimes, doing more leads to a better outcome for patients. And sometimes it does not." (General practitioner, A06).

Quotation: "Through this interview, I became aware again of the difficulties to define medical overuse. It is complex. (...) There will always be borderline cases with which it is difficult to decide between action and wait-and-see." (General practitioner, A09).

Regarding the debate on medical overuse, some of the interviewed GPs argued for a shift of emphasis to other health care problems such as under-supply in terms of health care financing, undertreatment, doctor shortage and bureaucracy in the health care system. One GP feared that the overuse debate could pave the way for rationing health care resources.

Quotation: "There are debates that the same number of cars could be produced in two factories instead of four factories. Nobody poses the question, whether we actually have a financing problem or not. Hospital beds are used to capacity, nurses complain about overwork, physicians grumble about too much bureaucracy." (General practitioner, A09).

3. The scope of medical overuse in primary care

3.1 Examples of medical overuse

The GPs were of the opinion that medical overuse in primary care is a topic broad in scope and relates to both over investigation and overtreatment. They observed that medical overuse takes place in all three reimbursement categories within the German health care system: Diagnostic and treatment procedures covered by the German statutory health insurance; health care for patients with a private health insurance that reimburses about twice as much as the statutory health scheme and accepts a broader range of investigations and treatment; and finally diagnostic and treatment procedures in the context of the so-called "individual health services" which are covered by direct payment. Table 1 shows examples of over investigation and overtreatment from the perspective of the interviewed GPs. The boundaries between the three main reimbursement categories are overlapping – the stated examples occur in all the three health schemes.

Table 1 The scope of medical overuse in primary care

Statutory health insurance ↔ Individual health services ↔ Private health insurance
Over investigation
Laboratory diagnostics
Holter-ECG/Long-term blood pressure control
Ultrasound (thyroid, abdomen)
General check-up in asymptomatic patients
PSA screening in asymptomatic patients
"Extended prevention investigation" in asymptomatic patients: Ultrasound, ECG, ergometry, spirometry, laboratory diagnostics
GP-recommended self-diagnostic devices (blood glucose/blood pressure)
Overtreatment
Polymedication in general (often discrepancies after hospital discharge)
Physical therapy covered by health insurance for new unspecific back pain
Broad-spectrum antibiotics for uncomplicated community acquired pneumonia (CAP)
Injections for back pain relief
Antibiotics for viral infections
Long-term prescription of benzodiazepines
Opioid therapy in chronic non-cancerous pain
Vitamine replacement therapy
Referrals to out-patient secondary care: GP-, specialist- or patient-driven
Specialist visits for basic medical problems: uncomplicated hypertonia, diabetes, new unspecific back pain
Referrals to MR Imaging for new unspecific back pain

A specific emphasis was placed on prevention and screening services such as medical check-ups and PSA-testing for screening of prostate cancer. In Germany, all patients with statutory health insurance coverage can make use of a biennial preventive check-up from the age of 35 (general medical examination). Some of the GPs criticised a lack of evidence regarding patient-centred outcomes for these examinations and a missing standardisation that leads to a varying check-up quality. Moreover, they frequently experienced an adverse selection of asymptomatic patients with a health-conscious, low-risk lifestyle, whereas patient groups with higher risks were underrepresented. Some also disapproved of PSA screening in asymptomatic patients, referring to clear evidence against screening.

Quotation: "As I said, a patient without previous medical history, without symptoms. In this case, I have never auscultated a lung and thought: "Thank god I listened to that lung." I mean, what do you expect from a healthy patient when you auscultate the lung? A healthy lung." (General Practitioner, A01).

3.2 Low priority of primary care and gate keeping in Germany – Medically unnecessary referrals?

In Germany, primary care has not been given much gate-keeping responsibility as this is the case in other health care systems. Secondary care is carried out not only in the in-patient, but also in the out-patient sector. Moreover, German patients have direct access to secondary out-patient care without seeing a GP first. The interviewed GPs reported on frequent presentation of patients to secondary care specialists (especially in the out-patient sector) either based on patient self-referral or GP referral without a clear medical indication as an important dimension of medical overuse (see Table 1 for examples). The interviewed GPs were pointing out various drivers for this aspect of unnecessary medicine. Direct factors related to GPs themselves were: The fear of making mistakes, little capacity of coping with residual uncertainty and finally the possibility of placing the responsibility for strenuous patients to other colleagues.

Quotation: "I've been grateful for my whole life that there are secondary care specialists. I have never wanted to be the last link in the chain, the one to decide about the final diagnosis. That's why I did not go into anaesthesiology, although I really liked it. Because I thought, there you are the last to decide, everything is up to me. That is not my personality. There is this insecurity, yes." (General Practitioner, A13).

The interview partners also pointed to reasons of medically unnecessary referrals which could not be influenced by the GPs themselves (indirect factors): So-called "circle referrals" made by secondary care specialists within the office-based ambulatory sector which undermine the role of the GP both as a family doctor and a gate-keeper; narrow follow-up intervals (every three months) in the out-patient secondary care sector; patients with a considerable need for reassurance; patients considering secondary care specialists as better qualified to deal with medical problems in general; and finally insufficient time for the individual patient due to an inadequate capitation fee per patient.

Quotation: "I have experienced so-called "circle referrals" [author's note: referrals between secondary care specialists in the out-patient sector]. There exist some kinds of networks. In this context, there is medical overuse based on a missing flow of information. And in this case, there is no overview over the patient's entire diagnostics, treatment and risks related to it, especially when medical problems occur outside of the specialist's focus." (General Practitioner, A11).

4. Drivers of medical overuse from a primary care perspective

The participating GPs were asked about their beliefs and observations regarding drivers of medical overuse. They reported on manifold drivers of unnecessary medicine (see Fig. 4), which could be related – from the GPs'

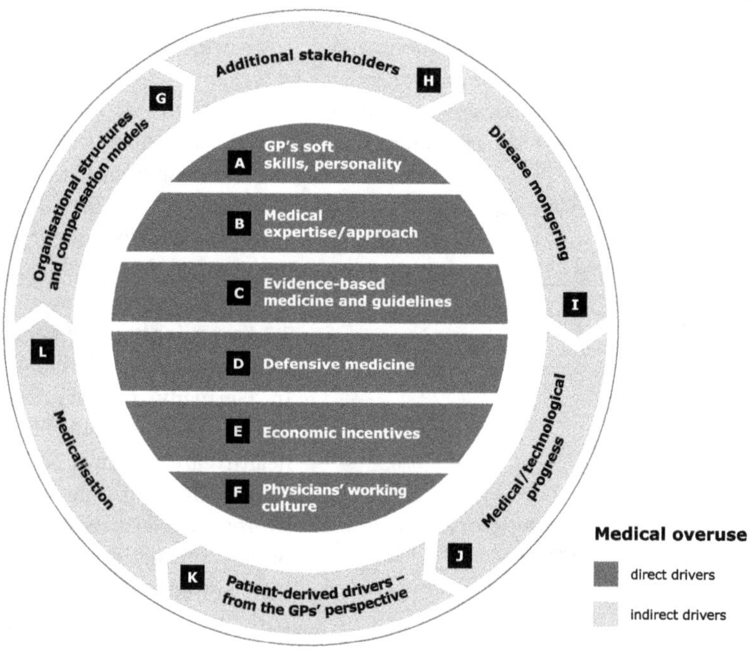

G Organisational structures and compensation models

- Direct access to secondary care for patients
- Lack of time for patients/insufficient capitation
- No consequences/impact analysis resulting from GPs' referrals to specialists
- Incentives for technical diagnostics
- Inefficient information management between sectors/providers
- Double structure of secondary care specialists in out-patient/in-patient sector
- Shortage of psychotherapists

H Additional stakeholders

- Health insurance companies: non-evidence based benefit packages/rewards programs
- Pharma/advocacy groups

I Disease mongering

- Re-definitions: shifting boundaries between health and disease
- Indication expansion
- Narrow patient re-evaluation intervals

J Medical/technological progress

- New technological devices
- New laboratory diagnostics

K Patient-derived drivers – from the GPs' perspective

- Customer-oriented role perception
- High number of consultations
- Belief: "good medicine" includes ultrasound/imaging
- Refusal of psychosomatic aspects of disease/illness
- Specialists preferred for basic medical problems
- Doctor shopping
- Insufficient sense of personal responsibility

L Medicalisation

- Pronounced health worries
- "Prevention dogma": more care/prevention is better
- Monocausal, mechanistic perception of salutogenesis
- Decreasing lay knowledge on medical issues
- Media influence
- More distinct in urban than rural areas

Fig. 4 Drivers of medical overuse in primary care

perspective – to a multilayer continuum of direct or indirect areas of influence (in dependence on Morgan's classification of direct and indirect drivers [2]). The study focus lay on aspects being located within the GPs' direct area of influence. These direct drivers are described in detail below, followed by a brief description of indirect drivers.

4.1 Direct drivers

A. GPs' soft skills and personality

Some of the interviewed GPs believed that a lack of empathy or communicative skills and a dysfunctional doctor-patient relationship that loses sight of the individual patient's needs could promote medical overuse. Additionally, many of the GPs were of the opinion that a missing ability to accept well-founded "wait and see" could lead to unnecessary medicine. In this context, they considered the following factors to be influential: A refusal of GPs to take on responsibility for the medical process, an insecure personality structure with low professional self-confidence and a low level of ambiguity tolerance in the sense of an inability of coping with residual uncertainty.

> *Quotation: "You have to be self-confident. Actually, being self-confident in taking actions is not the point. You have to be self-confident in not doing something." (General Practitioner, A12).*

B. Medical expertise/approach

Some GPs stated that they were prone to medical overuse in their first years on the job because of their uncertainty due to a lack of medical work experience. Many of the GPs pointed out that a low quality of medical education and training could result in diagnostic uncertainty and finally promote unnecessary medicine. A growing tendency towards (sub-)specialisation and a low priority of history taking and physical examination were also seen as major drivers for the maximisation of technical diagnostics. GPs criticised that the absence of a holistic patient assessment which includes overall morbidity, health-related quality of life and psychosocial factors promotes medical overuse.

> *Quotation: "The greatest challenge will be to put more emphasis on history taking and physical examination again. If a young physician learns how to observe clinical symptoms and adequately acts on it, he will feel secure. This is the prerequisite to avoid further unnecessary investigations." (General Practitioner, A02).*

C. Evidence-based medicine and guidelines

The interviewed GPs' approach to medical decision-making varied. Some held the opinion that medical decision-making should be based on evidence as a way to avoid medical overuse, allowing for deviations of guidelines in individual cases.

> *Quotation: "In an ideal world, GPs would cooperate. We would establish evidence-based guidelines for primary care, we would work together, we would work in group practices. Organise our practices according to the best guidelines available and care about us and for our patients." (General Practitioner, A04).*

Some answers showed a reasonable knowledge and approval of evidence-based medicine, but also revealed a lack in adherence. Either GPs did not feel responsible for managing an overall evidence-based care for their patients or they even appreciated medical overuse in inpatient care as a welcome diagnostic work-up and baseline for the subsequent outpatient care.

> *Quotation: "When a patient gets discharged from the hospital, I sometimes have the feeling that they did anything medically possible. But from the out-patient care perspective, I also appreciate that. (...) At the very moment a patient starts showing symptoms, I know, the patient has been in in-patient treatment recently. And then I am glad that I can refer to something. (...) And you could describe that as medical overuse to some extent. Because we are talking about tests which were not totally urgent or rather luxurious given the specific symptoms at that time. But it can be really helpful to have this reference point." (General Practitioner, A11).*

In some of the GPs, a lack of acceptance or willingness to reflect the principles of evidence-based medicine could be observed. Other GPs even spoke of a blind spot in this context. Contrary to current guidelines, some of the interviewed GPs overestimated the benefit of certain medical procedures and contributed to medical overuse. This was especially noticeable when talking of the benefits of PSA testing or general medical check-ups in asymptomatic persons. There were several reasons why physicians overruled current guidelines and insisted on their freedom of therapy and the individuality of each patient: First, the misinterpretation of statistical evidence; second, an "action" dogma of doing anything that is possible for the individual patient; third, a belief that screening and prevention is always something good; fourth, an over-reliance on (causal) treatment effects; and fifth, a low visibility of negative consequences of medical overuse.

> *Quotation: "In my opinion, it would make sense to allow general practitioners to do anything possible*

when carrying out a general medical examination. In terms of prevention. Intima-media thickness, for example. Ultrasound, too. Once in a while, you find renal tumours there. You only find them accidentally when looking for something else. Otherwise you would miss them. I think any patient you identify is a life saved." (General Practitioner, A08).

Quotation: "In my opinion, those things which help, those who cure the patient are right. And when there is a patient who tells me that my vitamin therapy helped him, I don't adhere to studies saying it is useless." (General practitioner, A13).

In general, all groups described problems arising with the development of evidence-based guidelines such as vested interests, limited applicability to the individual patient and a tendency to promote action rather than inaction. A timeline of interviews combined with a mapping of answers and categories to the topic of "Evidence-based medicine and guidelines" is provided in Additional file 2. It also shows theoretical saturation of information within the study population.

D. Defensive medicine

Some interview partners pointed to the fear of liability as an important reason for unnecessary diagnostic tests. Although none of them reported on personal experience of legal actions against them, this aspect played an important role from the GPs' point of view.

Quotation: "Another reason is that diagnostic tests are also carried out due to a fear of liability. To protect oneself from claims of compensation." (General Practitioner, A03).

E. Economic incentives

All interview participants referred to economic drivers of medical overuse. Some GPs reported that they themselves or colleagues carried out unnecessary tests and treatments for reimbursement reasons. The rationales given were located between necessary economic survival and profit maximisation. Some GPs described the existence of provider-induced demand that would lead to non-evidence-based care.

Quotation: "There is little transparency among general practitioners in terms of income. It was often presented as a basic economic necessity to increase turnover with these services [non-evidence based individual health services with direct payment; annotation by the author]. Personally, I am not dependent on that." (General Practitioner, A01).

F. Physicians' working culture

Some of the GPs stated that there is little individual scope for structural change. Eminence-based medicine, hierarchical structures and a lack in debate culture were also seen as drivers for medicine without patient benefit. In general, a paradigm shift from action to inaction in well-founded cases was assessed as essential but hard to achieve.

Quotation: "In the Anglo-Saxon countries they practice evidence-based medicine, we Germans carry out eminence-based medicine. It has been like this for a long time, when chief physicians were gods and everybody had to believe them." (General Practitioner, A04).

4.2 Indirect drivers (G-L)

The interviewed GPs also referred to drivers which were not located within their direct area of influence (see Fig. 4). From the GPs' perspective, these indirect aspects included (G) organisational structures and compensational models which could promote medical overuse; (H) additional stakeholders such as health insurance companies or pharmaceutical industry that primarily act on economic prerequisites instead of avoiding unnecessary medicine; (I) disease mongering [1], a process that shifts boundaries between health and disease; (J) the medical and technological progress expanding diagnostic and treatment options; (K) patient-derived drivers, relating to patient demands which arise from a multidimensional setting of personal belief systems, dysfunctional incentives and sociocultural developments; and (L) a general process of medicalisation of the society as a whole, affecting all stakeholders such as the public, politicians, doctors, patients, health insurances, pharma industry or other advocacy groups.

5. Vulnerable groups

The interviewed GPs identified various vulnerable groups who in their view are especially at risk of medical overuse: First, the so-called "worried well" [11], individuals with no or minor symptoms who frequently see a doctor; second, patients in a palliative situation who receive maximum investigations and treatment instead of a quality of life-focused symptom-oriented approach; third, patients with psychosomatic diagnoses who focus on somatic health care instead of psychotherapy; and fourth, old and multimorbid patients who are at risk of polypharmacotherapy potentially leading to severe side effects.

Quotation: "Patients in palliative situations are at risk of medical overuse. For them, it makes no sense to do anything that is medically possible." (General Practitioner, A05).

Quotation: "In primary care, we have many patients with diseases that are no diseases or only minor disturbances." (General Practitioner, A08).

6. Quaternary prevention: Strategies for reducing medical overuse

Derived from their perspective on the scope and drivers of medical overuse, the participating GPs came forward with a variety of recommendations to reduce medical overuse in primary care (see Table 2). These strategies could be related – from the GPs' perspective – to a multilayer continuum of direct, intermediate and indirect levels of influence.

In terms of a *direct* level of influence (A), they outlined manifold quaternary prevention strategies: Establishing a long-standing, trustful doctor-patient-relationship, based on shared-decision-making, an emphasis on communication and empathy for the patient and a holistic patient assessment could help downsizing unnecessary medical procedures. A focus on reducing diagnostic uncertainty through high-quality education and training, supervision especially for young GPs and carrying out stepwise diagnostics with a focus on anamnesis and physical examination and a well-founded "wait and see"-strategy instead of an early-stage shotgun testing were also seen as essential quaternary prevention strategies. On an *intermediate* level of influence (B), the promotion (through GP associations) of a more primary care-centred health care model and patient education were considered as important. On an *indirect* level of influence (C), the importance of improving health care structures and discussing health care priorities in society as a whole was emphasised.

The interviewed GPs also stressed their limited influence and the decisive power of various other stakeholders (health policy, statutory health insurance, media or the pharmaceutical industry).

Discussion

1. Principal findings

According to our main research questions, the interviewed GPs gave numerous definitions of medical overuse, comprising over investigation and overtreatment. They defined medical overuse as unnecessary investigations and treatment which lack benefit for patients or could even harm them in terms of morbidity, health-related quality of life or mortality. The interview partners were of the opinion that medical overuse occurs in all three reimbursement categories within the German health care system: the statutory health insurance, private health coverage and payments covered by the patients individually ("individual health services"). Especially PSA screening and medical check-ups were seen as controversial. GPs criticised the little acceptance of gate-keeping in German primary care and a low-threshold of referral, in particular the direct accessibility of secondary care. In their opinion, these special characteristics of the German health care system contribute to medical overuse, leading to (a) GP-driven referrals without clear medical indication, (b) "circle referrals" within the out-patient secondary care sector or (c) patient-driven direct visits to out-patient secondary care specialists.

Table 2 Quaternary prevention from a primary care perspective

Quaternary prevention strategies: Levels of influence		
A. DIRECT	B. INTERMEDIATE	C. INDIRECT
A1. Establishing a trustful doctor-patient-relationship	B1. Promotion of a primary care-centred health care model	C1. Improving health care structures
Focus on a long-term relationship between doctor and patient	Improvement of evidence-based primary care	Restriction of non-evidence-based individual health services (direct payment)
Shared-decision-making	GP as guide and coordinator	Population-based health care approach (instead of an extended high risk approach)
Improving soft skills (communication, empathy)	Distinction between primary and secondary care	Change in reimbursement paradigms: less incentives for technical diagnostics
Holistic patient assessment (including the patient's social background)	Better integration of primary care into medical school curriculum	
A2. Reducing diagnostic uncertainty	B2. Patient education	C2. Discussion in society as a whole
High quality, evidence-based medical education and training	Information on evidence for recommended or requested services	Identification of relevant stakeholders
Supervision for young GPs	Information on advantages of a wait-and-see-approach instead of immediate maximum diagnostics	Process of setting priorities in health care
Stepwise diagnostics: Focus on anamnesis and physical examination	Information on importance of health-conscious behaviour/personal responsibility	
Well-founded "wait and see"	Price/cost transparency	

They pointed to various drivers of medical overuse being associated either directly or indirectly with their areas of influence. Direct drivers promoting unnecessary medicine comprised a lack of consultation skills, such as empathy and an ability to communicate, insecure personality traits, a lack of medical experience, little acceptance of guidelines, a high degree of defensive medicine, economic incentives and the physicians' working environment with its lack of debating culture and inherent hierarchies in general. They also referred to indirect drivers of medical overuse, such as dysfunctional incentives in terms of organisational structures and compensation models, interests of additional stakeholders (health care companies or the pharmaceutical industry), disease mongering [1], medicalisation, patient demands and the medical and technological progress.

Four vulnerable patient groups who especially are at risk of medical overuse were identified: The so-called "worried well" [11] seeing a doctor frequently, patients in palliative care situations, patients with psychosomatic diseases and old, multimorbid patients who are at risk of polypharmacotherapy.

The interviewed GPs proposed a number of strategies to reduce medical overuse in primary care (quaternary prevention). Strategies which could be directly applied by GPs themselves (direct level of influence) comprised an improvement of the doctor-patient-relationship through shared-decision-making, communication and a holistic patient assessment. These strategies also included the reduction of diagnostic uncertainty through high-quality training for GPs, a well-founded wait-and-see approach and stepwise diagnostics with a focus on history taking and physical examination, for example. On an intermediate level of influence, strategies emphasised the development of a primary care-centred health model and the importance of patient education. On an indirect level of influence, adjusting health care structures and discussing health care priorities were seen as essential.

2. Findings in relation to other studies

The definitions, scope, drivers and also the outlined quaternary prevention strategies we found, coincided with international findings to a large extent. However, there were country-specific German particularities, especially the extensive use of ultrasound in general practices, the amount of referrals to specialists due to non-medical reasons or the uncontrolled direct access to secondary care for patients themselves.

The GPs' heterogeneous evaluation of check-up tests in asymptomatic individuals corresponded to findings from other countries such as Ireland [20]. In terms of reasons for medically unnecessary referrals made by GPs, our results coincided with Wammes et al. who also found a fear of making mistakes, lack of time and demanding patients to be major drivers [21].

The importance of drivers such as malpractice claims, financial incentives for diagnostic testing and too little time for patients corresponded to the findings of a representative study with US primary care physicians [22]. However, the impact of fear of malpractice claims on medical overuse is controversially discussed in literature. Levinson et al. reported on the importance of a well-functioning doctor-patient-relationship for the decrease of potential lawsuits [23].

Other findings showed the concerns the interviewed GPs raised over complex and potentially biased guidelines. A review of NHS clinical practice guidelines from 2010 and 2011 analysed that publications which formed the evidence basis for these guidelines were in 62% of uncertain relevance to the primary care setting [24]. There is also evidence that many primary care physicians are not trained well enough to interpret statistical information on screening and favoured it despite a lack of clear evidence [25]. These results were in line with something like a "dogma of prevention", which we observed in some of the interviewed GPs, suggesting that screening and prevention is always something valuable.

Some of the interviewed GPs partially explained the performance of unnecessary procedures with demanding patients. In a study with oncological patients, there are clues that GPs overrate patient expectations as a driver for medical overuse [26]. Further research in other patient populations is needed. Fenton et al. showed in a representative study that higher patient satisfaction not only reduces emergency department use as a positive consequence, but also correlates with "greater inpatient use, higher overall health care and prescription drug expenditures, and increased mortality" [27].

In a recent review, Chiolero et al. [28] summarised some major strategies for preventing medical overuse. However, there was no special focus on primary care or strategies that could be directly applied by GPs. The authors commonly called for a greater general awareness of medical overuse, a better training in assessing potential benefits and risks of medical procedures and watchful waiting strategies in situations with a high risk of over investigation and overtreatment.

3. Strengths and limitations of the study

Although medical overuse has a growing impact on health care research and policy, there has been little research from a primary care perspective so far. In this context, the strength of our study lay in its focus on the GPs' perspective on medical overuse. We particularly aimed at exploring a broad scope and set of drivers in terms of unnecessary investigations and treatment and also strategies to reduce it (=quaternary prevention). As this focus required a qualitative study design, it was not possible to link each context of medical overuse with its individual drivers and strategies. This question will be addressed in a subsequent quantitative study.

With regard to the principle of reflexivity [29], the authors started with the preliminary hypothesis that over investigation and overtreatment represent a serious problem in primary health care which ought to be reduced through quaternary prevention strategies. However, we particularly payed attention to negative cases (GPs who thought overuse to be of no or only minor importance) in order to deal with this potential research bias [18, 29]. Throughout the iterative research process, we also expanded our semi-structured interview guide with cross-checks for rivalling explanations [29].

We did not interview secondary care specialists, patients or other stakeholders, which could have added to internal validity [29]. We suggest further research to continue with building a comprehensive theory on the phenomenon of medical overuse, taking vulnerable groups, specific diagnostic and treatment processes into account. Due to the qualitative research design and theoretical sampling of a limited number of participating GPs, the study lacks representativeness and external validity [29] in terms of a quantitative research approach.

Conclusions

The findings of our study indicate that there are various aspects of medical overuse that can be addressed and improved in primary care itself. GPs are often located at the very starting point of a patient's diagnostic and treatment process. They can decide whether to trigger the cascade [16] of unnecessary medicine or not. If this avalanche is already set off, it will be far more difficult to stop it than at an earlier stage. In this context, a trustful doctor-patient-relationship, patient education and the promotion of a primary care-centred health care model could be helpful. High-quality training could empower GPs to cope with residual uncertainty and to accept well-founded "wait and see".

Research shows that GPs are open to feedback on their way of practicing [22]. This openness could be the basis of applying quaternary prevention strategies in primary care. Finally, the definition of low value health care requires precise definitions and decisions about cut-off points regarding a net benefit or a benefit-cost ratio. This requires a careful consideration of various complex underlying normative and social implications [30]. In this context, a process of setting priorities in health care could be helpful [8].

Endnotes

[1]The remainder consists of special programs (for soldiers, for example) and of persons without a health insurance.

Abbreviations

GP: General practitioner

Acknowledgements

We would like to thank all the general practitioners who took the time to be interviewed. Kathrin Alber performed the present work in (partial) fulfilment of the requirements for obtaining the degree "Dr. med."

Funding

We acknowledge support by Deutsche Forschungsgemeinschaft (DFG) and Friedrich-Alexander-University Erlangen-Nuernberg (FAU) within the funding programme Open Access Publishing.

Authors' contributions

KA and TK conceptualized and planned the study. All interviews were realized by KA. Data analysis was carried out by KA and TK (investigator triangulation). KA drafted the manuscript and TK, AS and SS critically revised it. All authors read and approved the final manuscript.

Author's information

Kathrin Alber was a student of medicine at Friedrich-Alexander-University Erlangen-Nuernberg (FAU) while conducting this study. Thomas Kuehlein, MD, PhD, is professor and head of the Institute of General Practice, Friedrich-Alexander-University Erlangen-Nuernberg (FAU). Angela Schedlbauer, PhD, and Susann Schaffer, PhD, are senior research fellows at the Institute of General Practice, Friedrich-Alexander-University Erlangen-Nuernberg (FAU).

Consent for publication

Not applicable.

Competing interests

The authors declare that they have no competing interests.

References

1. Carter SM, Rogers W, Heath I, Degeling C, Doust J, Barratt A. The challenge of overdiagnosis begins with its definition. BMJ. 2015; https://doi.org/10.1136/bmj.h869.
2. Morgan DJ, Brownlee S, Leppin AL, Kressin N, Dhruva SS, Levin L, et al. Setting a research agenda for medical overuse. BMJ. 2015; https://doi.org/10.1136/bmj.h4534.
3. Brody H. Medicine's ethical responsibility for health care reform - the top five list. N Engl J Med. 2010;362:283–5.
4. Chassin MR. Is health care ready for six sigma quality? Milbank Q. 1998;76:565–91.
5. Berwick DM, Hackbarth AD. Eliminating waste in US health care. JAMA. 2012;307:1513–6.
6. Djulbegovic B, Paul A. From efficacy to effectiveness in the face of uncertainty. Indication creep and prevention creep. JAMA. 2011;305:2005–6.
7. Heath I. Overdiagnosis: when good intentions meet vested interests. BMJ. 2013; https://doi.org/10.1136/bmj.f6361.
8. Starfield B, Hyde J, Gérvas J, Heath I. The concept of prevention: a good idea gone astray? J Epidemiol Community Health. 2008;62:580–3.
9. Pencina MJ, Navar-Boggan AM, D'Agostino RB, Williams K, Neely B, Sniderman AD, Peterson ED. Application of new cholesterol guidelines to a population-based sample. N Engl J Med. 2014;370:1422–31.

10. American Board of Internal Medicine Foundation (ABIM). Choosing Wisely Recommendations. 2015. http://www.choosingwisely.org/wp-content/uploads/2015/01/Choosing-Wisely-Recommendations.pdf. Accessed 02 Apr 2016.
11. Kuehlein T, Sghedoni D, Visentin G, Gérvas J, Jamoulle M. Quaternary prevention: a task of the general practitioner. PrimaryCare. 2010;10: 350–4.
12. Jamoulle M. Quaternary prevention, an answer of family doctors to overmedicalization. Int J Health Policy Manag. 2015;4:61–4.
13. Bentzen N (ed.). Wonca Dictionary for General/Family Practice. Wonca International Classification Committee. 2003. http://www.cff.org.br/userfiles/5%20-%20BENTZEN%20N_%20Wonca%20Dictionary%20of%20General%20Family%20Practice.pdf?winst=1415225987182&of=0&of=2488613. Accessed 07 Nov 2014.
14. Bluemel M, Busse R. The German Health Care System, 2015. In: Mossialos E, Wenzl M, Osborn R, Sarnak D (eds.). International profiles of health care systems 2015. The Commonwealth Fund 2016. http://www.commonwealthfund.org/publications/fund-reports/2016/jan/international-profiles-2015. Accessed 24 June 2017.
15. Schneider A, Dinant G, Szecsenyi J. Stepwise diagnostic workup in general practice as a consequence of the Bayesian reasoning [article in German]. Z Arztl Fortbild Qualitatssich. 2006;100:121–7.
16. Deyo R. Cascade effects of medical technology. Annu Rev Public Health. 2002;23:23–44.
17. Strauss A, Corbin J. Basics of qualitative research: grounded theory procedures and techniques [German edition]. Beltz Psychologie Verlags Union: Weinheim; 1996.
18. Corbin J, Strauss A. Grounded theory research: procedures, canons, and evaluative criteria. Qual Sociol. 1990;13:3–21.
19. Huang R. RQDA - Qualitative Data Analysis (Version 0.2–7). 2014. http://rqda.r-forge.r-project.org/. Accessed 23 Nov 2015.
20. Murphy M, McGloughlin M, Walkin S. The 'general check-up' in the asymptomatic adult - a study of GPs in the north west of Ireland. Eur J Gen Pract. 2015;21:58–62.
21. Wammes JJ, Jeurissen PP, Verhoef LM, Assendelft WJ, Westert GP, Faber MJ. Is the role as gatekeeper still feasible? A survey among Dutch general practitioners. Fam Pract. 2014;31:538–44.
22. Sirovich BE, Woloshin S, Schwartz LM. Too little? Too much? Primary care physicians' views on US health care: a brief report. Arch Intern Med. 2011; 171:1582–5.
23. Levinson W, Roter DL, Mullooly JP, Dull VT, Frankel RM. Physician-patient communication: the relationship with malpractice claims among primary care physicians and surgeons. JAMA. 1997;277:553–9.
24. Steel N, Abdelhamid A, Stokes T, Edwards H, Fleetcroft R, Howe A, Qureshi N. A review of clinical practice guidelines found that they were often based on evidence of uncertain relevance to primary care patients. J Clin Epidemiol. 2014;67:1251–7.
25. Wegwarth O, Schwartz LM, Woloshin S, Gaissmaier W, Gigerenzer G. Do physicians understand cancer screening statistics? A national survey of primary care physicians in the United States. Ann Intern Med. 2012;156:340–9.
26. Gogineni K, Shuman KL, Chinn D, Gabler NB, Emanuel EJ. Patient demands and requests for cancer tests and treatments. JAMA Oncol. 2015;1:33–9.
27. Fenton JJ, Jerant AF, Bertakis KD, Franks P. The cost of satisfaction: a national study of patient satisfaction, health care utilization, expenditures, and mortality. Arch Intern Med. 2012;172:405–11.
28. Chiolero A, Paccaud F, Aujesky D, Santschi V, Rodondi N. How to prevent overdiagnosis. Swiss Med Wkly. 2015; https://doi.org/10.4414/smw.2015.14060.
29. Malterud K. Qualitative research: standards, challenges, and guidelines. Lancet. 2001;358:483–8.
30. Blumenthal-Barby JS. "Choosing wisely" to reduce low-value care: a conceptual and ethical analysis. J Med Philos. 2013;38:559–80.

22

"It's complicated" - talking about gout medicines in primary care consultations

Caroline Morris*, Lindsay Macdonald, Maria Stubbe and Anthony Dowell

Abstract

Background: Gout is the most common form of inflammatory arthritis. It is associated with substantial co-morbidity and often managed in primary care. A greater understanding of the communication process between patients and healthcare professionals provides one way of improving the management of this condition. This paper describes communication about gout medicines and treatment between patients and primary care health professionals during routine consultations.

Methods: Video-recordings of 31 individual healthcare consultations between patients and a range of primary care practitioners (general practitioners, practice nurses, podiatrists, dietitians) from an archived database were reviewed. Consultations that encompassed any discussion about gout medicines and treatment were included ($n = 27$) and were not solely restricted to those where gout was the presenting complaint. Themes were derived from an inductive qualitative analysis, from clinical and linguistic perspectives, based on the conversation between patients and practitioners about medicines and visual observation of these interactions.

Results: A number of factors were identified that had the potential to impact on the optimal management of gout in primary care. These included level of patient knowledge, patient attitudes to medicines, and the attributes of practitioner communication with patients. The latter related to the style of delivery and content of the information provided, and the ability of practitioners to make use of opportunities that arose to discuss these issues.

Conclusions: Patients with gout communicate at varying levels of complexity with a diverse range of primary care healthcare professionals about the treatment of their condition. It is important that all practitioners engaging with gout patients in this setting are knowledgeable about the current management of gout, provide clear, consistent and accurate messages, remain aware that these messages may need repeating over time, and are supportive of patients' medicine-taking preferences.

Keywords: Communication, Consultation, Gout, Medicine, Primary care

Abbreviations: ARCH, Applied Research on Communication in Health; DS, Diabetes study; GP, General practitioner; IS, Interaction study; NS, Nurse; POD, Podiatrist; PT, Patient; TS, Tracking study

* Correspondence: caroline.morris@otago.ac.nz
Department Primary Health Care & General Practice, University of Otago, Wellington, 23a Mein Street, Wellington, New Zealand

Background

Gout is recognised as the most common form of inflammatory arthritis and is often associated with substantial co-morbidity [1]. This condition, usually managed in primary care, is closely linked with diabetes and chronic kidney disease and is an independent risk factor for cardiovascular mortality [2]. The clinical and economic burden of the disease is substantial [3, 4].

Some aspects of gout management appear straightforward and there is a plethora of management reviews and treatment guidelines in existence globally [1, 5–9]. Non-steroidal anti-inflammatory drugs (NSAIDs) are one of the main medicine groups used for the management of acute flares, with colchicine and steroids providing alternative treatment options. A target serum uric acid level of less than 0.36 mmol/L is aimed for and allopurinol and other urate-lowering therapies are indicated for the chronic management of gout.

The burden of the disease is rising, [3] and aspects of management remain challenging. Differences in primary care management strategies have been widely noted between routine practice and both reported management and recommended guidelines [10–15].

Differing patient and physician perceptions of gout have been identified as one of the challenges to management in primary care [16]. Issues identified include patients experiencing difficulty in obtaining information they perceive as directly relevant to them, [17] self-diagnosis and treatment by patients, [18] a lack of patient knowledge about gout medicines, [19–22] a lack of practitioner knowledge about treatment guidelines and recommendations [21] and a reluctance on the part of some practitioners to offer preventive medicines as a long-term solution, with some making an assumption that patients would prefer to be treated for an acute flare rather than take long-term medication [21].

While some previous studies have attempted to address views about gout treatment from both patient and practitioner perspectives, [21, 23] there is no research that investigates directly observed conversations in primary care consultations. Existing findings therefore rely on people's abstract perceptions or retrospective reports of healthcare encounters. We describe communication between patients and primary care practitioners about gout medicines and treatment in the context of routine consultations. We identify how patient and practitioner perceptions are brought into play in the course of natural interactions between them. The prevalence of gout, due to its association with cardio-vascular disease and diabetes, is likely to increase further. A greater understanding of the communication process will help determine how the management of this condition can be improved.

Methods

Data source

Data were derived from the Applied Research on Communication in Health (ARCH) Corpus at the University of Otago, Wellington, New Zealand [24]. This comprises a searchable digital collection of healthcare interactions and related data for use in interactional and narrative analysis. The data in the Corpus has been collected in the course of a series of funded projects since 2003. These studies include the 'Interaction Study' (IS), a study exploring clinical decision-making when rationing is explicit; the Tracking Study (TS), a study exploring communication processes throughout a single complete episode of care of patients referred from primary to secondary care; the Diabetes Study (DS), a longitudinal study tracking the contact of newly diagnosed patients with Type 2 diabetes with healthcare professionals over a six-month period. Data are permanently archived for use by authorised researchers.

As the data contained in the Corpus has been collected on a project-by-project basis it does not claim to be 'representative' in the statistical sense. It is, however, representative in the sense that the video-recordings were made in the course of 'practice as usual'. They are therefore typical of routine interactions occurring in the New Zealand healthcare setting.

Logging of data in the ARCH Corpus

The digital video-recording for each consultation is logged by a trained research nurse onto a template summarising key clinical content (e.g. presenting problem, other clinical issues discussed, treatment with medicines) and a time-coded sequence of key events and topics discussed. Each consultation is subsequently transcribed in full using linguistic transcription conventions to capture both the words spoken and selected non-verbal cues (e.g. typing of notes on the computer) to assist in interpretation of the transcribed speech. The Corpus has a custom-designed information management system.

Search strategy for identifying gout consultations

When sampled, the Corpus included 418 video-recorded interactions between patients and practitioners recorded between 2004 and 2011. Consultations occurring in primary care and consultations where patients had given consent for secondary analysis of their data were included, resulting in a subset of 337 eligible consultations. These comprised 247 individual patients, 30 general practitioners (GPs), 31 nurses and 15 other practitioners.

A query was then run on the information held within the database using the keyword "gout". A second search incorporating a list of key gout-related medicines was run, but did not yield any additional consultations.

Consultations included in the analysis

The search identified 31 consultations, 27 of which were included in the final analysis.

The majority of consultations identified came from those archived as part of the DS ($n = 20$). Gout was not, therefore, the primary focus of these encounters; many gout-related conversations stemmed from enquiries made by practitioners that resulted directly from application of the nationally agreed protocol for diabetes care. Despite this, discussion about gout medicines of varying length and complexity was a feature in the majority of these consultations ($n = 16$). In the remaining four, there was no mention of medicines in the context of gout; these consultations were therefore excluded from further analysis. As this study tracked patients over a six-month time-frame, the same patient was sometimes involved in more than one consultation in the sample and potentially more likely to discuss gout medicines with a practitioner if they had talked about them in a healthcare encounter in the recent past.

Contextual information about the 11 GP consultations derived from the IS study ($n = 5$) and the TS study ($n = 6$) is provided in Table 1.

Patient and practitioner demographic characteristics

The final dataset of 27 consultations used for analysis encompassed 17 individual patients (male $n = 12$, female $n = 5$; age-range 36 to 67 years) consulting with 15 different practitioners. The number of consultations per patient ranged from one to eight, with the majority of patients (14/17) having only one included consultation. Patients interacted with a diverse range of professionals (GPs $n = 9$, nurses $n = 3$, podiatrists $n = 2$, dietitian $n = 1$).

Data analysis

This was an exploratory descriptive study based on direct observation of gout-related interactions from both clinical and linguistic viewpoints. Our aim was to identify and report on the range of patient-practitioner models of engagement around medicines use as these emerged from the data, with no preconceived assumptions.

Themes identified from the overall dataset were derived via an iterative process of inductive qualitative analysis [25] of the medicine-related gout conversations between patients and practitioners, with visual observation of these interactions complementing the textual analysis of the transcripts. CM identified and coded all mentions or sequences of talk relating to the use of medicines in the management of gout in the transcripts. Video-recordings of consultations were then viewed to confirm and enrich the content analysis of the transcripts. Initial coding included the location within the consultation, who (patient or practitioner) initiated the conversation, the types and names of medicines discussed, the context in which that discussion took place and any significant non-verbal interactions. The video-recordings and transcripts were then re-reviewed to identify any other medicine-related conversation to help provide additional insights and context for the gout-related medicines communication. CM and AD reviewed and discussed the initial themes derived from data analysis and interpretation of data from their clinical perspectives (pharmacy and general practice), with disagreements resolved by consensus. LM and MS subsequently reviewed the data and themes derived from a linguistic and interactional perspective. All authors reviewed and agreed the final themes.

Table 1 GP consultations that were not part of the DS ($n = 11$)

Description	Number
Gout was the patient's presenting complaint	2
Gout was the presenting complaint in the patient's previous consultation (not part of the Corpus archive) and was followed up by the GP on this occasion	2
Gout discussed in the context of a medicine that had been previously prescribed for this condition	7

GP general practitioner

Results

Communication about gout medicines

Interactions about gout treatment occurred at various levels of complexity, taking many different forms. Some focused solely on the treatment of acute flares with NSAIDs, colchicine or steroid injections, some solely on preventive treatment with allopurinol, while others encompassed both acute and chronic management.

Three overarching themes emerged from our data. These themes (and sub-themes where applicable) are shown in Table 2 and described more fully below. Abbreviations used in the quotes are as follows: GP = general practitioner; NS = nurse; PT = patient; POD = podiatrist.

Level of patient knowledge

We identified a number of instances where patients displayed a lack of important knowledge about medicines used for gout. NSAIDs, a medicine class with significant potential to cause harm if inappropriately used, caused confusion for a number of patients. In this example a patient with a long-standing diagnosis of gout had been unsuccessfully self-treating an acute flare with an insufficient dose of a medicine purchased over-the-counter:

Table 2 Overarching themes and sub-themes identified from the data

- Level of patient knowledge
- Patient attitudes to medicines
- Attributes of practitioner communication
  - Delivery and content of information provided
  - Taking the opportunities presented

GP: so, you'd been taking lots of ... those 'mini' Voltarens™ [diclofenac 25 mg strength], and so we switched you on to the one hundreds [100 mg strength] ... and when you started on those initially you said there was a bit of improvement ..." (IS-GP02-14)

The GP then listens carefully and attentively to the patient as they describe the beneficial effect that this increase in dose has had on their symptoms over time.

In addition, some patients showed a lack of understanding of generic and brand (™) names, not realising that the same medicine could have two different names. In this consultation, a patient with a history of hip pain managed with an NSAID is newly diagnosed with gout. The GP spends considerable time explaining the causes and symptoms of gout before mentioning treatment with medicines:

GP: "... I'll give you some diclofenac, ... it's good for your gout and also for the other pain

PT: and can I have some Voltaren™ [diclofenac] please?

GP: It's the same thing as Voltaren™ [diclofenac]

PT: Is it?" (DS-GP29-01)

The following patient with a confirmed diagnosis of gout is already willingly taking a low dose of allopurinol as preventive therapy. However, this is not currently adequately managing their symptoms. The GP explains the reason why they are unable at this point to increase the dose:

Joint consultation with nurse and GP:

GP: "... now you know those allopurinol tablets for the gout, you still taking them?

PT: yep, cos I wanted to prevent the gout

GP: the problem [is] that's quite a low dose and we probably need to increase it, but I can't increase it when you've got acute gout because it gets worse so ... what we'll do is leave you on that dose and increase it in a couple of weeks when it's better." (DS-NS13-01c_GP18)

The patient smiles indicating that they are comfortable with this approach and understanding of the reasoning behind it. The following excerpts from subsequent consultations with this patient and other practitioners appear to show that a patient's understanding may evolve over time and that confusion may creep in as a result.

Consultation with dietitian two weeks later:

PT: "They haven't put me on [more] of the medication [allopurinol] because this can enhance more gout, so they just said to me to stick on what I've got and hopefully when I get rid of the gout they'll increase it, so it can lower the [number of] times I have gout." (DS-HP06-01b)

The patient had been given information by one practitioner (GP) and then recited that same information back to another practitioner (dietitian) a short time later. Two weeks after this, the patient recalls that they were to stay on the same dose, and reconsiders their situation in light of their worsening symptoms. While doing so they are also now questioning the possibility that allopurinol can exacerbate gout.

Consultation with podiatrist one month after the GP consultation:

PT: "It [gout] started from my toes round to my ankle and then it just stayed there for a while and it just slowly headed up ... [and] they told me to keep on it [allopurinol] ... so I stayed on that and I thought that was triggering it because that's the longest I've ever had gout ... [and] I wasn't quite sure ... and I was questioning myself 'Should I stop it?' cos I don't know if that was triggering it worse

POD: but it's a treatment for gout so you wouldn't think it would actually exacerbate your symptoms or pain ..." (DS-HP07-01b)

This consultation series also shows that in primary care teams with multiple healthcare professionals, advice about medicines may be given by professionals other than the prescriber. In this instance it would have been helpful if the podiatrist could have appropriately addressed the patient's understanding. However, in the final quotation, the podiatrist seems unaware of the action of allopurinol and inadvertently creates a further source of confusion potentially undermining the patient's knowledge and understanding of gout treatment.

Patient attitudes to medicines

It was clear that how patients perceived medicines sometimes impacted on the way in which their gout was treated. One patient with previously diagnosed gout identified "I don't like tablets" as a general statement at the beginning of a consultation and then segued straight into talking specifically about gout:

PT: "... and I said before, I told you with my gout I don't want to take any more tablets ...

GP: When did you last have a flare of gout?

PT: Well, sometimes I feel it is a little bit sore on my elbow but I don't take anything - it comes and goes ...

GP: "... your uric acid level in your blood, that's the one that's associated with gout is still high, so I think if you do start having regular flare-ups then we should look again at putting you back on allopurinol to bring that uric acid level down." (DS-GP19-02b)

While it was unclear what the patient's uric acid level was or whether allopurinol therapy at this point was justified, clinically, the impact of the condition on the patient's life appeared manageable without the use of medicines. It is possible that the GP may have judged the level of clinical severity against the patient's desire to be tablet-free and they appeared accepting of the patient's preference at this point in time. While there was no discussion about the reasons for the patient's reticence to take medicines, the possible future need for treatment with tablets was brought clearly into the open by the GP, with tacit approval from the patient indicated by a nodding of their head and a verbal acknowledgment in the form of "yeah, yeah".

Another patient was fully aware of the potential adverse impact that taking an NSAID for her long-term gout symptoms could have on a co-morbid condition. Although her specific circumstances dictated that she took the medicine anyway, she had developed a personal strategy in an attempt to minimise the risk:

NS: "What are you taking in terms of pain relief?

PT: Well, I actually ran out of what [the GP] gave me ... and all I had was diclofenac ... so what I was trying to do was half it [the dose] because I was in so much pain because I know that the diclofenac triggers my asthma" (DS-NS13-01d_GP18)

There is no discussion or negotiation about alternative options that may be more suitable for the patient, nor is the patient able to glean what the nurse may think by either verbal or non-verbal means. The consultation moves swiftly on to codeine, another medicine that the patient is taking for pain relief, and its tendency to cause constipation:

PT: "so then I had, what do you call it, codeine

NS: codeine doesn't help the constipation either" (DS-NS13-01d_GP18)

Attributes of practitioner communication

Delivery and content of information provided

Communication style varied across the consultations. Many practitioners asked open questions, clearly listened to the patient's view, provided clear, accurate information, and confirmed that the patient understood this information and was comfortable with the final decision. In this example the patient presented to the GP because they had run out medicines. This prompts a general discussion about their medicines leading to the patient describing symptoms they knew to be gout:

GP: "... getting a good dose of diclofenac would be probably the most useful thing; so this is your first gout attack for a long, long time isn't it? So I don't think we need to look at the allopurinol thing

PT: well, no cos I mean this attack, I totally knew [the cause], it just didn't occur to me at the time, it was just silly, but yeah this [attack] isn't a mystery" (TS-GP09-05)

There was clear agreement between them, with the GP smiling and both parties verbally acknowledging that they were happy with this approach by saying "mm mm".

In another consultation a substantial amount of discussion, initially raised by the GP, took place around the use of colchicine in a patient with gout that had previously proven difficult to manage. Effective clear communication with the patient occurred resulting in a clear management plan agreed by both parties. The only contentious issue here might be the use of the word "prophylaxis"; something that may not necessarily be understood by the patient:

GP: "... allopurinol is probably an option, but [the specialist] thought you should stay on colchicine ... which is what you've done isn't it? One tablet twice a day for the prophylaxis and I think if that's doing the trick and not giving you symptoms then that's fine ... if that turned [out] for any reason not to be suiting you in terms of prevention; either not effective enough or giving you side effects, then there are the other things that we can try

PT: I'm actually only taking one a day, it seems to be effective so then I guess I could

GP: if one a day is doing it that's fine [but] you can easily up it to two if you're getting any breakthrough - it would be fine." (IS-GP02-03)

The patient tacitly indicates by nodding his head that he agrees with the GP.

All of the podiatrist consultations ($n = 4$) were with patients with diabetes and featured practitioner engagement with the patient around medicines to some degree. These consultations were relatively lengthy (between 20 and 30 min) compared to GP consultations and talk about medicines was usually used as a time-filler following what seemed to be uncomfortably long gaps of silence for the practitioner. The following extract took place 10 min into a consultation where the podiatrist had been asking questions or providing information about diabetes with limited response from the patient:

> POD: "... [gout] that's a type of arthritis [that] tends to run in families ... it can be quite painful gout are you on medication for it?
>
> PT: Yes" (DS-HP10-02a)

Taking the opportunities presented

While a small number of 'lost' opportunities to discuss gout and gout medicines were identified across the dataset, there were many excellent examples of practitioners making good use of opportunities that presented themselves by responding to 'openings' provided by patients.

In this example the patient raises the issue of gout, identifying that he had been given an unnamed "injectable treatment" abroad in the past. Although the patient clearly articulates that gout is not currently a problem, the GP seamlessly picks up on the opportunity to explain the rationale for his current treatment approach offering reassurance that alternative options exist should the patient's circumstances change:

> PT: "...I do get gout ... but it normally goes away by itself. I think the last time would have been last year sometime ...
>
> GP: I feel we've got more than enough information right now to know what the next step should be and at this stage, because things are not that bad, I'm saying I'd quite like to be very conservative in this and not push you know lots and lots of treatment, but we've got it there waiting if things got a bit [clinically] worse or didn't improve as far as these [uric acid] numbers are concerned" (DS-GP01-04)

The patient listens carefully to the explanation, smiles, maintains eye contact and nods their head in acceptance.

Another example shows the potential benefit of coordinated multidisciplinary care. This patient had expressed concern about their gout pain to the nurse in an appointment the previous week. The nurse then reintroduces this issue in their second consultation, discussing the patient's symptoms with them and identifying that there was a need to involve the GP further in their gout-related care. In this instance, having been provided with information about a new treatment option for their symptoms the patient very clearly verbally articulates that this is something they would like to try.

> NS: "I had a wee chat with [GP's name] ... you had a concern about your toes about the gout ... and she says that if you're having more than two episodes in a year
>
> PT: oh yes definitely
>
> NS: oh okay, she said then you probably need some treatment which you carry on taking long-term because it helps to prevent [gout]
>
> PT: oh I would - it's always at the back of my ankle and ... it gets right here [pointing at foot] and I can't walk on it and stuff like that, six times maybe seven times a year easily and they all swell up and the other place I get it is on my side of my toes ...
>
> NS: have you got those symptoms at the moment? No okay, alright so I probably need to leave a message for [the GP]" (DS-NS13-01b)

However, not all patient-practitioner gout interactions resulted in any significant discussion about the condition. Sometimes another potentially more pressing problem or patient concern becomes the focus of that part of the consultation and the moment and the potential opportunity has passed.

Only one example of an opportunity being truly missed was identified from the dataset. This practitioner phrased her question about a gout medicine in a closed way that did not invite debate or discussion as she simultaneously turns her back to the patient and prints out a computer generated blood test form:

> NS: "your allopurinol, you know about it don't you? It's the same. So that's a fasting blood test [form], first thing in the morning for fasting ..." (DS-NS27-02)

There is silence while the form is printing and once this is done the nurse hands it to the patient, explains what fasting means, advises them when they should schedule their next visit and the consultation is closed.

Discussion

Our study is the first to describe communication about medicines for gout treatment in the context of routine consultations in primary care. We identified three overarching themes from the data; level of patient knowledge about gout medicines, patients' attitudes towards medicines, and the attributes of practitioner communication. Each of these inter-linking themes has the potential to impact either positively or adversely on the successful management of gout. Optimising the manner, and avenues, by which information is shared with patients has the potential to improve patient knowledge and understanding, and promote clinician-patient agreement. A link between good communication and positive health outcomes has been previously described in the literature [26].

The strength of our study is that it enabled us to see, hear and review the interaction between patients and their practitioner in real encounters, rather than relying on the abstract views or retrospective opinions of each party. As some of the included consultations formed part of a longitudinal study we were also able to review encounters with a range of practitioners and gain insight into how patients' knowledge and attitudes may alter over time. Although data were drawn from an archived database rather than a study specifically related to gout, the use of a video-recorder may have introduced an artificial bias, with participants behaving differently from 'normal' due to its presence. However, although all parties appear cognisant of a camera's presence early on in a consultation, this effect can be observed to wane as the business of the consultation progresses [27].

It was concerning that some patients lacked basic knowledge about the main medicines used for gout treatment. This has clear implications for the quality and safety of medicines use. In line with earlier work, [19, 20] this study revealed lack of knowledge related to the appropriate NSAID dosing for an acute gout flare and confusion around NSAID generic and brand names. Some patients also lacked a clear understanding of the specific and unusual issues around the initiation of allopurinol therapy; an area which has been previously identified as a source of patient confusion [19, 20, 28].

It was evident on following a single patient through a series of consultations that information may need repeated explanation to ensure that understanding remains consistent over time. Information that appeared to be unproblematic when initially given became less clearly understood by the patient as time progressed and other experiences intervened. All healthcare professionals that may interact with patients, including community pharmacists, have a potentially valuable role to play in facilitating patient understanding and hence the safe and effective use of medicines.

The level of knowledge about gout treatment may impinge on patients' attitudes towards gout medicines and the likelihood of patient-practitioner concordance [29]. There were examples in the present study of patients taking medicines 'differently' to the way the practitioner expected and a reticence expressed, by some, to taking preventive medicines long-term. To be considered for preventive treatment patients will have been previously symptomatic, although the level of pain experienced by an individual may vary widely. It is therefore not surprising that here, and in previous studies, [19, 23] patients have admitted to failing to take medicines both unintentionally (they were unaware of how it should be taken or simply forgot) and intentionally (they had no desire to take a medicine every day) [19, 23]. It is notable that one patient continued to take a medicine to treat gout despite the fact that it exacerbated a co-morbid condition, identifying that patient values and judgments around medicine side-effects may differ from their practitioner's.

Communicating in an open way and engaging the patient in a discussion about treatment options is likely to increase patient knowledge about the rationale behind their treatment and potentially promote agreement and adherence to a treatment plan that takes account of the patient's beliefs and wishes [29]. Although some patients may ultimately choose to defer a treatment decision to their healthcare professional, the majority desire some level of involvement in the decision-making process [30]. Patients are only able to make an informed and evaluated decision on how they personally wish to engage with medicine taking or sign-up to a suggested treatment plan if they have appropriate and accurate information on which to base their decision. It is therefore of note that gout patients have previously identified that they did not always understand the information that GPs provided and have suggested that practitioners should explicitly confirm their understanding [19]. Furthermore, as in our study, potentially important mismatches in perceptions between patients and healthcare providers (including doctors, nurses, podiatrists) about the effectiveness and place of specific medicines in gout management and the adequacy of information provided have been shown to exist [23].

The present study reviewed consultations with a range of different primary care health professionals. It was notable that medicines were a feature of consultations across all professional groups, although, not surprisingly, medicines-related talk occurred to a greater extent with GPs who are the prescriber of medicines. It is, however, vital that all practitioners engaging with gout patients are knowledgeable about the up-to-date management of this condition and provide clear, consistent and accurate messages to avoid the potential for misleading or confusing patients.

While our findings potentially have relevance to other musculoskeletal conditions, it is possible that communication between patients and practitioners about gout treatment may differ from, for example, osteoarthritis [31]. In contrast to this condition, gout can be effectively managed using preventive therapy and is far less likely to be perceived as a normal part of getting old.

Our study was undertaken in the context of routine clinical practice. It thus allowed us to view the communication process within the real time constraints under which practitioners undertake their daily work. Furthermore, consultations were not solely for gout providing, for the first time, an indication of how this issue is routinely raised in primary care practice. Overall, there were many examples of good communication; practitioners often use open questions, are supportive of their patients' medicines-related preferences and seize opportunities that present to discuss gout and its treatment.

The difficulty of managing patients with gout and its associated co-morbidities in a short consultation is a key challenge to the optimal management of gout in primary care [16]. Given that medicines are a key feature of gout management and that GP consultation time constraints are unlikely to be easily overcome, a multidisciplinary team approach to care via primary care gout clinics including pharmacist input has been recently reported [32].

Conclusions

Patients with gout communicate at varying levels of complexity with a range of primary care practitioners. All practitioners who interact with gout patients need to be able to provide patients with clear, consistent and accurate messages about gout treatment as the need arises, be aware that these messages may need repeating over time, and be supportive of patients' medicine-taking preferences for this condition.

Acknowledgments

The data archived in the Applied Research on Communication in Health Group (ARCH) Corpus of Health Interactions were originally collected as part of research projects funded by the New Zealand Health Research Council, the Royal Society of New Zealand Marsden Fund, the New Zealand Lotteries Health Research Fund and the University of Otago Research Committee. The authors thank all participants for generously allowing their consultations to be recorded and archived, and acknowledge the input of Lesley Gray, Rachel Tester and other colleagues and research assistants from the ARCH Group, Kevin Dew, another member of the ARCH group, from the School of Social and Cultural Studies, Victoria University of Wellington, New Zealand and Barbara Docherty, Devi-Ann Hall, Timothy Kenealy, Debbie Raphael and Nicolette Sheridan from the Faculty of Medical and Health Sciences, The University of Auckland, New Zealand

Funding

The funders of the studies from which these data are drawn (New Zealand Health Research Council, Royal Society of New Zealand Marsden Fund, New Zealand Lotteries Health Research Fund, University of Otago Research Committee) had no part in the design of the original studies that provided the data for secondary analysis that was used for this article. In addition, they had no involvement in the collection, analysis and interpretation of data for this article, the writing of this article or the decision to submit it for publication. No external funding source was secured for this work; all authors completed it in within their paid University employment time.

Authors' contributions

AD, LM and MS designed the studies from which these data are drawn. LM undertook fieldwork and data collection. CM viewed and reviewed video-recorded data and transcripts and with AD was responsible for the initial data analysis and interpretation. All authors contributed to the final interpretation. CM drafted the manuscript. All authors read and approved the final manuscript.

Authors' information

CM is a practising pharmacist with a pharmacy practice PhD. LM is a registered nurse with a postgraduate qualification in nursing and linguistics. MS is an experienced health communication researcher with a PhD in applied sociolinguistics. AD is a practising GP and Professor of Primary Health Care and General Practice.

Competing interests

The authors declare that they have no competing interests.

Consent for publication

Consent was obtained for the use of de-identified data and transcript excerpts in academic publications (as is the case here).

References

1. Roddy E, Mallen CD, Doherty M. Gout. Br Med J. 2013;347:f5648. doi:10.1136/bmj.f5648.
2. Kuo C-F, See L-C, Luo S-F, Ko Y-S, Lin Y-S, Hwang J-S, et al. Gout: an independent risk factor for all-cause and cardiovascular mortality. Rheumatology. 2010;49:141–6.
3. Kuo C-F, Grainge MJ, Mallen C, Zhang W, Doherty M. Rising burden of gout in the UK but continuing suboptimal management: a nationwide population study. Ann Rheum Dis. 2015;74:661–7
4. Wertheimer A, Morlock R, Becker MA. A Revised Estimate of the Burden of Illness of Gout. Curr Ther Res. 2013;75:1–4.
5. Anon. An update on the management of gout. Best Pract J. 2013;51:8–14.
6. Jordan KM, Cameron JS, Snaith M, Zhang W, Doherty M, Seckl J, et al. British Society for Rheumatology and British Health Professionals in Rheumatology Guideline for the Management of Gout. Rheumatology. 2007;46(8):1372–4.
7. Zhang W, Doherty M, Bardin T, Pascual E, Barskova V, Conaghan P, et al. EULAR evidence based recommendations for gout. Part II: Management. Report of a task force of the EULAR Standing Committee For International Clinical Studies Including Therapeutics (ESCISIT). Ann Rheum Dis. 2006;65: 1312–24.
8. Khanna D, Fitzgerald JD, Khanna PP, Bae S, Singh MK, Neogi T, et al. 2012 American College of Rheumatology guidelines for management of gout. Part 1: Systematic nonpharmacologic and pharmacologic therapeutic approaches to hyperuricemia. Arthritis Care Res. 2012;64:1431–46.
9. Auckland region clinical pathway for gout - acute in adults ≥16 years. http://www.healthpointpathways.co.nz/gout-acute/. Accessed 25 Feb 2016.
10. Mikuls TR, Farrar JT, Bilker WB, Fernandes S, Saag KG. Suboptimal physician adherence to quality indicators for the management of gout and asymptomatic hyperuricaemia: results from the UK General Practice Research Database (GPRD). Rheumatology. 2005;44:1038–42.
11. Annemans L, Spaepen E, Gaskin M, Bonnemaire M, Malier V, Gilbert T, et al. Gout in the UK and Germany: prevalence, comorbidities and management in general practice 2000–2005. Ann Rheum Dis. 2008;67:960–6.
12. Singh JA, Hodges JS, Toscano JP, Asch SM. Quality of care for gout in the US needs improvement. Arthritis Care Res. 2007;57:822–9.
13. Kuo C-F, Grainge MJ, Mallen C, Zhang W, Doherty M. Eligibility for and prescription of urate-lowering treatment in patients with incident gout in England. JAMA. 2014;312:2684–6.

14. Roddy E, Zhang W, Doherty M. Concordance of the management of chronic gout in a UK primary care population with the EULAR gout recommendations. Ann Rheum Dis. 2007;66:1311–5.
15. Harrold LR, Mazor KM, Negron A, Ogarek J, Firneno C, Yood RA. Primary care providers' knowledge, beliefs and treatment practices for gout: Results of a physician questionnaire. Rheumatology. 2013;52:1623–9.
16. Dalbeth N. Management of gout in primary care: challenges and potential solutions. Rheumatology. 2013;52:1549–50.
17. Richardson JC, Liddle J, Mallen CD, Roddy E, Prinjha S, Ziebland S, et al. "Why me? I don't fit the mould… I am a freak of nature": a qualitative study of women's experience of gout. BMC Womens Health. 2015; doi:10.1186/s12905-015-0277-z
18. Liddle J, Roddy E, Mallen CD, Hider SL, Prinjha S, Ziebland S, et al. Mapping patients' experiences from initial symptoms to gout diagnosis: a qualitative exploration. BMJ Open. 2015. doi:10.1136/bmjopen-2015-008323.
19. Martini N, Bryant L, Karu LT, Aho L, Chan R, Miao J, et al. Living with gout in New Zealand: An exploratory study into people's knowledge about the disease and its treatment. J Clin Rheumatol. 2012;18:125–9.
20. Te Karu L, Bryant L, Elley CR. Maori experiences and perceptions of gout and its treatment: a kaupapa Maori qualitative study. J Prim Health Care. 2013;5:214–22.
21. Spencer K, Carr A, Doherty M. Patient and provider barriers to effective management of gout in general practice: A qualitative study. Ann Rheum Dis. 2012;71:1490–5.
22. Lindsay K, Gow P, Vanderpyl J, Logo P, Dalbeth N. The experience and impact of living with gout: a study of men with chronic gout using a qualitative grounded theory approach. J Clin Rheumatol. 2011;17:1–6.
23. Harrold LR, Mazor KM, Velten S, Ockene IS, Yood RA. Patients and providers view gout differently: a qualitative study. Chronic Ill. 2010;6:263–71.
24. ARCH Corpus of Health Interactions. University of Otago, Wellington. http://www.otago.ac.nz/wellington/research/arch/corpus/ Accessed 25 Feb 2016.
25. Boyatzis R. Thematic Analysis and Code Development: Transforming Qualitative Information. London: Sage Publications; 1998.
26. Street Jr RL, Makoul G, Arora NK, Epstein RM. How does communication heal? Pathways linking clinician–patient communication to health outcomes. Patient Educ Couns. 2009;74:295–301.
27. Dowell A, Macdonald L, Stubbe M, Plumridge E, Dew K. Clinicians at work: What can we learn from interactions in the consultation? N Z Fam Physician. 2007;34:345–50.
28. Harrold L, Mazor K, Peterson D, Naz N, Firneno C, Yood R. Patients' knowledge and beliefs concerning gout and its treatment: a population based study. BMC Musculoskelet Disord. 2012. doi:10.1186/1471-2474-13-180.
29. Stevenson FA, Cox K, Britten N, Dundar Y. A systematic review of the research on communication between patients and health care professionals about medicines: the consequences for concordance. Health Expect. 2004;7: 235–45.
30. Politi MC, Dizon DS, Frosch DL, Kuzemchak MD, Stiggelbout AM. Importance of clarifying patients' desired role in shared decision making to match their level of engagement with their preferences. Br Med J. 2013. doi:10.1136/bmj.f7066.
31. Paskins Z, Sanders T, Croft PR, Hassell AB. The identity crisis of osteoarthritis in general practice: a qualitative study using video-stimulated recall. Ann Fam Med. 2015;13:537–44.
32. Goldfien RD, Ng MS, Yip G, Hwe A, Jacobson A, Pressman A, et al. Effectiveness of a pharmacist-based gout care management programme in a large integrated health plan: results from a pilot study. BMJ Open. 2014. doi:10.1136/bmjopen-2013-003627.

Permissions

All chapters in this book were first published in FP, by BioMed Central; hereby published with permission under the Creative Commons Attribution License or equivalent. Every chapter published in this book has been scrutinized by our experts. Their significance has been extensively debated. The topics covered herein carry significant findings which will fuel the growth of the discipline. They may even be implemented as practical applications or may be referred to as a beginning point for another development.

The contributors of this book come from diverse backgrounds, making this book a truly international effort. This book will bring forth new frontiers with its revolutionizing research information and detailed analysis of the nascent developments around the world.

We would like to thank all the contributing authors for lending their expertise to make the book truly unique. They have played a crucial role in the development of this book. Without their invaluable contributions this book wouldn't have been possible. They have made vital efforts to compile up to date information on the varied aspects of this subject to make this book a valuable addition to the collection of many professionals and students.

This book was conceptualized with the vision of imparting up-to-date information and advanced data in this field. To ensure the same, a matchless editorial board was set up. Every individual on the board went through rigorous rounds of assessment to prove their worth. After which they invested a large part of their time researching and compiling the most relevant data for our readers.

The editorial board has been involved in producing this book since its inception. They have spent rigorous hours researching and exploring the diverse topics which have resulted in the successful publishing of this book. They have passed on their knowledge of decades through this book. To expedite this challenging task, the publisher supported the team at every step. A small team of assistant editors was also appointed to further simplify the editing procedure and attain best results for the readers.

Apart from the editorial board, the designing team has also invested a significant amount of their time in understanding the subject and creating the most relevant covers. They scrutinized every image to scout for the most suitable representation of the subject and create an appropriate cover for the book.

The publishing team has been an ardent support to the editorial, designing and production team. Their endless efforts to recruit the best for this project, has resulted in the accomplishment of this book. They are a veteran in the field of academics and their pool of knowledge is as vast as their experience in printing. Their expertise and guidance has proved useful at every step. Their uncompromising quality standards have made this book an exceptional effort. Their encouragement from time to time has been an inspiration for everyone.

The publisher and the editorial board hope that this book will prove to be a valuable piece of knowledge for researchers, students, practitioners and scholars across the globe.

List of Contributors

Rebecca Reynolds, Iqbal Hasan, Jan Slewa, Winnie Chen, David Tian and Sangeetha Bobba
UNSW, Sydney, Australia

Nicholas Zwar
UNSW, Sydney, Australia
School of Medicine, University of Wollongong, Wollongong, NSW 2522, Australia

Sarah Dennis
University of Sydney, Camperdown, Australia

R. Nisenbaum
Centre for Urban Health Solutions, Li Ka Shing Knowledge Institute, St. Michael's Hospital, 30 Bond Street, Toronto, ON M5B 1W8, Canada
Dalla Lana School of Public Health, University of Toronto, Health Sciences Building, 155 College Street, 6th Floor, Toronto, ON M5T 3M7, Canada

Kathrin Alber, Thomas Kuehlein, Angela Schedlbauer and Susann Schaffer
Institute of General Practice, Friedrich-Alexander-University Erlangen-Nuernberg (FAU), Universitaetsstr. 29, 91054 Erlangen, Germany

Franziska D. Welzel and Janine Stein
Institute of Social Medicine, Occupational Health and Public Health, Medical Faculty, University of Leipzig, Philipp-Rosenthal-Straße 55, 04103 Leipzig, Germany

Steffi G. Riedel-Heller
Institute of Social Medicine, Occupational Health and Public Health, Medical Faculty, University of Leipzig, Philipp-Rosenthal-Straße 55, 04103 Leipzig, Germany
Institute of General Medicine, University of Leipzig, Leipzig, Germany

André Hajek and Hans-Helmut König
Department of Health Economics and Health Services Research, University Medical Centre Hamburg-Eppendorf, Hamburg, Germany

Patricia J. Lucas
School for Policy Studies, University of Bristol, 8 Priory Road, Bristol BS8 1TZ, UK

Justine Strand de Oliveira
Barts and The London School of Medicine and Dentistry, Queen Mary University of London, London, UK

Grete Moth, Linda Huibers, Astrid Ovesen, Morten Bondo Christensen and Peter Vedsted
Research Unit for General Practice, Department of Public Health, Aarhus University, Bartholins Alle 2, 8000 Aarhus, Denmark
Section for General Medical Practice, Department of Public Health, Aarhus University, Bartholins Alle 2, 8000 Aarhus, Denmark

Mirella Carolin Uhl, Christiane Muth, Ferdinand Michael Gerlach and Beate Sigrid Müller
Institute of General Practice, Goethe University Frankfurt, Theodor-Stern-Kai 7, 60590 Frankfurt am Main, Germany

Goentje-Gesine Schoch
Scientific Institute for Benefit and Efficiency in Health Care (WINEG), Techniker Krankenkasse (TK), Bramfelder Straße 140, 22305 Hamburg, Germany

Hannah Thornton, Christie Cabral and Alastair D. Hay
Centre for Academic Primary Care, Population Health Sciences, Bristol Medical School, University of Bristol, Canynge Hall, 39 Whatley Road, Bristol BS8 2PS, UK

Sophie Turnbull
Centre for Academic Primary Care, Population Health Sciences, Bristol Medical School, University of Bristol, Canynge Hall, 39 Whatley Road, Bristol BS8 2PS, UK
Centre for Academic Primary Care, School of Social and Community Medicine, University of Bristol, Bristol BS8 2PS, UK

Brandi Leach, Perri Morgan, Sharon Hull, Truls Østbye and Christine Everett
Department of Community and Family Medicine, Duke University School of Medicine, Durham, NC, USA

Niamh M. Redmond
National Institute for Health Research Collaborations for Leadership in Applied Health Research and Care West (NIHR CLAHRC West), University Hospitals Bristol NHS Foundation Trust, 9th Floor, Whitefriars, Lewins Mead, Bristol BS1 2NT, UK

Hannah Christensen
Population Health Sciences, Bristol Medical School, University of Bristol, Oakfield House, Oakfield Grove, Bristol BS8 2BN, UK

Peter S. Blair
Population Health Sciences, Bristol Medical School, University of Bristol, Level D, St Michael's Hospital, Southwell St, Bristol BS2 8EG, UK

Brendan C. Delaney
Department of Surgery and Cancer, Imperial College London, St Mary's Hospital, W2 1NY, London, UK

Matthew Thompson
Department of Family Medicine, University of Washington, Seattle, WA 98195-4696, USA

Paul Little
Primary Care and Population Sciences Unit, University of Southampton, Aldermoor Health Centre, Aldermoor Close, Southampton SO16 5ST, UK

Tim J. Peters
School of Clinical Sciences, University of Bristol, 69 St Michael's Hill, Bristol BS2 8DZ, UK

Franca G. H. Ruikes, Willem J. J. Assendelft and Henk J. Schers
Radboud Institute for Health Sciences, Department of Primary and Community Care, Radboud university medical centre, Nijmegen, the Netherlands

Raymond T. C. M. Koopmans
Radboud Institute for Health Sciences, Department of Primary and Community Care, Radboud university medical centre, Nijmegen, the Netherlands
Joachim and Anna, Centre for specialized geriatric care, Nijmegen, the Netherlands

Eddy M. Adang
Radboud Institute for Health Sciences, Department for Health Evidence, Radboud university medical centre, Nijmegen, the Netherlands

Sytse U. Zuidema
Department of General Practice and Elderly Care Medicine, University of Groningen, University Medical Centre Groningen, Groningen, Netherlands

Jane M. Garbutt
Departments of Medicine and Pediatrics, Washington University School of Medicine, St. Louis, MO, USA

Sherry Dodd and Katharine Kulka
Department of Pediatrics, Washington University School of Medicine, Campus 660 S. Euclid Ave, St. Louis, MO 63110, USA

Emily Walling
Department of Pediatrics, Washington University School of Medicine, Campus 660 S. Euclid Ave, St. Louis, MO 63110, USA
Department of Pediatrics, Michigan Medicine, C.S. Mott Children's Hospital, Ann Arbor, USA

Amanda A. Lee and Rebecca Lobb
Department of Surgery, Washington University School of Medicine, St. Louis, MO, USA

Erik L. Werner
Department of General Practice, Institute of Health and Society, Faculty of Medicine, University of Oslo, Oslo, Norway

Ida Løchting and Kjersti Storheim
Research and Communication Unit for Musculoskeletal Health (FORMI) Clinic for Surgery and Neurology, Oslo University Hospital, Oslo, Norway

Margreth Grotle
Department of Physiotherapy, Oslo Metropolitan University/FORMI, Clinic for Surgery and Neurology, Oslo University Hospital, Oslo, Norway

Eivind Meland, Øystein Hetlevik, Thomas Mildestvedt and Sturla Gjesdal
Department of Global Public Health and Primary Care, University of Bergen, Bergen, Norway

Luckson Dullie
Department of Global Public Health and Primary Care, University of Bergen, Bergen, Norway
Partners In Health, Neno, Malawi
University of Malawi College of Medicine, Blantyre, Malawi

Debbie Cavers, Natalia Calanzani, David Weller and Christine Campbell
The Usher Institute of Population Health Sciences and Informatics, Medical School, University of Edinburgh, Doorway 1, Teviot Place, Edinburgh EH8 9AG, UK

Sheina Orbell
Department of Psychology, University of Essex, Wivenhoe Park, Colchester CO4 3SQ, UK

Gabriele Vojt
Department of Psychology, Social Work and Health Sciences, Glasgow Caledonian University, 70 Cowcaddens Road, Glasgow, UK

Robert J. C. Steele
Division of Cancer Research, Ninewells Hospital and Medical School, Mailbox 4, Level 6, Dundee DD1 9SY, UK

Linda Brownlee
Scottish Bowel Screening Centre, Kings Cross Hospital, Clepington Road, Dundee DD3 8EA, UK

Steve Smith
NHS Bowel Cancer Screening Midlands and North West Programme Hub, St. Cross Hospital, Barby Road, Rugby CV22 5PX, UK

Julietta Patnick
Cancer Epidemiology Unit, Oxford University, Richard Doll Building, Roosevelt Drive, Oxford OX3 7LF, UK

Janet Hanley
School of Health and Social Care, Edinburgh Napier University, Sighthill Campus, Sighthill Court, Edinburgh EH11 4BN, UK

Hilary Pinnock
Allergy and Respiratory Research Group, Usher Institute of Population Health Sciences and Informatics, University of Edinburgh, Teviot Place, Edinburgh EH8 9AG, UK

Mary Paterson and Brian McKinstry
E-Health Research Group, Usher Institute of Population Health Sciences and Informatics, University of Edinburgh, Nine Edinburgh BioQuarter, Edinburgh EH16 4UX, UK

Lars Bruun Larsen, Anders Larrabee Sonderlund, Jens Sondergaard, Janus Laust Thomsen, Niels Christian Hvidt, Elisabeth Assing Hvidt and Trine Thilsing
Department of Public Health, Research Unit of General Practice, University of Southern Denmark, Odense, Denmark

Line Bjornskov Pedersen
Department of Public Health, Research Unit of General Practice, University of Southern Denmark, Odense, Denmark
Department of Business and Economics, COHERE, University of Southern Denmark, Odense, Denmark

Anders Halling
Department of Clinical Sciences, Center for Primary Health Care Research, Lund University, Lund, Sweden

Troels Mønsted
Department of Informatics, University of Oslo, Oslo, Norway

Ewa M. Roos
Department of Sports Science and Clinical Biomechanics, Research Unit for Musculoskeletal Function and Physiotherapy, University of Southern Denmark, Odense, Denmark

Pia Vivian Pedersen
National Institute of Public Health, University of Southern Denmark, Copenhagen, Denmark

Andree Rochfort, Sinead Beirne, Gillian Doran, Patricia Patton and Claire Collins
Irish College of General Practitioners, 4-5 Lincoln Place, Dublin 2, Ireland

Jochen Gensichen
Institute of General Practice and Family Medicine, University Hospital, LMU, Munich, Germany

Ilkka Kunnamo
University of Helsinki, EBM Guidelines, Duodecim Medical Publications Ltd, Helsinki, Finland

Susan Smith
Royal College of Surgeons in Ireland, Dublin, Ireland

Tina Eriksson
GP Copenhagen, Copenhagen, Denmark

Deanna M. Hoelscher
Michael & Susan Dell Center for Healthy Living, University of Texas Health Science Center at Houston (UTHealth) School of Public Health in Austin, Austin, TX, USA

Meliha Salahuddin
Michael & Susan Dell Center for Healthy Living, University of Texas Health Science Center at Houston (UTHealth) School of Public Health in Austin, Austin, TX, USA
University of Texas Health Science Center at Tyler, Tyler, TX, USA
Population Health, Office of Health Affairs, University of Texas System, Austin, TX, USA

Sarah E. Barlow
Texas Children's Hospital, Baylor College of Medicine, Houston, TX, USA
UT Southwestern Medical Center, Dallas, TX, USA

Stephen J. Pon
Texas Center for the Prevention and Treatment of Childhood Obesity, Dell Children's Medical Center, University of Texas at Austin Dell Medical School, Houston, TX, USA

Nancy F. Butte
USDA/ARS Children's Nutrition Research Center; Department of Pediatrics, Baylor College of Medicine, Houston, TX, USA

Meirong Wang, Shuang Shao, Yingjie Liu, Xiaojingyuan Xu and Juan Du
School of General Practice and Continuing Education, Capital Medical University, No.10 Xitoutiao, You An Men, Beijing 100069, China

Jing Li
Dongfeng Community Health Service Center, Chaoyang District, Beijing, China

Mary Ann O'Brien, Andrea Carson, Rabiya Siddiqui and Saddaf Syed
Department of Family and Community Medicine, University of Toronto, 500 University Avenue, Fifth Floor, Toronto, ON M5G 1V7, Canada

Frank Sullivan
Department of Family and Community Medicine, University of Toronto, 500 University Avenue, Fifth Floor, Toronto, ON M5G 1V7, Canada
North York General Hospital, Toronto, ON, Canada
Medical School, University of St Andrews, Scotland, UK
Institute for Clinical Evaluative Sciences, Toronto, ON, Canada

Lawrence Paszat
Sunnybrook Research Institute, Toronto, ON, Canada
Institute for Clinical Evaluative Sciences, Toronto, ON, Canada

Ladson Hinton
Department of Psychiatry and Behavioral Sciences, University of California Davis, 2230 Stockton Blvd., Sacramento, CA 95618, USA

Andrés F. Sciolla
Department of Psychiatry, University of California Davis, 2230 Stockton Blvd., Sacramento, CA 95618, USA

Jürgen Unützer
Department of Psychiatry and Behavioral Sciences, 1959 NE Pacific Street, Seattle, WA 98195, USA

Edward Elizarraras
Department of Biology, San Francisco State University, 1600 Holloway Avenue, San Francisco, CA 94132, USA

Richard L. Kravitz
Division of General Internal Medicine, University of California Davis, 4150 V Street, Sacramento, CA 95817, USA

Ester Carolina Apesoa-Varano
Betty Irene School of Nursing, University of California Davis, 4610 X Street, Sacramento, CA 95817, USA

Ginetta Salvalaggio, Christopher Meaney, Rahim Moineddin, Eva Grunfeld and Donna Manca
Ginetta Salvalaggio, University of Alberta, Edmonton, Canada

S. Davie and M. Slater
Department of Family & Community Medicine, St. Michael's Hospital, 30
Bond Street, Toronto, ON M5B 1W8, Canada

N. Persaud
Department of Family & Community Medicine, St. Michael's Hospital, 30 Bond Street, Toronto, ON M5B 1W8, Canada
Department of Family & Community Medicine, University of Toronto, 500 University Avenue, 5th Floor, Toronto, ON M5G 1V7, Canada
Centre for Urban Health Solutions, Li Ka Shing Knowledge Institute, St. Michael's Hospital, 30 Bond Street, Toronto, ON M5B 1W8, Canada

A. Schuler
Department of Family & Community Medicine, St. Michael's Hospital, 30 Bond Street, Toronto, ON M5B 1W8, Canada
Centre for Urban Health Solutions, Li Ka Shing Knowledge Institute, St. Michael's Hospital, 30 Bond Street, Toronto, ON M5B 1W8, Canada

A.D. Pinto
Department of Family & Community Medicine, St. Michael's Hospital, 30 Bond Street, Toronto, ON M5B 1W8, Canada
Department of Family & Community Medicine, University of Toronto, 500 University Avenue, 5th Floor, Toronto, ON M5G 1V7, Canada
Centre for Urban Health Solutions, Li Ka Shing Knowledge Institute, St. Michael's Hospital, 30 Bond Street, Toronto, ON M5B 1W8, Canada
Dalla Lana School of Public Health, University of Toronto, Health Sciences Building, 155 College Street, 6th Floor, Toronto, ON M5T 3M7, Canada

T. Kiran
Department of Family & Community Medicine, St. Michael's Hospital, 30 Bond Street, Toronto, ON M5B 1W8, Canada
Department of Family & Community Medicine, University of Toronto, 500 University Avenue, 5th Floor, Toronto, ON M5G 1V7, Canada
Centre for Urban Health Solutions, Li Ka Shing Knowledge Institute, St. Michael's Hospital, 30 Bond Street, Toronto, ON M5B 1W8, Canada
Institute for Clinical Evaluative Sciences, 2075 Bayview Avenue, Toronto, Ontario M4N 3M5, Canada

A.K. Lofters
Department of Family & Community Medicine, St. Michael's Hospital, 30 Bond Street, Toronto, ON M5B 1W8, Canada
Department of Family & Community Medicine, University of Toronto, 500 University Avenue, 5th Floor, Toronto, ON M5G 1V7, Canada
Centre for Urban Health Solutions, Li Ka Shing Knowledge Institute, St. Michael's Hospital, 30 Bond Street, Toronto, ON M5B 1W8, Canada
Dalla Lana School of Public Health, University of Toronto, Health Sciences Building, 155 College Street, 6th Floor, Toronto, ON M5T 3M7, Canada
Institute for Clinical Evaluative Sciences, 2075 Bayview Avenue, Toronto, Ontario M4N 3M5, Canada

N.N. Baxter
Dalla Lana School of Public Health, University of Toronto, Health Sciences Building, 155 College Street, 6th Floor, Toronto, ON M5T 3M7, Canada
Department of Surgery, Li Ka Shing Knowledge Institute, St. Michael's Hospital, 30 Bond Street, Toronto, ON M5B 1W8, Canada

E. Kucharski
Cancer Care Ontario, 620 University Avenue, Toronto, ON M5G 2L7, Canada

Caroline Morris, Lindsay Macdonald, Maria Stubbe and Anthony Dowell
Department Primary Health Care & General Practice, University of Otago, Wellington, 23a Mein Street, Wellington, New Zealand

Index

www.ingramcontent.com/pod-product-compliance
Lightning Source LLC
LaVergne TN
LVHW080720210926
848485LV00003B/496

* 9 7 8 1 6 3 9 2 7 4 5 2 9 *